VASCULAR DISORDERS of the UPPER EXTREMITY

Third Revised Edition

edited by

Herbert I. Machleder, M.D.

Professor of Surgery
Section of Vascular Surgery
UCLA Medical School
Los Angeles, California

**Futura Publishing
Company, Inc.**
Armonk, NY

Library of Congress Cataloging-in-Publication Data

Vascular disorders of the upper extremity / edited by Herbert
   I. Machleder. — 3rd rev. ed.
       p.   cm.
     Includes bibliographical references and index.
     ISBN 0-87993-409-3 (alk. paper)
      1. Extremities. Upper—Blood-vessels—Diseases. I. Machleder,
Herbert I. (Herbert Ivan), 1937–   .
    [DNLM: 1. Vascular Diseases. 2. Extremities—blood supply. WG
500 V33146 1998]
   RC951.V37   1998
   617.5'7—DC21
   DNLM/DLC
   for Library of Congress   98-21934
                                                      CIP

Copyright © 1998
Futura Publishing Company, Inc.

Published by
Futura Publishing Company, Inc.
135 Bedford Road
Armonk, New York 10504

LC #: 98-21934
ISBN #: 0-87993-409-3

Every effort has been made to ensure that the information in this book is as up
to date and accurate as possible at the time of publication. However, due to the
constant developments in medicine, neither the author, nor the editor, nor the
publisher can accept any legal or any other responsibility for any errors or omis-
sions that may occur.

Printed in the United States of America on acid-free paper.

Contributors

Samuel S. Ahn, MD
Associate Clinical Professor of Surgery
Section of Vascular Surgery
UCLA
Los Angeles, California

Allan Belzberg, BSc, MD
Assistant Professor of Neurosurgery
The Johns Hopkins School of Medicine
Baltimore, Maryland

Patricia E. Burrows, MD
Chief, Division of Cardiovascular/Interventional Radiology
Children's Hospital
Boston, Massachusetts

James M. Edwards, MD
Professor of Surgery
Division of Vascular Surgery
Oregon Health Sciences University
Portland, Oregon

Antoinette S. Gomes, MD
Associate Professor of Radiology
Chief, Section of Cardiovascular Radiology
UCLA Medical Center
Center for the Health Sciences
Los Angeles, California

J. Patrick Johnson, MD
Section of Spinal Neurosurgery
UCLA
Los Angeles, California

Sheldon E. Jordan, MD
Neurological Associates of West Los Angeles
UCLA Department of Neurology
Santa Monica, California

David J. Klashman, MD
Assistant Professor of Medicine
UCLA School of Medicine
Division of Rheumatology
Los Angeles, California

Dwight H. Kono, MD
Scripps Clinic and Research Foundation
Department of Immunology
La Jolla, California

Gregory J. Landry, MD
Resident, Division of Vascular Surgery
Oregon Health Sciences University
Portland, Oregon

Tal Laor, MD
Staff Radiologist
Children's Hospital
Boston, Massachusetts

Herbert I. Machleder, MD
Professor of Surgery
Section of Vascular Surgery
UCLA Medical School
Los Angeles, California

Swee Cheng Ng, MD
Registrar, Department of Medicine IV
Tan Tock Seng Hospital
Singapore

Marc R. Nuwer, MD, PhD
Professor, Department Neurology, UCLA School of Medicine
Department Head, Clinical Neurophysiology Department
UCLA Medical Center
Los Angeles, California

Emil F. Pascarelli, MD
Department of Medicine
Cumulative Trauma Disorders
Columbia University College of Physicians & Surgeons
New York, New York

Harold E. Paulus, MD
Professor of Medicine
UCLA School of Medicine
Division of Rheumatology
Los Angeles, California

John M. Porter, MD
Professor of Surgery
Chief, Division of Vascular Surgery
Oregon Health Sciences University
Portland, Oregon

Ledford L. Powell, MD
Surgery Department
University of California at Irvine
Orange, California

Kyung M. Ro, BS
Section of Vascular Surgery
UCLA
Los Angeles, California

David B. Roos, MD
Clinical Professor of Surgery
University of Colorado
Health Sciences Center
Presbyterian Professional Plaza
Denver, Colorado

Jacob P. Schwartz, BA
The Johns Hopkins School of Medicine
Baltimore, Maryland

David S. Sumner, MD
Distinguished Professor of General Surgery
Chief, Section of Peripheral Vascular Surgery
Director of Noninvasive Vascular Laboratories
Program Director, Vascular Fellowship
Southern Illinois University School of Medicine
Springfield, Illinois

Lloyd M. Taylor, Jr, MD
Professor of Surgery
Division of Vascular Surgery
Oregon Health Sciences University
Portland, Oregon

Kent Williamson, MD
   Resident, Division of Vascular Surgery
   Oregon Health Sciences University
   Portland, Oregon

Samuel E. Wilson, MD
   Chairman, Department of Surgery
   University of California at Irvine
   Orange, California

Preface

With publication of the third edition of *Vascular Disorders of the Upper Extremity*, the subjects of the first and second editions have been extensively rewritten and updated. The decade since the preparation of the second edition has been witness to major developments in the evaluation and treatment of upper extremity dysfunction. These developments have been concomitant with a recognition that upper extremity disorders are now among the most common industrial injuries and sources of disability occurring in young working people. The rapid development of keyboard-based industries has in many regards superceded the previous generation's exposure to heavy manual labor. The third edition now provides a valuable resource for physicians dealing with the new work place.

Part I focuses on the vascular evaluation, as well as diagnostic and interventional angiography, and reflects the extensive development of endovascular techniques. Newer diagnostic methods such as magnetic resonance angiography are discussed in relation to upper extremity diagnosis.

Part II is a new section dealing with the Cumulative Trauma Disorders. The chapters on the Thoracic Outlet Compression Syndromes now include the most recent electrophysiologic evaluations including electromyographic guided selective blocks. Surgical options and methodology are described in detail. The new chapters on arterial and venous manifestations of the compression syndrome are comprehensive and reflective of contemporary understanding of these problems, and review the most recent advances in therapy. A new chapter deals with the evaluation and treatment of the repetitive motion disorders found in office workers and musicians. Explanations of the pathophysiology are followed by discussion of sophisticated assessment methodologies and conservative management regimens. This chapter represents the current approach of one of the most innovative and successful clinics for these disorders. Part II concludes with a chapter on the management of chronic upper extremity pain. This includes current theories of chronic pain as well as strategies for conservative and pharmacological management, electrophysiological intervention, and surgical management techniques.

Part III has been augmented with an extensive chapter that deals comprehensively with the categorization, diagnosis, and management of Arteriovenous Malformations. The conceptual framework and the extensive illustrations make this one of the most useful references for these often perplexing and challenging conditions. The discussion on Small Vessel

Disease represents a logical and effective approach to the evaluation and management of the varying disorders that present with digital ischemia or Raynaud's phenomenon. This chapter is developed from a large clinical experience augmented by extensive long-term investigative efforts. The vascular specialist and nephrologist will find an excellent treatise on the various manifestations of Vascular Access dysfunction.

Part IV deals again with the unique approach of the second edition, in describing the upper extremity manifestations of systemic vascular disorders. Vasculitis and collagen-vascular disorders are reviewed in the context of current diagnostic methods and management techniques. The section is expanded by a description of the extraordinary development of the endoscopic approach to the autonomic disorders of the upper extremity.

The more than 225 illustrations and tables provide the reader with an excellent reference source for almost all of the myriad disorders that present with upper extremity pain and dysfunction. The radiologic and morphological appearances are both displayed in a comprehensive manner.

The design of the third edition is once again focused on a multidisciplinary approach to the upper extremity. The authors are drawn from a multitude of disciplines, reflecting the reality of current practice. The vascular specialist; whether internist, cardiologist, interventional radiologist, angiologist, or vascular surgeon will find this a most useful reference when approaching the upper extremity. The disability and industrial medicine specialist will have a reliable basis for evaluating the vascular and cumulative trauma component of upper extremity complaints. The same holds true for the orthopedist and plastic surgeon dealing with hand and arm complaints that often derive from cumulative trauma and have a significant vascular component. The internist, primary care specialist and rheumatologist will appreciate the framework for appraising these often unusual disorders, and for developing a coherent algorithm for assessment. Specialists in pain management and rehabilitation will find useful information on the evolution of chronic pain in the cumulative trauma and industrial disabilities, with a well outlined methodology for accurate evaluation.

Herbert I. Machleder, MD

Contents

PART III   INTRINSIC AND ACQUIRED DISORDERS OF THE UPPER EXTREMITY VESSELS

PART IV   VASCULAR MANIFESTATIONS OF SYSTEMIC DISORDERS

Part I
The Vascular Evaluation

1

The Initial Clinical Examination

Herbert I. Machleder, MD

The upper extremities are subject to a variety of unique intrinsic arterial and venous disorders, as well as the peripheral manifestations of systemic collagen vascular diseases. The extensive use of the upper extremities for venous and arterial vascular access also results in a host of problems that require recognition and management by the vascular specialist.

Patients who develop arterial insufficiency of the upper extremities will generally demonstrate one of three different clinical patterns: (1) attacks of Raynaud's disease symptoms; (2) digital ischemia and gangrene; or (3) crampy pain on exercise, often referred to (with disregard for the word origin) as claudication. The uniformity of clinical symptoms belies the multiplicity of underlying diseases, which range from relatively simple cases of trauma to complex autoimmune and connective tissue disorders. This complexity of underlying disease requires a methodical approach to ensure expeditious diagnosis and an effective therapeutic plan.

A peculiar blanching and cyanosis of the fingertips characterizes upper extremity vascular insufficiency. Raynaud put it rather succinctly in the introduction to his second treatise on vasospastic syndromes affecting the upper extremity:

> In the slight cases the ends of the fingers and toes become cold, cyanosed, and livid, and at the same time more or less painful. In grave cases the area affected by cyanosis extends upwards for several centimeters above the roots of the nails; . . . finally, if this state is prolonged for a certain time, we see gangrenous points appear on the extremities; the gangrene is always dry, and may occupy the superficial layers of the skin from the extent of a pin's head up to the end of a finger, rarely more.

From Machleder HI, (ed): *Vascular Disorders of the Upper Extremity*. Third Revised Edition. Futura Publishing Company, Inc., Armonk, NY, © 1998.

The initial evaluation should enable differentiation of arterial and venous obstruction, the recognition of chronological elements of the obstructive phenomena (such as repetitive events versus a single isolated and progressive event) and whether or not the ischemic symptom is related to vasospasm or true arterial occlusion. It is also important to recognize at the outset whether the vascular manifestations in the upper extremity are symmetrical, part of a generalized process, or are confined to an isolated event in the affected extremity.

Raynaud's phenomenon, which is characteristic of the early onset of many types of vascular occlusive phenomena, is generally quite evident to the patient and is noticed as a blanching of a single digit,

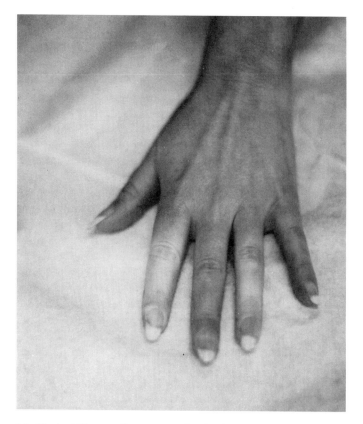

Figure 1A. Typical Raynaud's pattern of selective digital ischemia, occurring to the metacarpal phalangeal joint. This stage is usually characterized by numbness of the involved digits.

perhaps symmetrically disposed to both upper extremities. The phenomenon is usually precipitated by a drop in temperature that may, however, be quite slight (of only several degrees magnitude). The blanching becomes cadaveric in appearance and the finger becomes numb; within seconds to minutes, and occasionally longer, the blanching is replaced by a mottled, deeply cyanotic, and ruborous appearance. The return of capillary filling is generally accompanied by dysesthesia and occasionally frank burning pain (Figures 1A and 1B). The symptoms may spread to other digits as time progresses, and in fact may involve the entire hand unilaterally or both hands symmetrically. Occasionally this sequence of events can be seen in traumatic situations, which although not specifically linked to temperature changes, may well be exacerbated by exposure to cold.

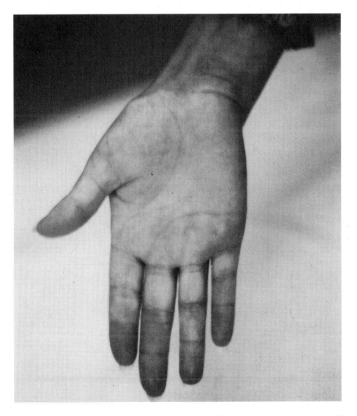

Figure 1B. Within a few minutes, the blanching gives way to rubor, usually accompanied by a throbbing dysesthesia.

Vascular Examination of the Upper Extremity

The initial examination of the upper extremity should begin with inspection for color changes; areas of gangrene; discoloration such as blanching, cyanosis, and livido reticularis; or areas of erythema. A note should be made of abnormal distention of veins, particularly related to positional changes of the upper extremity. Ordinarily prominent veins on the dorsum of the hand and antecubital fossa should become flat as the arms reach the cardiac position. Observation of marked collateral vessels, particularly around the shoulder, should be noted, particularly if they are asymmetrical. When venous obstruction is suspected, measurement of recumbent venous pressure in an antecubital vein can be easily done with a spinal manometer filled with saline (Figures 2A and 2B).

Palpation should follow inspection and should involve palpation of the carotid arteries bilaterally, and for prominent pulsations in the supra-clavicular area, as well as assessment of the axillary, brachial, radial, and ulnar pulses. The Allen's test should be routinely performed for assessing the arterial competence of the palmar arch. The test is performed in the following manner, one hand at a time. With the patient facing the examiner, palmar surface of the hand up, both the radial and ulnar arteries are compressed. The examiner's thumb is placed on the arteries and the remaining digits are placed along the back of the patient's wrist. The arteries are compressed while the patient clenches his fist to evacuate blood from the hand. When the hand is opened, the palm has a pale,

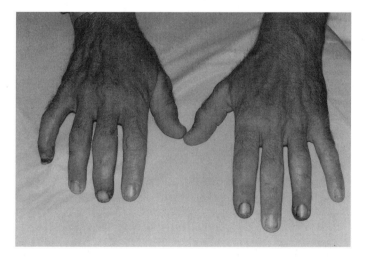

Figure 2A. Fingertip gangrene, seen with systemic collagen vascular disorders or with digital artery occlusion.

mottled appearance. Radial artery compression is released first, whereupon prompt color or even reactive hyperemia should appear on the entire palmar surface of the hand. In the presence of radial artery occlusion, the pallor remains and mottling continues. When there is insufficient collateral flow across the palmar arch, only the radial portion of the hand will be perfused, and the ulnar part of the hand will remain blanched and mottled. When the ulnar artery is then released, color will return to the ulnar aspect of the hand. The examiner next repeats the test by compressing the radial and ulnar artery with the thumbs while the patient clenches his hand, and then opens it, revealing the blanched, mottled appearance. Compression is then released from the ulnar artery, and again, if normal, prompt blushing of the hand or even reactive hyperemia should occur. In the event of ulnar artery occlusion, the hand remains white and mottled; if there is insufficient collateral circulation across the palmar arch, perfusion of only the ulnar aspect of the hand will be apparent. The test is then repeated on the contralateral extremity. When properly performed, this test is extremely accurate, with a high degree of sensitivity and specificity (Figure 3). In patients with neurovascular compression at the thoracic outlet, there is often tenderness to palpation over the anterior scalene muscle and a positive tinnels sign when tapping over the brachial plexus.

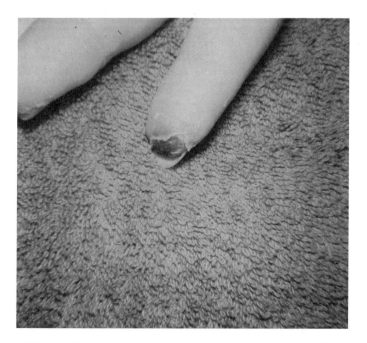

Figure 2B. Digital and nail fold infarcts seen with vasculitis.

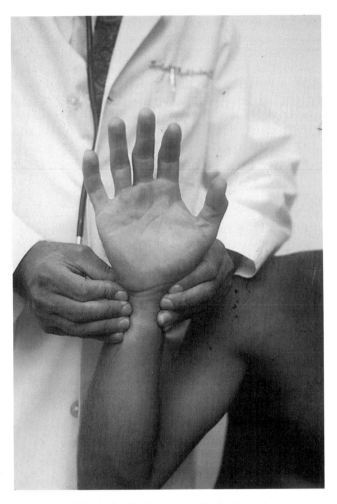

Figure 3. Performance of Allen's test.

In this situation there is also characteristically, hypersensitivity to percussion on the clavicle (Figure 4).

Auscultation is an important part of upper extremity examination and should begin in the supraclavicular fossa. Subclavian bruits often begin just lateral to the palpable carotid pulse at the base of the neck and will radiate toward the acromioclavicular joint and below the middle third of the clavicle toward the axilla. Auscultation should be done bilaterally with the arm in the neutral position, and then with Adson's maneuver. Auscultation should then be performed with the diaphragm of the stethoscope placed just beneath the middle third of the clavicle as the arm is gradually brought into the abducted and externally rotated position (Figure 5). This is done while palpating the radial pulse, and if obliteration of the radial pulse occurs, careful auscultation should be then augmented by moving the stethoscope laterally in the infraclavicular area, then medially in the supraclavicular area in an attempt to detect any site of compressive occlusion. Bruits in this area are typically obliterated over a few degrees of the abduction and external rotation arc, and the maneuver must be performed slowly so that the point of maximum bruit can be ascertained. Placing the arm in a full abducted and externally rotated position may totally obliterate the pulse, and the bruit may be overlooked.

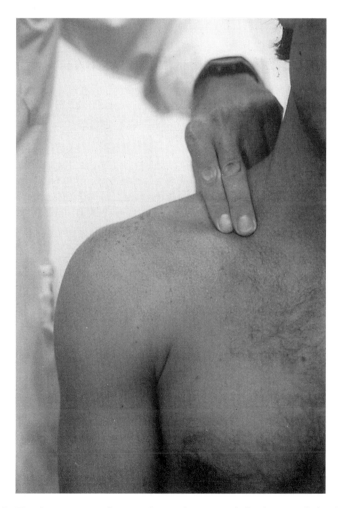

Figure 4. Tenderness over the anterior scalene muscle is characteristic of patients with neurovascular compression syndrome at the thoracic outlet.

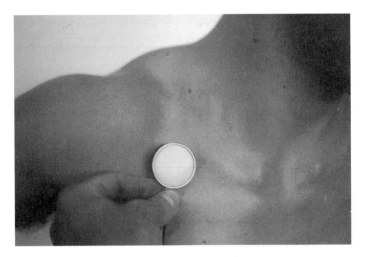

Figure 5. Proper position of the stethescope when auscultating for a bruit at the thoracic outlet. This location is particularly sensitive when performing Adson's maneuver, or abduction and external rotation maneuver (see Chapter X).

The bell and diaphragm of the stethoscope should be used to auscultate over any abnormal group of veins or angiomatous malformation. Arteriovenous fistulas will often be identified in this manner, and this technique is highly accurate in identifying this type of lesion.

Vascular Laboratory Diagnosis

Noninvasive vascular testing can be utilized to further document disorders that may be suggested by symptoms or subtle physical findings. The systolic pressure should be measured at the brachial artery and at the radial or ulnar artery with the patient supine and the arm in the neutral position. This is done by placing the blood pressure cuff around the upper arm in a manner identical to that used in assessing the standard blood pressure using auscultation for Korotkoff's sounds. The vascular examination uses the Doppler flow detector to assess the exact point of initiation of systolic flow. The flow detector is placed over the antecubital brachial artery, and the pressure cuff is inflated until arterial signals are obliterated. Pressure is slowly released, and the pressure is noted at which the initial thumping arterial sound resumes. By doing this first over the brachial artery and then over the radial and ulnar with the cuff moved to the forearm, segmental pressures can be recorded that may further indicate a site of obstruction if this should be the case. If thoracic outlet obstruction is a possibility, the test should be repeated with the patient in the sitting position. It is difficult to elicit vascular compressive signs of thoracic outlet compression when the patient is recumbent.

The sensitivity of all tests must be well recognized by the examiner, and it should be specifically understood that reductions of cross-sectional area in an artery less than 75% or reductions of cross-sectional diameter less than 50% will rarely result in a pressure drop unless specific measures are used to reduce peripheral resistance and increase flow rates (such as reactive hyperemia or specific ergometric testing).

A specific and detailed history of positional characteristics that bring on symptoms of arterial or venous obstruction must be documented and these positions utilized when performing a variety of arterial and venous tests. The extensive collateralization of the upper extremity may lead to a paucity of signs and symptoms at rest, in the face of severe disability when specific muscle groups are called on during work or recreational activity.

As in the lower extremity, the more distal the obstruction (especially in the presence of tandem lesions), the more severe will be the pressure drop appreciated peripherally. Occasionally, differences of up to 15 mm Hg between the two upper extremities may be within the normal range and can be accounted for by the extreme sensitivity of the upper extremity vessels to sympathetic innervation and minute changes in peripheral resistance. In general, an occlusion at the level of the subclavian artery will result in a pressure drop of between 30 and 40 mm Hg. When evaluating upper extremity pressures that are symmetrical, particularly in the presence of other evidence of vascular insufficiency, an ankle-brachial index should be assessed in an attempt to recognize symmetrical occlusions of the major aortic branches, as occur in some varieties of arteritis. When suspicion is high, oculopneumoplethysmography can also be used in an attempt to assess the true central arterial pressure in the event of symmetrical subclavian occlusive disease.

An abnormal Allen's test on the initial examination should always be further assessed by measuring segmental pressures with the probe placed over the radial as well as the ulnar artery in an attempt to establish the level of occlusive disease. In more sophisticated testing, small finger cuffs can be used to assess individual digital artery pressures. This can be done either with a Doppler flow probe or with a mercury strain gauge or digital photoplethysmograph.

The significant reactivity of the digital vessels to sympathetic stimulation should alert the examiner to changes in ambient temperature as well as changes in the patient's apprehension during the examination. Insensitivity to these factors may often yield results that, in retrospect, become difficult to interpret. Many individuals have a dramatic response to smoking, which may last from 1 to 8 hours after even a single cigarette. Before embarking on these sensitive arterial evaluations, the history of recent smoking must be noted.

Digital plethysmography can be useful in differentiating proximal from distal arterial obstructive phenomena, and the effect of reactive hyperemia on the pulse wave pattern will also differentiate primary Raynaud's disease from Raynaud's phenomenon associated with collagen vascular diseases. When vasodilatation is effected by immersing the hand in warm water or applying a cuff to maintain ischemia for 5 minutes, patients with primary vasospastic syndromes will demonstrate a normal return of pulse volume and curve characteristics. Those with collagen diseases, however, have vascular obstructive phenomena secondary to intimal proliferation or deposition of immune complexes and will have fixed lesions that demonstrate minimal, if any, change after reactive hyperemia. These tests are extremely useful in assessing the potential response to vasodilating or sympatholytic therapies.

When addressing the upper extremity arterial circulation, the examiner should become familiar with the normal and abnormal Doppler signal, which is obtained from peripheral vessels. The ordinary signal is described as triphasic, but can be appreciated only by assiduous listening, to establish a good baseline for recognition. Although tracings can be subjected to more sophisticated analysis, this should rarely be necessary in all but the most extensive of upper extremity vascular evaluations. The normal high-frequency short burst of systolic flow, followed by a short low-pitched diastolic component, is easily recognized and can be detected in other peripheral vessels that clinically do not seem involved in the disease process. The abnormal flow sound is usually described as monophasic, is of lower frequency and longer duration, and is more undulant in quality. At times, it approaches the venous signal, which can be utilized as a reference. Segmental auscultation with the Doppler flowmeter can often reveal the site of obstruction without more sophisticated testing.

The need for sequential performance of these tests cannot be overemphasized, because the Allen's test will often identify an obstruction in the radial or ulnar artery, whereas nondirectional Doppler assessment may reveal a relatively normal flow pattern in both vessels. The flow, however, may be reversed in the obstructed vessel because of the extensive collateralization across the palmar arch. It should be quite obvious that the Allen's test, although based on a visual interpretation, can be further documented by performance using the Doppler flow detector to assess signal changes during compression.

Some specific noninvasive assessment procedures aid in the diagnosis of venous obstruction. The presence of swelling should be documented by segmental girth measurements. Occasionally, there will be distention of the superficial veins and mild cyanosis. Patients usually complain of heaviness and pressure or a distensive feeling with exercise. Although venous collateral vessels develop rapidly and extensively, symptoms abate slowly, if at all, and are particularly exacerbated by exercise. Edema that is present from primary lymphatic obstruction, may occasionally be difficult to differentiate from venous obstruction, but often can be clarified by measurement of antecubital vein pressures using the saline-filled manometer, or a pressure transducer.

Flow in the upper extremity is paradoxically related to venous flow in the lower extremity, and these facts must be kept in mind when assessing upper extremity venous outflow. Often, outflow in the upper extremities will be decreased with deep inspiration related to changes in intrathoracic pressure. The upper extremity venous return tends to be more pulsatile than that demonstrated in the lower extremities. Velocity changes in the antecubital and axillary veins can be assessed with the Doppler flowmeter, much as they can be assessed in the lower extremities when these important differences are kept in mind.

Surgically constructed arteriovenous fistulas will be dealt with in more detail in later chapters. Several characteristics should be appreciated, however, referring to the previously described examinations. The arterial flow distal to a surgically constructed arteriovenous fistula may well be retrograde in the artery distal to the fistula. Additionally, flow in the distal vein of a side-to-side arteriovenous fistula is commonly reversed such that the flow is traveling in a distal direction. Dramatic augmentation of flow will be appreciated in the donor artery to the arteriovenous fistula. Compression of the fistula would generally restore normal flow patterns in the distal, arterial, and venous vessels.

2

Noninvasive Vascular Laboratory Assessment

David S. Sumner, MD

Introduction

The multiplicity and complexity of the vascular disorders that afflict the upper extremity often tax the diagnostic acumen of even the most astute clinician.[1-3] Although much can be learned from the history and physical examination, simple noninvasive tests can contribute to a more accurate diagnosis and to a more precise evaluation of the severity of the circulatory impairment.[4-6] Frequently, they point the way toward further investigations, such as arteriography, nerve blocks, or extensive blood work. They may also suggest etiologies and the appropriate treatment. Finally, they provide a valuable method for objectively assessing the results of surgical or medical treatment.

Among the questions to be answered by the vascular laboratory are: whether there is arterial or venous obstruction; whether the obstruction is intermittent or continuous; whether there is a vasospastic component to the obstruction; and whether the obstruction is diffuse, symmetrical, or isolated.

Arterial Disease

Included under the heading of arterial disease are all entities that continuously or intermittently obstruct the lumen of the large and small

From Machleder HI, (ed): *Vascular Disorders of the Upper Extremity*. Third Revised Edition. Futura Publishing Company, Inc., Armonk, NY, © 1998.

arteries or arterioles. This broad classification encompasses a wide variety of dissimilar conditions—ranging from thoracic outlet syndromes to primary Raynaud's disease, from atherosclerotic or embolic obstructions to autoimmune disorders, and from blunt trauma to toxic damage. Applicable to all of these conditions are the following basic tests: measurement of systolic blood pressure, studies of arterial flow patterns, and analysis of plethysmographic pulses. When vasospasm is suspected, the effects of cold and sympathetic activity must be examined.

Physiology of Arterial Obstruction and Cold Sensitivity

The rational use of noninvasive testing for arterial disease of the upper extremity requires a basic understanding of hemodynamics and knowledge of the pathophysiology of cold sensitivity. As a rule, stenoses in major arteries do not become hemodynamically significant (that is, they do not affect pressure or flow appreciably) unless they reduce the cross-sectional area of the artery by 75% or more. This corresponds to a 50% or greater reduction in diameter. In response to a hemodynamically significant lesion, collateral channels enlarge to carry blood around the stenotic or occluded artery, and the arterioles of the peripheral vascular bed dilate to compensate for the increased resistance imposed by the diseased artery and its collaterals. How well these compensatory mechanisms work is a function of the location of the obstruction, the availability of pre-existing collaterals, and the rapidity with which the obstruction develops.

An isolated chronic obstruction of the subclavian, axillary, or brachial arteries is ordinarily fairly well compensated. Under resting conditions, peripheral blood flow will be normal, but peripheral pressure will be reduced due to the increased proximal resistance. Exercise, with its increased metabolic demands, may not be well tolerated, resulting in claudication of the forearm and hand.

Chronic and even some acute lesions of the arteries of the forearm, hand, or fingers may produce remarkably few hemodynamic changes. The multiple interconnections between the parallel and roughly equal-sized radial and ulnar arteries account for the ability of either one of these arteries to carry blood relatively unimpeded around an obstruction in the other. A similar situation exists in the fingers, where there are parallel proper digital arteries, and, to a lesser extent, in the hand, where there is a superficial and deep palmar arch.

Acute occlusions, such as those that result from trauma or emboli, are usually more devastating. Collaterals do not have time to develop, and emboli have a tendency to lodge at bifurcations, where they obstruct not only the main channel but also the input to major collateral channels. Arterial pressure distal to an acute occlusion is often severely reduced and may not even be detectable. Resting blood flow may be inadequate to sustain tissue viability.

Multiple occlusions, even when they develop gradually, may be so extensive or critically placed that they overtax the compensatory mechanisms, resulting in ischemia. This can occur at any level, but especially in the fingers. Occlusions of end arteries, such as the common digital, may also result in ischemia.

Unless collaterals are extremely well developed, an arterial occlusion will reduce the peripheral pressure, alter the flow pulse, and distort the contour of the digit volume pulse. These changes are all easily recognized with simple noninvasive tests. Proximal to the site of occlusion, the pressure will remain unchanged and flow pulses may be normal, or if recorded close to the obstruction, diminished flow and increased wave reflections may be observed. Intermittent extrinsic compression will produce similar changes during the period of arterial obstruction, but pressure and flow patterns will be normal when the obstruction is relieved.

Arteriolar diameter is subject to control by the sympathetic nervous system. Emotional stimuli, respiratory reflexes, and cold exposure all cause the peripheral arterioles to constrict. This is a normal response, experienced by all; but when it is superimposed on a fixed obstruction in the digital or more proximal arteries, the resulting transient ischemia can be severe (Figure 1).[7,8] Raynaud's phenomenon secondary to collagen diseases, Buerger's disease, or other forms of arterial obstruction are explained by this mechanism.[9] Even when the fingers are warm, digital pressure may be reduced and flow patterns and digit pulses will be abnormal.

Primary Raynaud's disease is caused by abnormally marked constriction of the digital arteries in response to cold or emotional stimuli.[8-13] Reflex and direct arteriolar constriction superimposed on the digital artery constriction further restricts blood flow, augmenting the ischemia (Figure 1).[11,14-16] The digital arteries themselves show no anatomic abnormalities,[17] and flow patterns and digital pressures are normal when the hands are warm.[7] At room temperature, however, finger blood flow may be somewhat less than normal, implying the presence of increased sympathetic activity.[16,18] Whereas local application of cold induces constriction of both the digital arteries and the arterioles, remote cold exposure (the effects of which are mediated through the sympathetic nervous system) causes constriction of only the digital arterioles. Consequently, local cold causes a reduction in both digital pressure and flow, but remote cold exposure only causes a reduction in flow.[16]

In a recent study, ultrasonically measured diameters of digital arteries in normal subjects were observed by Singh et al[19] to vary linearly with skin temperatures of 15° to 35°C. Above 25°, digital artery diameters in patients with primary Raynaud's disease and secondary Raynaud's phe-

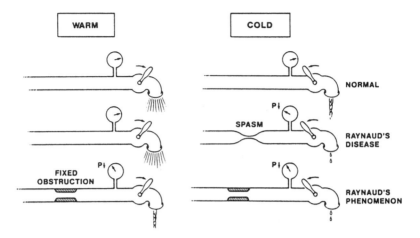

Figure 1. Effect of cold exposure on blood flow (output of faucet) and blood pressure (gauges) in normal fingers, fingers with primary Raynaud's disease, and fingers with Raynaud's phenomenon secondary to a fixed arterial obstruction. Faucets represent arteriolar sphincters (handle to the right = dilatation; handle to the left = constriction). From Summer DS: Evaluation of acute and chronic ischemia of the upper extremity. In: *Vascular Surgery* (4th ed), Rutherford RB (ed), W.B. Saunders Co., Philadelphia, 1995, pp. 918–935.

nomenon responded in a similar fashion; but below this temperature marked vasoconstriction occurred with spasm resulting in complete closure at 17°C. Thus, there appears to be a temperature threshold that triggers pathological vasoconstriction in cold sensitive arteries.

In many cases, the distinction between primary Raynaud's disease and secondary Raynaud's phenomenon is blurred. Patients in one category not infrequently manifest responses consistent with those of the other. For example, spasm of the digital arteries can occur in patients with histological features of autoimmune disease; and autoimmune phenomena may play a role in sensitizing the apparently normal digital arteries of patients with primary Raynaud's disease. It is well known that many patients who have all the clinical features of primary Raynaud's disease eventually develop scleroderma or other autoimmune disorders.

Segmental Pressure Measurements

The initial procedure in any examination for upper extremity ischemia should be measurement of systolic blood pressure. Pneumatic cuffs are placed around the brachial area, upper forearm, and just above the wrist. Segmental pressures at these levels are most conveniently measured by using a Doppler velocity detector to sense the return of flow in the radial or ulnar arteries when the cuff is slowly deflated. With the cuff at the wrist level, it is often easier to place the probe over the palmar arch. In the rare event that a Doppler signal cannot be obtained, a mercury-in-Silastic rubber strain gauge or a photoplethysmograph attached to a finger may be used to detect the return of flow.

Pressures at each of the three levels are compared with the pressure obtained at the comparable level in the opposite arm. At any given site, there seldom should be more than a 15 mm Hg difference between the two arms (Table 1). In normal limbs, an index of upper arm pressures, obtained by dividing the lower of the two pressures by the higher, averages 0.96 ± 0.03 (Table 1).[20] The pressure gradient between any two levels in the same arm is ordinarily less than 15 mm Hg (Table 2). Normally, the mean index (pressure at the specified level divided by the upper arm pressure) is 0.97 ± 0.06 (range 0.87 to 1.06) at the upper forearm and 0.99 ± 0.06 (range 0.89 to 1.15) at the wrist. As these figures indicate, systolic pressures measured in this way may be higher at the distal sites than they are at the brachial area.[20]

A low brachial pressure signifies the presence of occlusive disease in the ipsilateral upper brachial, axillary, subclavian, or innominate artery (Table 3).[21,22] An abnormally large gradient between any two levels in the arms indicates that the intervening arterial segment is severely stenosed or occluded (Table 4).[23] However, when the ipsilateral brachial pressure

Table 1
Pressure Data—Normal Arms
(Pressures in One Arm Compared to Those in the Other Arm at the same Level)*

	Difference—mm Hg Higher Pressure - Lower Pressure	
	Mean ± SD	(Range)
Brachial	5.4 ± 4.6	(0–16)
Forearm	7.6 ± 4.6	(2–16)
Wrist	7.2 ± 6.1	(0–22)
	Index Lower Pressure/Higher Pressure	
	Mean ± SD	(Range)
Brachial	0.96 ± 0.03	(0.88–1.00)
Forearm	0.93 ± 0.04	(0.85–0.98)
Wrist	0.94 ± 0.05	(0.83–1.00)

* Data derived from Sumner et al., 1979.[20]

Table 2
Pressure Data—Normal Arms
(Pressures at Different Levels Compared in the
Same Arm)*

	Gradient - mm Hg	
	Mean ± SD	(Range)
Brachial - Forearm	5.0 ± 4.8	(−6 to +15)
Forearm - Wrist	6.6 ± 4.6	(−19 to +14)
	Index	
	Mean ± SD	(Range)
Forearm/Brachial	0.97 ± 0.06	(0.87–1.06)
Wrist/Brachial	0.99 ± 0.06	(0.89-1.15)

* Data derived from Sumner et al., 1979.[20]

Table 3
Pressure Data—Upper Brachial, Axillary,
Subclavian, or
Innominate Arterial Obstruction*

	Difference—mm Hg	
	Obstructed - Nonobstructed	
	Mean ± SD	(Range)
Brachial	52 ± 33	(20–124)
	Index	
	Obstructed/Nonobstructed	
	Mean ± SD	(Range)
Brachial	0.65 ± 0.15	(0.38–0.81)

* Data derived from Sumner et al., 1979.[20]

Table 4
Pressure Data—Lower Brachial, Antecubital, Radial
or Ulnar Arterial Obstruction*

	Gradient—mm Hg	
	Mean ± SD	(Range)
Brachial - Forearm or Wrist	42 ± 30	(12–114)
	Index	
	Mean ± SD	(Range)
Forearm or Wrist/Ipsilateral Brachial	0.68 ± 0.16	(0.37–0.86)

* Data derived from Sumner et al., 1979.[20]

is also reduced, the gradient down the arm may not be greatly increased, even in the presence of significant distal disease. Wrist or forearm pressures obtained with the Doppler probe over the radial artery may differ from those obtained with the probe over the ulnar artery. A distinct disparity serves to identify which of these two arteries is more severely involved.

Digital Pressure Measurements

Systolic blood pressure in the fingers can be measured with a technique analogous to that used to determine arm pressure.[8,24,25] A pneumatic cuff, having a width that exceeds 1.2 times the diameter of the finger, is placed around the base of the digit.[24] Return of flow as the cuff is slowly deflated is sensed with a Doppler flow probe applied to the volar digital artery at the distal interphalangeal (DIP) joint. Alternatively, a mercury strain gauge or a photoplethysmograph placed over the distal phalanx may be used (Figure 2). Return of flow is indicated by a rise in the baseline of the tracing or by the return of detectable pulsation—whichever occurs first (Figure 3). The pressure, measured in this way, reflects the pressure in the common and proximal proper digital arteries.

All studies should be performed in a warm (about 25°C), draft-free room with the patient relaxed. Efforts should be made to allay apprehen-

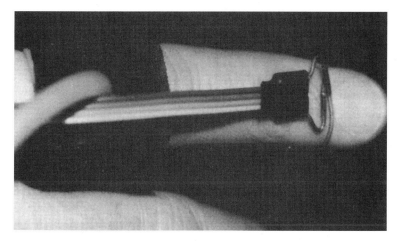

Figure 2. Mercury strain gauge and Velcro-backed pressure cuff used to measure blood pressure in the finger. A photoplethysmograph could be substituted for the strain guage. From Sumner DS: Measurement of segmental arterial pressure. In: *Vascular Surgery* (2nd ed), Rutherford RB (ed), W.B. Saunders Co., Philadelphia, 1984.

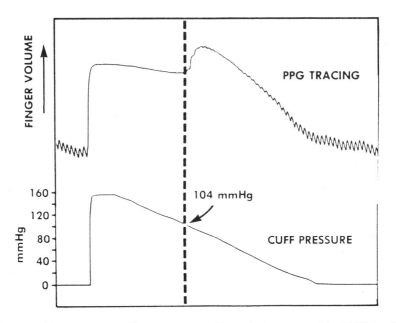

Figure 3. Measurement of finger pressure. Photoplethysmographic (PPG) tracing from digital tip is shown in upper tracing, and the cuff pressure is shown in the lower tracing. Pulses disappear when the cuff is inflated. As the cuff is deflated, the PPG tracing suddenly rises and pulses reappear at a pressure of 104 mm Hg.

sion. In this way, vasoconstriction, which makes the determinations much more difficult, can be avoided.

In normal limbs, the digital pressure index (digital systolic pressure divided by the ispilateral brachial systolic pressure) averages 0.97 ± 0.09 (range 0.78 to 1.27).[20] The mean digital pressure index in 21 patients with cold sensitivity, who seemed by all other criteria and laboratory tests to fit into the category of primary Raynaud's disease, was 0.96 ± 0.11 (range 0.60 to 1.23) (Figure 4).

Measurement of digital pressure is particularly important when symptoms and signs point toward ischemia of the hand and the brachial, forearm, and wrist pressures are normal. If all finger pressures are approximately equally reduced, the obstruction must involve the palmar arch and/or both terminal radial and ulnar arteries. When the arch is incomplete or occluded at some point, the pressure may be reduced only in those digits on the radial or on the ulnar side of the hand, implying obstruction of the terminal branches of the ipsilateral arteries. Isolated obstruction of a common digital artery is indicated by decreased pressure in the involved digit and normal pressures in adjacent digits. Finger pressures may be normal when only one of the two volar digital arteries is involved.[26,27] Obviously, many combinations are possible.

In 26 patients with evidence of digital or palmar arterial obstruction but without evident disease in the subclavian, axillary, brachial, or forearm arteries, the mean digital pressure index was 0.56 ± 0.27 (range 0.0 to 0.95) (Figure 4). Fingers of both hands were affected in 57% of 23 patients in whom data were available for all 10 digits. Only 1 finger was

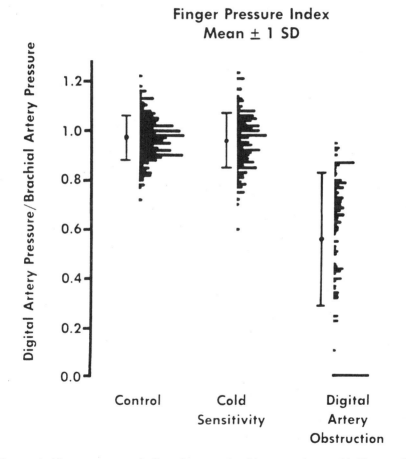

Figure 4. Finger pressure indices in control subjects, patients with Raynaud's disease, and in patients with digital or palmar arterial obstructions. Horizontal length of bars indicates number of fingers. Means ± one standard deviation are indicated by dots and vertical bars. From Sumner DS, Lambeth A, Russell JB: Diagnosis of upper extremity obstructive and vasospastic syndromes by Doppler ultrasound, plethysmography, and temperature profiles. In: *Hemodynamics of the Limbs,* Puel P, Boccalon H, Enjalbert A (eds), GEPESC, Toulouse, France, 1979.

involved in 17% of the hands, 2 fingers in 11%, 3 fingers in 22%, 4 fingers in 17%, and 5 fingers in 33%. All 10 fingers were affected in 26%.[20]

According to one report of finger pressures in patients with connective tissue disease, the mean digital pressure index was 0.62 in patients with rheumatoid arthritis, 0.53 in patients with systemic lupus erythematosus, and 0.38 in patients with scleroderma.[28] Indices of zero were observed only in patients with scleroderma.

When the pressure in the upper arm, forearm, or wrist levels is reduced, a similar reduction occurs in the digital pressure. If all the digital pressures are similarly and appropriately affected, one can assume that the disease is localized to the arm arteries and that the digital arteries are spared. If, however, one or more digital pressures are much lower than the others, the disease has evidently produced palmar or digital arterial obstruction as well.

In some conditions, obstructions may be confined to the more distal portions of the digital arteries, in which case the pressure measured with the cuff around the proximal phalanx may be normal.[26] Pressures can be measured at the level of the middle phalanx by moving the pneumatic cuff to that level and using a photoplethysmograph as the flow sensor.[27,29] Other methods are less satisfactory, because inflation of the cuff often interferes with proper placement of the Doppler probe and may distort the tracing obtained with a mercury strain gauge. It is even possible to obtain pressures at the very end of the finger by wrapping the pneumatic cuff around the distal phalanx, enclosing both the finger and the photoplethysmograph within the cuff. Although this technique seems crude, the results compare favorably with those obtained when the cuff is positioned at the level of the proximal phalanx. A bladder-free cuff has been devised by Hirai and associates specifically for measuring pressures in the terminal phalanx.[30]

Plethysmographic Studies

Digit volume pulses are most conveniently recorded with a mercury strain gauge or photoplethysmograph applied to the distal phalanx (Figure 2). Although the actual percent volume change that occurs with each pulse can be measured with the mercury strain gauge, for most purposes it is necessary only to define the contour of the pulse. In order to obtain good tracings, all studies are performed in a warm room (approximately 25°C). Even under these conditions, some patients may remain vasoconstricted. Soaking the hands in warm water for a few minutes will usually produce the required vasodilation. Another ploy is to record the pulses during the period of reactive hyperemia that follows restoration of flow after the hand has been ischemic for 3 to 5 minutes. Ischemia can be produced by inflating a pneumatic cuff, placed around the wrist or fore-arm, to super systolic pressures.[31]

The normal digit pulse has a rapid systolic upslope, a sharp systolic peak, and a downslope that bows toward the baseline. A dicrotic wave is usually present about midway on the downslope (Figure 5C). Obstructive pulses have a delayed upslope, a rounded peak, and a downslope that bows away from the baseline (Figure 5B). Pulses that do not fit into either of these categories are commonly observed in patients with digital is-chemia.[32,33] One variety—which we have called a *peaked-pulse*—has a rapid ascending limb, an anacrotic notch (or an abrupt bend) that termi-nates in a sharp systolic peak, and a dicrotic notch high on the downslope (Figure 5A). Another form is characterized by a relatively normal contour except that the dicrotic notch is quite high.[33,34]

Obstructive pulses are caused by attenuation of the high-frequency components of the pulse wave as it passes through a stenotic artery or is forced to traverse a series of high-resistance collaterals. Consequently, these pulses imply that there is a significant obstruction in the arterial tree somewhere proximal to the distal phalanx. The obstruction can be localized to the digital arteries or palmar arch or may involve the forearm, brachial, axillary, or subclavian arteries.

The exact physiological meaning of the peaked-pulse is unknown, but it may represent an intermediate form between the normal and obstructive pulse.[9,34] Because the dicrotic wave represents that portion of the pulse wave that is reflected from the terminal arteries and arterioles, it is possi-ble that its earlier occurrence, high on the downslope, indicates increased peripheral resistance or decreased compliance of the terminal vascula-ture.[34,35] It is also possible that the transit times of the various harmonic components of the pulse wave are altered by changes in the viscoelasticity of the arterial conduits. Normal pulses can sometimes be converted to peaked pulses by cold exposure, even in subjects with no history of cold sensitivity.[34] Whatever the cause of the peaked pulse, it is commonly seen in the fingers of patients with autoimmune (collagen) diseases, who do not have major proximal arterial obstruction.[32,36,37] As a corollary, finding peaked pulses in a patient with cold sensitivity should alert the physician to the possible diagnosis of collagen disease or Buerger's disease. In our experience, 92% of patients with collagen diseases have peaked or obstruc-tive pulses.[32]

Normal pulses are found in the absence of fixed or permanent arterial obstruction. When the hands of patients with primary Raynaud's disease are vasodilated, the digit pulses are normal (Figure 6). Moderate vasocon-striction changes the volume of the pulse but not the contour of the pulse. Severe vasoconstriction, on the other hand, will modify the contour of the pulse and may even render it undetectable.[35]

Total absence of the digit pulse even after warming or reactive hyper-

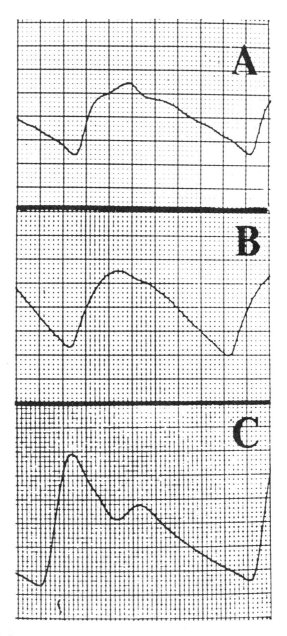

Figure 5. Plethysmographic pulse contours. **(A)** peaked, **(B)** obstructive, **(C)** normal. From Summer DS, Strandness DE Jr: An abnormal finger pulse associated with cold sensitivity. *Ann Surg* 175:294–298, 1972.

Control

Reactive
Hyperemia

Normal
Response

Abnormal
Response

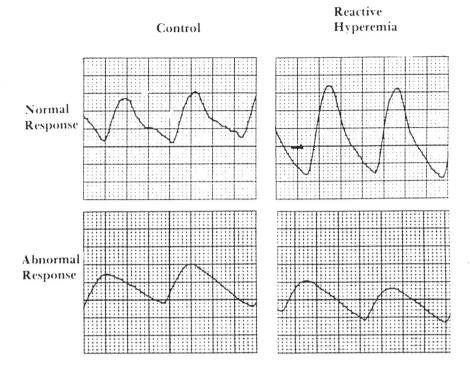

Figure 6. Normal and abnormal reactive hyperemia response. **Upper panels:** patient with Raynaud's disease. **Lower panels:** patient with scleroderma who had normal pressures at the proximal phalanx. From Sumner DS, Lambeth A, Russell JB: Diagnosis of upper extremity obstructive and vasospastic syndrome by Doppler ultrasound, plethysmography, and temperature profiles. In: *Hemodynamics of the Limbs,* Puel P, Boccalon H, Enjalbert A (eds), GEPESC, Toulouse, France, 1979.

emia indicates the total or near total absence of blood flow and, therefore, is indicative of severe ischemia.[38]

Observing the effects of cold and spontaneous rewarming on the amplitude of the finger pulse provides additional diagnostic information.[39] The pulse amplitude in normal subject decreases markedly when the fingers are exposed to temperatures below 20°C. Upon rewarming, the amplitude rapidly and steadily returns to pre-exposure levels. In patients with secondary Raynaud's phenomenon, the pulse disappears or becomes greatly attenuated in response to cold exposure; recovery to pre-exposure levels is steady but delayed. In contrast, patients with primary Raynaud's disease exhibit critical closure—an intense vasospasm that occurs at a specific reduction in finger temperature. Pulses disappear entirely and remain undetectable until the finger temperature rises above 24° to 26°C, whereupon a normal waveform suddenly reappears.

Investigators in France advocate the use of digital pulse volume to grade reactivity to cold.[40] Studies are performed with the patient in a 24° to 26°C room. A vasodilated pulse is first recorded after the hands have been warmed by 3-minute immersion in 45°C water. Maximal vasoconstriction is then produced by using a fan to blow air on the wet thorax of the patient and by immersing the patient's hand in 11°C water. The vasoconstricted pulse volume is then divided by the vasodilated pulse volume to obtain an index of reactivity. A type 1 response indicates "low reactivity" and has an index exceeding 0.20. Type 2 (mild reactivity) and type 3 (major reactivity) have indices of 0.05 to 0.20 and >0.0 to ≤0.19, respectively. Types 4 and 5 (severe reactivity) have ratios of 0.0 (no plethysmographic tracing) and are distinguished by spontaneous recovery of the pulse in less than or greater than 5 minutes, respectively. The authors found significant correlations between the reactivity index and the severity of cold sensitivity as indicated by the incidence of thumb involvement and the frequency of attacks during winter.[40] They also noted that mild to major reactivity was associated with primary Raynaud's disease and severe reactivity was more likely to be associated with scleroderma.

McLafferty et al[41] have devised a "plethysmographic digital obstruction index" (P-DOI) for evaluating hands of patients with moderate or severe hand ischemia. Patients with moderate pain with Raynaud's attacks that required lifestyle modifications to avoid cold exposure were classified in the "moderate" category and patients with finger ulcers associated with severe pain or those who were unable to use their hands when exposed to cold were classified in the "severe" category. For each finger, a score of 8 points was assigned if the digital waveform was normal, 4 points if the upstroke time was greater than 0.2 seconds and the dicrotic notch was lost, 2 points if minimal waveform activity was detected, and 0 if there was no digital waveform. To obtain the index, the scores of all five fingers of each hand were added and the result divided by 40 (a perfectly normal score). They observed that the P-DOI corresponded well with a similar index based on arteriography and that the P-DOI (0.75 ± 0.15) of hands with moderate ischemia was significantly greater than that of hands with severe ischemia (0.51 ± 0.20). A P-DOI less than 0.65 in patients with connective tissue disorders predicted digital ulceration with a sensitivity of 77%, a specificity of 100%, a positive predictive value of 100%, and a negative predictive value of 73%. On the basis of these observations, the authors concluded that digital photoplethysmography is the test of choice for evaluating patients with hand ischemia. Arteriography is required only for ruling out a source for emboli and for patients with no evident systemic illness that explains the hand ischemia.

Reactive Hyperemia

The ability of the digital arterioles to vasodilate can be ascertained by noting the response of the digital pulse to warm water or to reactive hyperemia.[20,31] As described above, reactive hyperemia is produced by inflating a pneumatic cuff placed around the arm to a pressure well above systolic pressure, allowing the cuff to remain inflated for 5 minutes, and then suddenly deflating the cuff. Maximum vasodilation usually develops within 30 seconds. In normal fingers or in those with primary Raynaud's disease, the pulse volume will more than double (Figure 6). Because of the fixed nature of the microvasculature associated with collagen diseases, many of these patients will display little or no vasodilation in response to a period of ischemia (Figure 6). Also, when the proximal obstruction is so severe that the arterioles have dilated maximally to compensate for the increased proximal resistance, there will be little response. Digits that show little or no reactive hyperemia would not be expected to benefit from surgical sympathectomy or from vasodilator drugs.

Sympathetic Nerve Activity

In the presence of an intact sympathetic nerve supply to the fingers, the digit pulse volume and fingertip volume will increase and decrease periodically, coinciding with respiratory activity (Figure 7). These respiratory waves are superimposed on larger, but less frequent, alpha, beta,

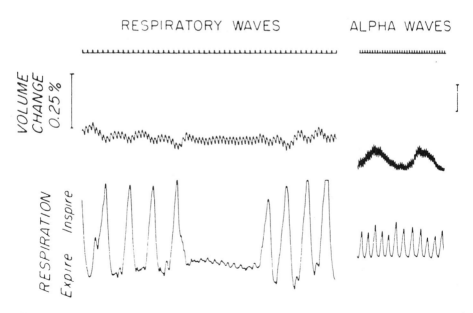

Figure 7. Respiratory waves and alpha waves recorded with a mercury strain gauge plethysmograph from a normal finger tip. From Strandness DE Jr, Sumner DS: *Hemodynamics for Surgeons*, Grune and Stratton, New York, 1975.

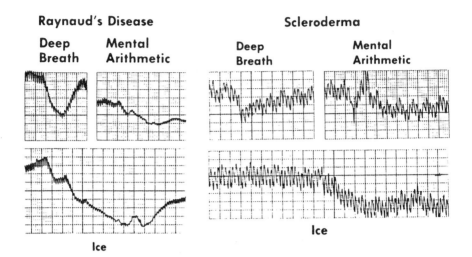

Figure 8. Effect of sympathetic stimuli on digit pulse volume and finger volume in a patient with Raynaud's disease (**left**) and a patient with scleroderma (**right**). Note that the sensitivity of the tracing is greater in the right hand panels than in the left. The patient with scleroderma demonstrates little or no response. From Sumner DS, Lambeth A, Russell JB: Diagnosis of upper extremity obstructive and vasospastic syndromes by Doppler ultrasound, plethysmography, and temperature profiles. In: *Hemodynamics of the Limbs.* Puel P, Boccalon H, Enjalbert A (eds), GEPESC, Toulouse, France, 1979.

gamma waves—all of which are attributed to periodic variations in sympathetic outflow.[9,42,43] A perfectly stable tracing, with little or no change in the volume of the finger or in the pulse volume is, therefore, abnormal and implies the absence of sympathetic activity.

Sympathetic innervation can also be monitored by recording the response of the digit pulse volume and fingertip volume to a deep breath, mental arithmetic, or to ice placed on the chest or forehead (Figure 8).[20] Normally, these maneuvers cause significant vasoconstriction in the presence of an intact sympathetic nerve supply.[14,44,45] Reduction in pulse volume reflects a comparable reduction in digit blood flow, and a reduction in fingertip volume reflects both a reduction in arterial inflow and constriction of the terminal arteries and veins.

These responses may be reduced or absent in patients with collagen diseases (Figure 8). Sympathectomy is unlikely to be beneficial in patients in whom there is little evidence of sympathetic activity.

In order to observe changes in fingertip volume, it is necessary to use the DC input of the recorder. Although changes in pulse volume will be evident on AC recordings, the slower, but larger changes in fingertip volume will be obscured by the ability of the AC circuitry to adjust the baseline.[31]

Doppler Arterial Survey

The Doppler flow signal recorded from a normal peripheral artery is characterized by a rapid systolic upstroke, a sharp peak, frequent reversal of flow in early diastole, and a low-level forward flow signal in late diastole (Figure 9). Obstruction proximal to the site of the probe produces a signal in which the high-frequency elements are attenuated. The resulting tracing shows a slow upslope, a rounded peak, and a downslope that continues throughout diastole (Figure 9). There is no reverse flow phase. Absence of a flow signal implies total occlusion of the underlying artery.

The experienced observer can recognize these patterns from the audible signal alone, obviating the need for recordings. Typically, the normal

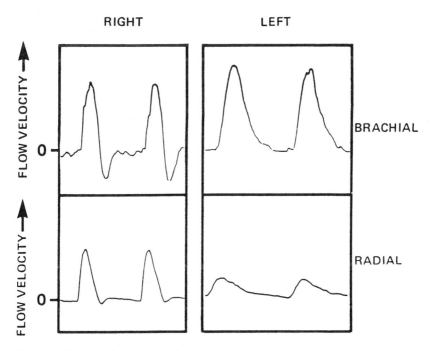

Figure 9. Doppler flow signals from right and left brachial and radial arteries in an 89-year-old female with subclavian arterial obstruction. Brachial pressure: right, 164 mm Hg; left, 101 mm Hg. Wrist pressure: right, 154 mm Hg; left, 77 mm Hg.

audible signal is biphasic or triphasic with a clearly distinguishable high-frequency sound of short duration early in systole. The obstructive signal, on the other hand, is of lower frequency and is monophasic.

By listening in serial fashion to the subclavian, axillary, brachial, radial, ulnar, and proper digital arteries on both sides of the fingers at both the proximal (PIP) and DIP interphalangeal joints, the examiner can often locate the site of arterial obstruction.[6,21,46] It is not unusual to find a signal at the DIP joint in the absence of an ipsilateral PIP signal.[20,46] In this event, compression of the contralateral digital artery at the base of the finger will obliterate the DIP signal, indicating proximal obstruction of the ipsilateral artery with crossover collaterals derived from the contralateral artery. Comparison of the signals obtained from one finger with those from the other fingers will often reveal variable degrees of obstruction that are not evident from the pressure recordings. It is especially important to conduct these finger-flow studies only when the hands are warm in order to avoid false positive results that might occur as a result of vasoconstriction.[46]

The status of the palmar arch can be ascertained quite easily by noting the effect of serial ulnar and radial artery compression on the mid-palmar signal.[47] In a similar fashion, the source of the blood supply to the individual fingers can be determined by noting the effect of radial and ulnar artery compression on the digital signal. In warm normal fingers, a flow signal can usually be heard over the volar surface of the distal phalanx. Absence of a signal in this area implies vasoconstriction or fixed arterial obstruction.

Because of the extensive collateral network available in the hand and forearm, normal or nearly normal arterial signals obtained from the ulnar or radial arteries at the level of the wrist do not always establish the proximal patency of these vessels. For example, both the palpable pulse and the Doppler signal from the radial artery were judged to be normal in a man who, several weeks previously, had undergone an end-to-end repair of a severed radial artery in the proximal forearm. However, the Doppler signal disappeared when the ulnar artery was compressed. Also, it was noted that the Doppler signal at wrist level was reversed, indicating that flow was traveling up the arm, rather than down the arm, toward the hand, as it normally would. Clearly, in this case, a casual observer might have been led to the erroneous conclusion that the proximal repair was patent.

Ultrasonic Imaging

Real-time color-coded duplex imaging of the upper extremity can be accomplished in much the same fashion as scanning of the lower extremity arteries.[48–51] Now that these sophisticated instruments are widely available and technologists have become skilled in their operation, duplex scanning is rapidly assuming an indispensable role in the noninvasive evaluation of subclavian, axillary, brachial, and forearm arteries. Unlike other noninvasive methods, duplex scanning provides precise anatomic information, locates stenotic or occlusive lesions and evaluates their extent and severity, identifies collateral pathways, and defines the patency of arteries distal to an occlusion. In addition, duplex scanning is very helpful in the diagnosis of other lesions such as aneurysms and arteriovenous malformations.[51]

The large vessels of the arm are easily located with the B-mode scan and, with the exception of the subclavian artery, can be scanned in their entirety. Their flow patterns are initially assessed with the color-flow mapping feature, which readily distinguishes between arteries and veins. By convention, arterial flow is labeled as red and venous flow, blue. As the arteries are scanned longitudinally down the arm, changes in color from red to white (sometimes to yellow or green, depending on the labeling convention) identify sites of increased velocity, which correspond to the location of stenoses. Absence of color (a black image) in a vessel seen on the B-mode scan implies total occlusion.

The B-mode and color-flow image allow precise placement of the Doppler sample volume in the region of interest. Spectral analysis of the signal provides velocity data and displays the contour of the flow pulse. Doubling of the velocity at the site of stenosis compared to that measured in a "normal" arterial segment a few centimeters above or below suggests a 50% diameter stenosis. Velocity ratios exceeding 3.0 are characteristic of more severe, hemodynamically significant stenoses. Absence of a flow signal in an interrogated vessel indicates total occlusion and confirms the significance of a black image on the color-flow map.

In normal arteries, recorded frequencies tend to parallel the envelope of the flow pulse, leaving a "window" free of signals in the Doppler frequency spectrum (provided the sample volume is small relative to the diameter of the artery). Loss of the window (spectral broadening) is an early finding suggesting the presence of a low-grade stenosis (<50% diameter reduction). As the stenosis becomes more severe, flow disturbances become more pronounced, and the "window" disappears entirely. Changes in the contour of the flow pulse are interpreted in the same way as those observed with the continuous-wave Doppler (see *Doppler Arterial Survey*).

Direct evaluation of the subclavian artery is necessarily incomplete, owing to its origin in the thorax and to the "blind spot" imposed by its passage under the clavicle. However, lesions in these areas can be detected and their severity evaluated, albeit indirectly, by examining flow patterns in accessible portions of the subclavian artery above or below the clavicle.

Because of their small size, finger arteries are the most challenging of the upper extremity vessels to study.[50] Encouraging results, however, have been reported recently by Langholz et al,[52] who compared color duplex scans of 450 digital arteries in 45 hands of 41 symptomatic patients with conventional hand arteriograms. Of 160 arteries with occlusions, 138 (86%) were correctly diagnosed by color duplex scanning. Of 290 arteriographically patent arteries, 270 (93%) were correctly identified. The positive predictive value of the color duplex interpretations was 87% and the negative predictive value was 93%. In terms of the whole hand, 39 (95%) of the diagnoses were accurate.

False-positive studies were largely due to incomplete visualization of the entire length of the finger arteries. False-negative studies were attributed to segmental occlusions that were overlooked by the ultrasonic scan and to misidentifying collateral vessels as the native artery.

Successful examination of the digital arteries is made possible by the use of advanced instrumentation that is sensitive to slow flow. Probe frequencies of 7 to 10 MHz produce the best images (15-MHz probes, when available, would be even better). Studies should be conducted in a warm room (22°C) to minimize vasospasm. If the finger arteries are inadequately demonstrated, immersion of the hand in 36°–40°C water for 15 minutes or spraying the fingers with topical nitroglycerin may be tried. Digital arteries on both sides of each finger are scanned from proximal to distal. A complete study requires 30 minutes to 1 hour.[52]

Cold-Induced Vasoconstriction

All who have attempted to reproduce vasoconstriction in the laboratory by exposing the hands to cold realize how frustrating such efforts may be. Even though the patient gives a typical history of Raynaud's phenomenon, it may be impossible to duplicate the characteristic color changes. Yet, it is desirable to have an objective method of documenting, grading, and following cold-induced vasospasm.

In our laboratory, we use a simple cold-tolerance test, described by Porter and his associates.[53] Thermistors are taped to the fingertips, preexposure temperatures are noted, the hands are immersed in ice water for 20 seconds, and postexposure temperatures are recorded for 20 minutes. The patients are fully clothed and the room temperature is maintained at about 25°C. Because blood flow to the fingertip bears a direct, though curvilinear, relation to finger temperature, this simple test affords a rough approximation of changes in digital blood flow in response to cold exposure.[9,54]

As shown in Figure 10, the finger temperatures of 19 control subjects (38 fingers) averaged 32° ± 3°C.[18] Twenty minutes after the hands had

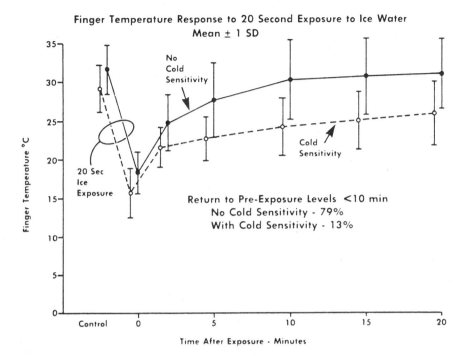

Figure 10. Cold tolerance tests: digital temperature response of control subjects (solid line) and patients with cold sensitivity (broken line) to a 20-second immersion in ice water. From Sumner DS, Lambeth A, Russell JB: Diagnosis of upper extremity obstructive and vasospastic syndrome by Doppler ultrasound, plethysmography, and temperature profiles. In: *Hemodynamics of the Limbs*, Puel P, Boccalon H, Enjalbert A (eds), GEPESC, Toulouse, France, 1979.

been removed from the ice water, the average digital temperature of the controls was 31° ± 4°C but that of the patients with cold sensitivity was only 26° ± 4°C. The average temperatures of the two groups were statistically different ($P < 0.001$) before cold exposure, immediately after, and at 2, 5, 10, and 15 minutes after exposure. Within 10 minutes, digital temperatures had returned to pre-exposure levels in 79% of the control subjects; but only 13% of those with cold sensitivity had attained their initial finger temperature.

A more complex but perhaps more accurate test has been devised by Nielsen and Lassen.[15,55,56] This test measures the systolic blood pressure in a finger cooled to a predetermined temperature. A double inlet cuff, placed around the middle phalanx of the finger being tested, is used first to cool the finger and the underlying arteries and then to measure the systolic blood pressure at that level. To ensure rapid cooling, a second cuff is placed around the proximal phalanx and inflated above systolic pressure, thereby creating an ischemic finger. Cooling solution is circulated through the double inlet cuff until a thermistor indicates that the desired temperature has been reached, a process requiring about 5 to 7 minutes. The double lumen cuff is then pressurized, the proximal occluding cuff is released, and the systolic pressure in the middle phalanx is determined by noting the point at which blood flow resumes as the double lumen cuff is gradually deflated. Return of blood flow is sensed by a mercury strain gauge (or photoplethymograph) applied to the distal phalanx. The process is repeated at progressively lower skin temperatures down to a level of 10°C. *Reopening pressure* is estimated at each temperature by subtracting the pressure in the cooled finger from that in another (uncooled) finger of the same hand.[15,55]

In normal fingers, the systolic blood pressure decreases as the skin temperature decreases; but even at 10°C, the average pressure is only 16% ± 3% less than it is when the fingers are warm. As the finger temperature is reduced in patients with primary Raynaud's disease, the digital artery pressure begins to drop rapidly and then more precipitously until no pressure can be detected. Although the point of complete closure of the digital arteries varies from patient to patient (<10° to 22°C), it is reproducible in the same patient when studies are conducted under standardized conditions. By noting the temperature at which complete closure occurs or by measuring the *reopening pressure* at a specified temperature, one can assess the efficacy of a vasodilator drug and determine the duration of its effect.[57] It is also possible to grade the severity of the cold sensitivity.

According to Alexander and associates,[37] this test has a sensitivity of 100% and a specificity of 79% for identifying the presence or absence of digital artery vasospasm in patients with primary Raynaud's disease or secondary Raynaud's phenomenon. It appears to be more accurate in patients with secondary Raynaud's phenomenon than it is in patients with primary Raynaud's disease.[13,58] The test is most sensitive when sympathetic activity is enhanced by total body cooling.[13]

Maricq et al,[59] using a modification of the Nielsen method, concluded that digital artery pressures may be helpful for differentiating between primary Raynaud's disease and Raynaud's phenomenon associated with scleroderma. Studies were conducted with the patients in a cool room (18°C) to maximize vasospasm. The ratio of digital to brachial pressure in patients with scleroderma averaged about 60% at a finger temperature of 30°C, a figure significantly lower than that in patients with primary Raynaud's disease, which averaged about 80%. The ratio in normal fingers at this temperature was over 90%. At finger temperatures of 10°–15°C, mean digital/brachial pressure ratios in scleroderma patients approached zero, while ratios in patients with primary Raynaud's disease were significantly higher (30%). Both were much lower than ratios in normal patients

(75%–80%) and in patients with "cold sensitivity" that did meet the clinical criteria for Raynaud's phenomenon (60%–70%). Although a pressure ratio less than 70% at a finger temperature of 10%–15°C was 97% sensitive for identifying patients with secondary Raynaud's phenomenon due to scleroderma, the specificity for identifying primary Raynaud's disease was only 25%. Predictive values were poor.

Recently, Naidu et al[60] described a more direct test for detecting digital artery spasm. Their method uses a 20-MHz ultrasonic probe to measure the diameter of finger arteries at room temperature (25°C) and then again after the hand has been immersed in cold water (10°C) for 5 minutes. Twenty-two normal controls and 60 patients with cold sensitivity were studied (40 with primary Raynaud's disease and 20 with secondary Raynaud's phenomenon). At room temperature, the average diameter of the normal control arteries (1.18 ± 0.17 mm) was only slightly greater than the average diameter of the cold sensitive arteries (1.06 ± 0.26 mm). After cold exposure, the diameter of the normal arteries decreased by only 8.7% ± 11.5% to 1.07 ± 0.15 mm. In contrast, the average diameter of the cold sensitive arteries decreased by 92.4% ± 16.4% to 0.09 ± 0.21 mm. When a cold-induced decrease in diameter of 45% was used as a cutoff point, arteries subject to vasospasm were identified with a sensitivity of 97% and normal arteries with a specificity of 100%. These results, while encouraging, need to be corroborated in other laboratories.

Although these techniques provide clinical scientists with valuable objective methods for investigating cold sensitivity, they are too cumbersome and technically demanding to be used in the routine evaluation of patients with Raynaud's phenomenon.

Capillary Microscopy

Capillaries in the nail folds are oriented parallel to the skin surface and can be examined with a microscope at a magnification of 20 to 40 times. To make the skin transparent, immersion oil is placed over the base of the nail. In the absence of a microscope, an ophthalmoscope may suffice. Normal capillary loops are uniformly distributed in parallel fashion and are similar in size and morphology. Capillaries in patients with connective tissue diseases may be enlarged, dilated, or otherwise distorted. Dropout of adjacent capillaries and areas of avascularity may also be present. Megacapillaries are not normally present in patients with rheumatoid arthritis, systemic lupus erythematosus, or polymyositis, but are found in 90% to 100% of patients with scleroderma.[61,62] According to a recent report, megacapillaries were observed in 86% of patients with dermatomyositis, 73% of patients with CREST syndrome, and 56% of patients with mixed connective tissue disease.[62]

Abnormal nail fold capillaries may be the first indication that patients with the clinical diagnosis of primary Raynaud's disease will eventually be found to have an underlying connective tissue disease.[63] In a prospective study of patients classified as having primary Raynaud's disease, Fitzgerald et al[64] found that the presence of abnormal nail fold capillaries was the variable most closely associated with the subsequent identification of a connective tissue disease (odds ratio, 27:1).

Capillary microscopy, therefore, may be best noninvasive method for confirming the presence of an underlying connective tissue disease.

Laser Doppler

Laser Dopplers are useful for evaluating blood flow in the capillaries and subpapillary plexus of a small volume of skin (several cubic millimeters). Because the Doppler shifted frequency of laser light is proportional to both the number and velocity of red blood cells in the sample volume, calibration in terms of volume or velocity of flow is not possible; rather, the output signal (red blood cell flux) is expressed in millivolts. The probe can be attached to the volar surface of the fingertip, where it may be used to assess changes in red blood cell flux or to measure digital blood pressure by detecting the return of flow when a pneumatic cuff placed on a more proximal phalanx is deflated.

Observations parallel those obtained with the noninvasive methods previously described.[65] For example, complete or partial closure of digital arteries in response to finger cooling (as indicated by decreased or absence flux or by markedly reduced or zero pressure) has been shown to differentiate between normal subjects and patients with Raynaud's syndrome.[66] Attempts to correlate digital flux parameters with capillary microscopic findings have met with some success, suggesting a role for laser Doppler in predicting which patients with what appears to be primary Raynaud's disease will eventually turn out to have scleroderma.[67] Others have found that, because of overlapping flux values, the laser Doppler is less discriminating than capillary microscopy for this purpose.[68]

The relative increase in laser Doppler flux observed in the fingertips after 5 minutes of digital artery occlusion (produced by inflating a pneumatic cuff placed around the proximal phalanx) has been investigated as a method for differentiating between primary Raynaud's disease and secondary Raynaud's phenomenon.[69] As expected, the reactive hyperemic response of normal fingers and of fingers of patients with primary Raynaud's disease is similar and is much larger than that in fingers of patients with fixed digital arterial obstruction. Although this test does not discriminate adequately among subgroups of patients with secondary Raynaud's phenomenon, it may be of some value in defining the degree of arterial obstruction.

Application

It is not necessary to perform all of the tests discussed above on every patient in whom arterial disease of the upper extremity is suspected. In the interest of time, economy, and diagnostic accuracy, it is better to be selective. Often, a comprehensive history and a careful physical examination will suggest the diagnosis or at least eliminate a number of categories of disease, permitting one to choose those tests that will be most productive.

Different tests are required depending on the suspected location of the disease, whether the condition is acute or chronic, the presence or absence of cold sensitivity, and whether the complaints are constant or intermittent. The simple algorithm in Figure 11 outlines an approach to the diagnosis of upper extremity ischemia that has been found useful in our laboratory.[70] Attention is first given to the detection of fixed obstruction proximal to the hand. In the event that no proximal disease is discovered, the subsequent examinations are focused on the hands and fingers.

Proximal Obstruction

Complaints suggesting ischemia of the entire arm imply an obstruction involving the brachial, axillary, or subclavian arteries. The diagnosis of obstruction somewhere within these arteries is established quite simply by measuring the brachial pressure in both arms. Pressure data also indicate the severity of the circulatory deprivation. Use of the Doppler flow detector will frequently permit the obstruction to be localized to one or more of the arteries, and sometimes the point of obstruction can be determined. Even more precise localization is possible with duplex scanning, which has the added advantage of delineating the lumen of the runoff vessels. In the event that the obstruction is constantly present, other noninvasive tests are seldom required.

Sudden, acute obstruction—especially in a patient with atrial fibrillation or a recent myocardial infarction—suggests an embolus. Precise location of the clot may help the surgeon decide whether to use a brachial or an antecubital approach. Arteriography is not necessary to make the diagnosis but is helpful for determining distal patency after the embolus has been removed.

In the case of penetrating trauma with suspected arterial injury, finding a decreased brachial pressure will clinch the diagnosis. Sometimes, if the site of entry is low in the upper arm, a forearm pressure measurement will be required. However, it should be emphasized that a normal or near-normal pressure in an arm with an extensive hematoma or history

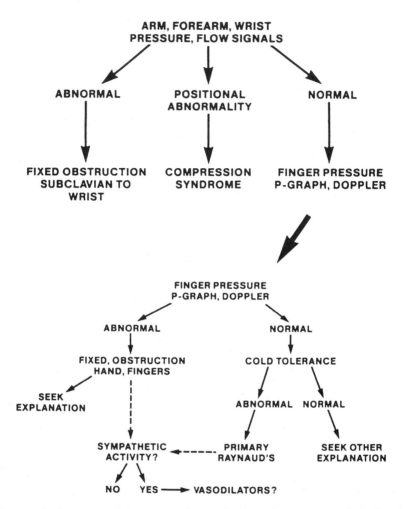

Figure 11. An approach to noninvasive evaluation of upper extremity ischemia. From Sumner DS: Noninvasive assessment of upper extremity and hand ischemia. *J Vasc Surg* 3:560–564, 1986.

suggesting arterial bleeding does not rule out arterial injury. In such cases, an arteriogram should be performed and the wound explored surgically.

Acute obstruction from blunt trauma, prolonged pressure, or *crutch-type* injuries can be assessed noninvasively. If the pressure in the brachial area is in the ischemic range (<40 mm Hg) or if no distal flow is obtained with the Doppler, arteriography should be performed immediately, barring extenuating circumstances. But if the pressure is well above 40 mm

Hg and there is no evidence clinically or noninvasively (finger pressure >40 mm Hg, digital plethysmographic pulses present, peripheral Doppler signals adequate) of severe ischemia, it is permissible to temporize.

Chronic obstruction from arteriosclerosis, neglected trauma, retained emboli, or more rarely from giant cell arteritis of Takayasu's disease should be evaluated with an approach analogous to that used for arterial disease of the legs. Arteriography is necessary only if surgery is planned, and the decision to perform surgery should be based primarily on symptoms and to a lesser extent on the results of noninvasive tests. If a patient complains of arm claudication and the brachial pressure is reduced, it is almost certain that the symptoms are related to arterial obstruction. If the symptoms are excessively troublesome or incapacitating, an operation should be considered. A normal arm pressure makes claudication due to arterial obstruction unlikely, but would not completely rule it out, especially if the patient's complaints develop only during intense exercise. Although inducing postexercise pressure drops in the arm is more difficult than it is in the leg, it can be done.[21,22] Another technique for detecting subtle degrees of arterial obstruction in the arm is to measure the pressure during the period of reactive hyperemia that follows reinstitution of flow after 5 minutes of ischemia produced by inflating a pneumatic cuff. When the pressure drop after exercise or after ischemia is significantly greater (>20 mm Hg) in the symptomatic arm than it is in the asymptomatic arm, the symptoms are probably related to arterial obstruction—even though the pressure in the involved arm under resting conditions is normal.

Noninvasive studies of the upper extremity may be useful in ruling in or out the subclavian steal syndrome.[71–73] It is probably impossible for the patient to have a subclavian steal if the ipsilateral brachial pressure is normal. Bilateral subclavian obstructions can be confusing; but in these cases, examination of the brachial flow patterns with the Doppler will indicate the presence of proximal obstruction. However, a low-brachial arterial pressure does not necessarily imply obstruction of the subclavian artery proximal to the origin of the vertebral, because it can also be due to obstruction of the distal subclavian, axillary, or brachial arteries. On the other hand, finding an abnormal Doppler signal in the infraclavicular space is compatible with the diagnosis of subclavian steal. A description of the noninvasive methods applicable to the vertebral artery is beyond the scope of this chapter; it is sufficient to say that when the Doppler detects reversed flow in the vertebral artery—especially when the volume of flow is increased during reactive hyperemia of the ipsilateral arm—there is a good chance that the patient has a subclavian steal.[71,72] Demonstration of reversed flow in the ipsilateral vertebral artery is best accomplished with the duplex scanner, which is capable of distinguishing the vertebral artery from other arteries in the vicinity.

Obstructions in the Forearm

When the brachial pressure is normal and the forearm pressure is reduced, the obstruction is located in the distal brachial or antecubital arteries. The pressure measured from the radial and ulnar arteries at the wrist will also be reduced, commensurate with the reduction at the forearm level. An excessively large gradient from forearm to wrist (>20 mm Hg) implies additional disease of the radial and ulnar arteries. As pointed out earlier in this chapter, localized obstructions confined to either the radial or ulnar arteries may be more difficult to detect because of the extensive collateral circulation.[27] A palpable pulse of good quality may be present and the pressure measured from the distal portion of the artery may be only slightly reduced even when the artery is obstructed higher up in the forearm. However, the diagnosis may be established with the Doppler, which will show abnormal flow signals that may even be traveling in the wrong direction, or with the duplex scanner, which will enable the obstruction to be visualized.

Most of the problems affecting the forearm arteries are similar to those affecting the brachial and axillary arteries. Emboli and trauma are more serious when they involve the antecubital rather than the more distal arteries, and this is reflected in the pressure data. Arteriosclerosis is less common and Buerger's disease is more common in the forearm than in the proximal arteries.

Iatrogenic trauma to the antecubital or lower brachial arteries is not uncommon following cardiac catheterization procedures.[23,74] Thrombi forming at the site of entry are frequent causes of total obstruction. Again, pressure data and Doppler flow surveys will establish the diagnosis and evaluate its severity.

The possibility of *spasm* is sometimes considered in these cases. In most cases of true spasm, there will be little or no reduction of blood pressure despite the fact that the radial and ulnar pulses are not distinctly palpable. A marked reduction in pressure implies mechanical obstruction. When the pressure at the forearm or wrist level is only moderately reduced, it may be wise to delay further investigation for an hour or so. If the cause was indeed spasm, the pressure will invariably return to normal levels. A number of cases of spasm undoubtedly represent thrombi that may lyse or break up and be dissipated to silent areas of the forearm or hand.

Hand and Fingers

Localized arterial obstruction of the hand and fingers are not difficult to demonstrate noninvasively, but because of the multiple possible etiologies, the rarity of some of the diseases, and the uncertainty regarding their pathophysiology, the diagnosis may remain obscure. As with proximal obstructions, the mode of onset of the complaint (sudden or gradual), the duration of the problem, its location and distribution, and its tendency to be constantly present or intermittent are important clues that enable the investigator to choose with more precision what noninvasive tests to use.

In all cases, the minimum Doppler survey should include testing the integrity of the palmar arch.[47] Because examining the flow patterns in each finger is time consuming and may not be productive, this test should be used selectively when indicated by the history and physical examination.

When all or several fingers of both hands are involved, digital pressures should be measured in all 10 fingers.[27] However, when the complaints are confined to only 1 finger or to adjacent fingers of one hand, it is sufficient to measure the blood pressure in the symptomatic fingers and in the comparable fingers of the opposite hand, which serve as a control. Proximal disease must be ruled out with brachial and forearm pressures.

It is especially important to obtain plethysmographic pulses when the digital pressures are normal, when collagen vascular diseases are suspected, and when the activity of the sympathetic nervous system needs to be assessed. The number of fingers that need to be tested depends on the distribution of disease. At a minimum, the pulses of the involved fingers and suitable controls should be examined.

A discussion of several of the most common pathological entities helps to illustrate the use of these tests. For example, an incomplete palmar arch could be congenital or could be due to trauma, arteriosclerosis, emboli, collagen diseases, Buerger's disease, etc. If there is no decrease in digital pressure and the plethysmographic pulses are normal, the condition is probably congenital. Trauma to the arch and to the ulnar artery—as in the hypothenar hammer syndrome—usually causes some decrease in pressure in the fingers on the ulnar side of the hand and obstructive changes in the plethysmographic pulses.[1,75-77] Doppler signals in the involved fingers will be obstructive and will be obliterated by compression of the radial artery at the wrist. Compression of the ulnar artery would have no effect. Because some of these patients may be suitable candidates for microvascular surgery, it is important to record the extent of the circulatory deprivation and to determine whether any of the peripheral (common digital) arteries are open.[76,78] Doppler surveys of the involved fingers, assessment of pulses, and measurement of digital pressures will help determine the need for surgery and its feasibility. When pressures are above ischemic levels and the digit pulses have a good volume, it is safe to wait to see whether spontaneous improvement occurs. Often this can be documented objectively with these noninvasive methods, thus avoiding surgery. Arteriography is required only when there is no improvement and the patient remains symptomatic or when the initial pressures are so low that the function of the fingers will be impaired. Again, duplex scanning may identify the site of obstruction and provide some clues to its etiology.[49–52]

The development of ischemic symptoms or signs in a single finger suggests emboli or localized trauma. This diagnosis is reinforced by finding normal pressures and plethysmographic pulses in the adjacent fingers. If there is no history to suggest trauma, an arteriographic search for an embolic source may be indicated even when there are no findings to suggest proximal disease. Likewise, when pulses are abnormal or pressures are reduced in the asymptomatic fingers of the same hand but are normal in the other hand, one must again consider multiple emboli or trauma. In such cases, the palmar arch is frequently involved. However, when abnormal findings are distributed widely in the asymptomatic fingers of both hands, the diagnosis is more likely to be a collagen disease, Buerger's disease, or bilateral trauma (eg, vibration-induced occlusions in patients using jackhammers).[79] Similar diagnoses should be entertained in the presence of symptomatic involvement of several fingers of both hands.

When the proximal digital pressures are normal but the pulse obtained from the distal phalanges is abnormal, the obstruction(s) must be confined to the digital arteries. Collagen diseases often present in this way.[32,80]

The level of the digital pressure and the volume of the digital pulse provide valuable prognostic information. These studies can help ascertain whether the treatment should be conservative or whether amputation or sympathectomy should be considered. Ischemia may fluctuate in severity, and the finger circulation often improves spontaneously.[81] Following the pulses and pressures will enable one to determine objectively how effective the treatment has been. The success of a sympathetic block is easily assessed by observing changes in the volume of the plethysmographic pulse. Ordinarily, if the proper nerves have been anesthetized and if the peripheral vasculature retains the ability to vasodilate, the plethysmographic pulse will double in volume.

Intermittent Digital Ischemia

Episodic ischemia of the fingers occurring in response to cold exposure or emotional stimuli is a frequent complaint of patients referred to the vascular laboratory.[82] This condition, which is commonly referred to as Raynaud's phenomenon, is a manifestation of many different disease entities. As discussed earlier in this chapter, the condition lends itself to two general pathophysiological classifications: *primary Raynaud's disease,* in which there is no identifiable arterial obstruction, and *secondary Raynaud's phenomenon,* in which there is a substrate of fixed arterial obstruction.[83,84]

Fixed arterial obstruction is present whenever there is any reduction in digital pressure or any abnormality in the plethysmographic pulse, provided these studies are conducted when the hands are warm and there is no vasoconstriction.

The typical patient with Raynaud's disease is usually young, the majority are female, the complaints are bilateral and symmetrical, and there are no skin changes. In these patients, the cold tolerance test will be abnormal (Figure 10); but the digital pressures and the plethysmographic pulses will be normal.[8,32,85] Vasodilatation in response to warmth or to reactive hyperemia is normal and sympathetic responses are active (Figures 6 and 8). In my experience, none of these patients have had any demonstrable abnormalities in their blood tests.

At the opposite extreme are patients with secondary Raynaud's phenomenon. These patients are usually older than those with Raynaud's disease. Although both hands may be affected, digital involvement is seldom symmetrical. Fingertip ulcers, gangrene, and atrophic skin changes are common, pain may be severe, and cold sensitivity is a less demanding complaint. Plethysmographic pulses are invariably abnormal,[32] the contour is usually peaked or obstructive, and the pulse volume may be reduced or absent (Figure 5). Characteristically, the extent to which the pulses are affected varies from finger to finger. Proximal digital pressures may be normal—even in the presence of obstructive or absent plethysmographic pulses—but are usually reduced and may not be recordable.[8,20,28] The quality of the Doppler flow signals will vary from finger to finger and from proximal to distal on the same finger. Evidence of collateral circulation from one side of a finger to the other is common. In these patients, it is frequently possible to establish a diagnosis. Mechanical factors (vibration-induced injury), toxic factors (industrial exposure), or Buerger's disease may be responsible. Blood tests or biopsies for collagen diseases are often positive.

Between these two extremes, there is a group of patients whose histories and physical examinations are compatible with primary Raynaud's disease but whose noninvasive tests suggest some underlying problem.[32,79,80,83] Some of the digital artery pressures may be moderately reduced, some or all of the plethysmographic pulses may be peaked or obstructive,[80,83] and the Doppler signals may display abnormalities. Occasionally, these patients will have abnormal blood tests (eg, an elevated sedimentation rate, a positive ANA, or some abnormality of the serum immunoelectrophoresis) that point toward a specific diagnosis.[86] Others will have no detectable abnormalities. It is likely that many, perhaps all, of these patients will eventually be diagnosed as having scleroderma or some other similar connective tissue disorder.[79] At present, abnormal capillary microscopy appears to be the best predictor of connective tissue disease.[63,64]

Noninvasive tests will help determine the extent of circulatory deprivation and can aid in selecting therapy. They also provide an objective method for assaying the benefits of any therapeutic regimen that is adopted.[57,87–91]

Thoracic Outlet Syndromes

Intermittent, positionally related obstruction of the subclavian artery as it emerges from the thorax can be detected by noninvasive means. A reduction of the brachial pressure and digital volume pulse when the arm is subjected to the various thoracic outlet maneuvers constitutes a positive test (Figure 12).[21,92,93] When the arm is elevated with the patient in a sitting position, the brachial blood pressure will always be reduced by an amount proportional to the vertical distance from the cuff to the heart. The extent of this hydrostatic effect in millimeters of mercury can be calculated by multiplying the distance in centimeters by 0.735. Therefore, for a hyperabduction test to be positive, the pressure reduction must exceed that due to the hydrostatic effect. Hydrostatic effects are minimal during the Adson's and costoclavicular maneuvers, but these tests are less useful and less specific than the hyperabduction maneuver. If the hyperabduction

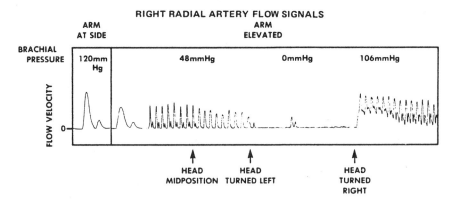

Figure 12. Doppler flow signals from the right radial artery of a 34-year-old man with thoracic outlet syndrome. Signals decrease with arm elevation and are obliterated when the head is turned to the left. Hyperemia occurs when the head is turned to the right. Brachial blood pressure is similarly affected.

maneuver is performed with the patient in a supine position, the hydrostatic effect does not exist.

Bilateral studies should always be performed. A reduction in pressure of more than 20 mm Hg on one side compared with that experienced on the other side is evidence of ipsilateral obstruction.

Doppler flow signals, monitored at the radial artery, will also demonstrate obstructive changes when the subclavian artery is compressed; however, they may not disappear completely even when the subclavian artery is totally occluded due to the extensive collateral network around the neck and shoulder.[21]

If the maneuvers do not reduce the cross-sectioned area of the subclavian artery by 75% or more, there will be little or no hemodynamic evidence of compression at the thoracic outlet. Therefore, negative tests do not rule out the thoracic outlet syndromes. Significant compression of the brachial plexus may be, and often is, present without interfering with the arterial blood flow. On the other hand, arterial compression may occur in the absence of evident nerve compression.

In my experience, physical examination consisting of palpation of the radial pulse and listening for infraclavicular bruits when the arm is being manipulated is usually positive in the same cases that have positive noninvasive studies. The noninvasive tests merely add a dimension of objectivity. Of more importance is the use of noninvasive tests to detect circulatory disturbances in the arm, hand, or fingers. Evidence of peripheral obstruction in an arm subject to intermittent subclavian compression should alert the physician to the possibility of emboli arising from a post-stenotic dilatation of the subclavian artery.

Venous Disease

Thrombotic obstruction of the subclavian or axillary veins can occur spontaneously or develop as a result of trauma, extrinsic compression, or most frequently in association with catheters used for venous access. Brachial veins may clot for similar reasons. Deep venous thromboses in these areas typically produce swelling of the arm and hand, a slight cyanotic discoloration, and some distention of the superficial veins. Pain, tenderness, or a sensation of heaviness may be present. With long-standing obstruction, patients sometimes experience fatigue or tightness in the affected area, particularly after exercise (venous claudication). Symptoms and signs depend on the location and extent of the clot, the rapidity with which it developed, how long it has been present, and the adequacy of the venous collaterals.

Swelling of the area can also result from lymphatic obstruction, trauma, infiltration of intravenous fluids, injections of toxic substances, and infection. Although it may be easy to distinguish clinically among the various possibilities, the picture is all too often confusing. Adding to the confusion is the fact that any of the possible causes listed above may exist in conjunction with deep venous thrombosis.

Noninvasive tests are often diagnostic. Venograms may be avoided altogether or the decision to obtain venograms or lymphangiograms can be made with more assurance that the results will be positive.

Superficial venous thromboses in the arm are usually caused by intravenous infusions or by catheter trauma. They are easily diagnosed clinically and do not require noninvasive evaluation except to rule out concomitant deep venous disease.

Pathophysiology

The dynamics of venous blood flow in the arm varies somewhat from that in the leg. In the leg of a supine individual, venous blood flow is reduced during inspiration and augmented during expiration, due to changes in intra-abdominal pressure caused by the contraction and relaxation of the diaphragm. Because there is no high-pressure area corresponding to the abdomen between the thorax and the arm, blood flow in the arm veins may increase with inspiration and decrease with expiration (Figure 13). These variations in flow reflect the alterations in intrathoracic pressure that develop during the respiratory cycle. However, during a rapid deep inspiration, the marked decrease in intrathoracic pressure may exhaust the volume of blood in the subclavian vein leading to its collapse,

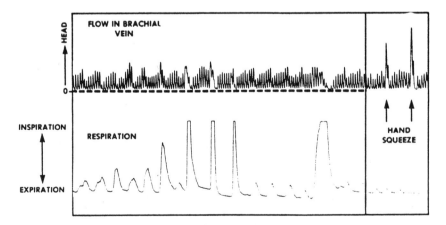

Figure 13. Effect of respiration on venous flow patterns in the arm. Note pulsatility, variable effect of respiration on flow, and effect of hand squeeze.

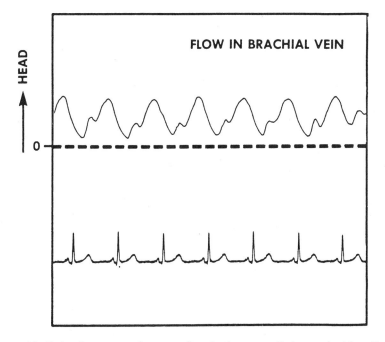

Figure 14. Pulsatile nature of venous flow in the arms. Pulses coincide with the cardiac cycle.

much as rapid suction on a limp straw in a soft drink may cause it to collapse. Thus, venous flow from the arm may actually be impeded during inspiration. In other words, two patterns can be observed: with slow inspiration, an increase in blood flow, and with rapid deep inspiration, a decrease in blood flow.

Moreover, venous blood flow at all levels in the arm tends to be pulsatile, the pulses occurring at the same rate as the heartbeat (Figure 14). (Pulsatile flow is seldom very evident in the lower extremity unless the central venous pressure is elevated as in cases of right heart failure.) Pulsatile flow is most marked in the axillary and subclavian veins but can easily be detected in the superficial veins of the hand. Accompanying each heartbeat, there are variations in the pressure within the right atrium and superior vena cava. When the pressure in these central vessels is increased, venous outflow from the arm is decreased; and when the central pressure is decreased, venous outflow is increased.

Squeezing the hand and contraction of the forearm musculature will evacuate the associated deep and superficial veins causing an augmentation of venous outflow in the proximal portion of the arm and in the subclavian area. Similarly, manual compression of the forearm will augment venous outflow. Competent valves in the deep and superficial veins prohibit reflux of venous flow down the arm when the proximal portions of the arm are compressed.

Obstruction, extrinsic or intrinsic, interferes with the flow pattern, providing the rationale for the use of the Doppler in the diagnosis of venous disease. Respiratory effects and pulsations will be reduced in the arm peripheral to the site of obstruction. The velocity of flow may also be decreased. The magnitude of these changes depends on the location and extent of the thrombus and on the capacity of the collateral circulation.

Doppler Venous Survey

In my experience, the Doppler velocity meter has been a most useful noninvasive instrument for detecting the presence of venous obstruction in the arm. (The accuracy in two small series was reported to be 100%.[94,95]) Either the 5- or 10-MHz probe may be used, but the former is better in the subclavian and proximal axillary areas and the latter is better for superficial veins. It is not necessary to record the signals because the audible signal is adequate and avoids the encumbrance of additional electronic gear. In all cases, the flow pattern should be studied in the jugular vein, the axillary vein below the clavicle, the brachial and antecubital veins, and in the radial veins at the wrist. Prominent superficial veins in the shoulder region and across the upper chest should also be examined. The studies should always be bilateral because at each level the flow patterns in the veins of one arm are compared with those of the other. Only in this way will subtle differences be detected.

The procedure is analogous to that used in studying the veins of the lower extremity. First, the adjacent artery is located to ensure accurate identification of the proper vein, and then the Doppler probe is shifted slightly to obtain the optimum signal. Some time must be spent listening to the spontaneous flow patterns. As discussed under *Pathophysiology*, the spontaneous signal should vary with respiration and show pulsations reflecting the contractions of the right atrium. Any decrease in the volume of the signal or damping of the respiratory waves or pulses suggests the presence of an obstruction in a more centrally located vein. Obviously, if the probe is situated over the site of obstruction, no flow will be detected. After the spontaneous signals have been adequately studied, the examiner augments the flow by squeezing the forearm. Alternatively, the patient may be asked to forcibly make a fist. Normally, these maneuvers will increase the flow of blood through the veins underlying the probe, thereby augmenting the signal. In the event that the obstruction lies between the site of the probe and the point where the arm is squeezed, there will be little or no augmentation. If both the probe and the point of squeeze are peripheral to the obstruction, there may be some augmentation of the signal, but the augmented signal will have a characteristic abrupt quality. Sometimes it is difficult to obtain good augmentation even when all the veins are normal. This is due to an inadequate volume of blood in the forearm veins and may occur when the arm is cold.

An increase in the velocity of flow in the superficial veins of the upper arm or chest is excellent evidence that these veins are serving as collateral channels. This finding, in conjunction with abnormalities in the deep venous flow pattern, establishes the diagnosis of venous obstruction.

Although precise location of the point or extent of the venous obstruction may not be possible, it is usually possible to narrow it down to the brachial area or the axillary subclavian region. Obstruction of the innominate vein not only alters the flow pattern in the ipsilateral axillary and brachial veins but also distorts or obliterates the signal in the jugular vein. I have observed this in a number of cases where the obstruction was originally thought to be limited to the subclavian vein. Ordinary venograms, performed through the arm, seldom permit one to diagnose innominate vein obstruction.

Intermittent obstruction of the subclavian vein at the thoracic outlet may be detected by comparing the Doppler signals with the arm in various positions.

Venous Imaging

Color duplex imaging has become the preferred method for noninvasive diagnosis of upper extremity venous thrombosis. This is the only noninvasive technique that can locate the clot and define its extent.

Examination methods are similar to those used in the lower extremity, with the exception that the proximal subclavian veins and the innominate veins cannot be compressed to ascertain patency. The clavicle is also an impediment to compression and to complete visualization of the subclavian vein. Color images indicate the direction of flow and permit direct observation of the effects of augmentation maneuvers and respirations. Changes in flow parameters are interpreted as described under *Doppler Venous Survey* and may be useful for diagnosing thrombi in blind segments of the subclavian or axillary veins. In most areas, however, venous thrombosis is readily identified by the absence of color in a vein imaged on the B-mode scan. In regions where probe compression is possible, incomplete collapse of the vein substantiates the presence of a thrombus. Encroachment on the color-flow image is suggestive of a stenosis or a partially occlusive thrombus. Although fresh clot may not be visible within the lumen, older clots are echogenic and are usually easily seen.

Patents are examined in the supine position. Surveys begin in the infraclavicular region, where the distal subclavian and the proximal axillary veins are imaged through the pectoral muscles. Scanning is continued along the inner aspect of the arm, beginning with the distal axillary vein followed by the brachial, radial, ulnar, basilic, and cephalic veins. A supraclavicular approach is used to examine the internal jugular, proximal subclavian, and distal innominate veins. Scanning is done in the longitudinal direction with cross-sectional images being obtained when necessary.

Despite the widespread use of color duplex imaging, there are relatively few reports of studies in which venography has been used to confirm its accuracy for identifying thrombi of the upper extremity veins. In a series of 22 patients with suspected thrombosis of the upper extremity or thoracic inlet veins, Knudson et al[96] found that color duplex had a sensitivity of 78%, a specificity of 92%, a positive predictive value of 88%, and a negative predictive value of 86%. The false-negative results occurred in two patients with proximal subclavian thrombosis and the single false-positive study was due to extrinsic compression. Others have reported 100% sensitivity and specificity for subclavian and axillary vein thrombosis.[97,98] In one study, the innominate vein was visualized in seven of eight cases, five of which were confirmed to be thrombosed.[97]

Color duplex is also very useful for "mapping" superficial arm veins to determine their diameter and anatomic course prior to lower extremity bypass grafting.[99]

Plethysmography

Although phleborheography and impedance plethysmography were reported to be reasonably accurate for diagnosing deep venous thrombosis of the upper extremity, these tests have now been superseded by duplex scanning and are now rarely used clinically.[94,100]

Arteriovenous Fistulas

Arteriovenous fistulas are of two basic types: acquired and congenital. The acquired variety is by far the simpler of the two. Formerly, most were the result of penetrating trauma, but now the vast majority are surgically constructed to provide vascular access. Unlike acquired arteriovenous fistulas, where there is usually only one connection between the artery and vein, congenital fistulas are far more complex, usually having multiple arteriovenous communications.

The clinical manifestations of arteriovenous fistulas are well known and need not be repeated here. Although in most cases, the signs, symptoms, and history clearly point to the diagnosis; occasionally the diagnosis may be obscure. Noninvasive tests are helpful in substantiating the diagnosis and in establishing the degree of peripheral circulatory deprivation caused by the fistula. In addition, they are valuable tools for assessing the function of surgically created arteriovenous fistulas.

Pathophysiology

Basically, an arteriovenous fistula creates a short-circuit between one or more arteries and veins.[9,101] This increases the volume of arterial inflow to the arm proximal to the fistula and similarly augments the venous outflow from the arm. However, peripheral to the fistula, arterial blood flow and arterial pressure may be reduced, occasionally to the point of causing ischemia. Peripheral venous pressure is usually increased, sometimes markedly so. The extent of the peripheral circulatory deprivation is a function of the size of the fistula and the magnitude of the resulting collateral circulation.

Arterial collaterals originate above the fistula and carry blood to some point distal to the fistula. Depending upon the relative resistances of the fistula and that of the collateral arteries, the collateral arteries may serve as the only source of blood to the peripheral tissues. They may also contribute blood to the fistula via the distal artery, where the direction of flow may be reversed, traveling retrograde up the arm toward the fistula rather than in the normal antegrade direction toward the hand. Reversed flow in the distal radial artery is commonly seen in limbs with a surgically constructed radial artery-cephalic vein fistula.

Venous collaterals develop in response to the relatively high pressure generated in the veins situated peripheral to the fistula. They serve to return blood to the central veins by circumventing the high-pressure areas. Flow in the distal vein of a side-to-side fistula is commonly reversed, that is, it is directed peripherally toward the hand rather than up the arm.

Noninvasive Tests

Examination of arterial and venous blood flow patterns with the Doppler velocity detector is perhaps the best method for instituting the investigation of a suspected arteriovenous fistula.[102]

The demonstration of increased blood flow in the arteries and veins proximal to the site of a presumed arteriovenous fistula establishes the diagnosis. Although inflammation will also increase both arterial inflow and venous outflow, erythema, swelling, and other signs will point to the correct diagnosis. No other disease and certainly no other vascular lesion results in isolated augmentation of arterial flow. Manual compression applied to the site of the presumed fistula will markedly reduce the flow, returning it to normal levels.

A Doppler survey of the arteries and veins distal to the fistula will demonstrate normal or reduced flow velocities. Blood flow in the distal artery and veins may be reversed. Frequently, compression of the fistula will augment peripheral arterial flow and may restore normal antegrade flow (Figure 15). Again, no other lesion behaves in this fashion.

Measurement of blood pressure in the arm, wrist, or fingers distal to a fistula enables the clinician to determine the magnitude of the circulatory deprivation produced by the steal (Figure 15). A normal distal blood pressure indicates that the fistula is small or is well compensated by collateral development. Depending upon the size of the fistula and the adequacy of arterial collaterals, compression of the fistula may actually increase the

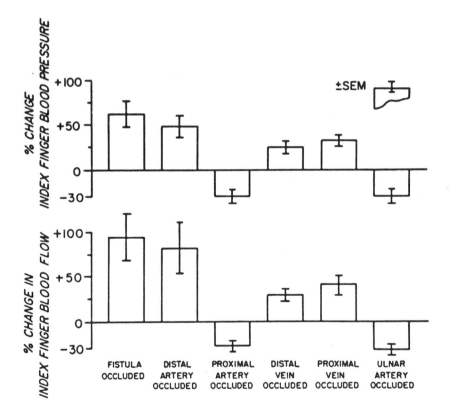

Figure 15. Effect of manual compression of various portions of radial artery–cephalic vein fistulas on index finger blood pressure and blood flow. Average values from 24 limbs are illustrated. From Strandness DE Jr, Sumner DS: *Hemodynamics for Surgeons*, Grune and Stratton, New York, 1975.

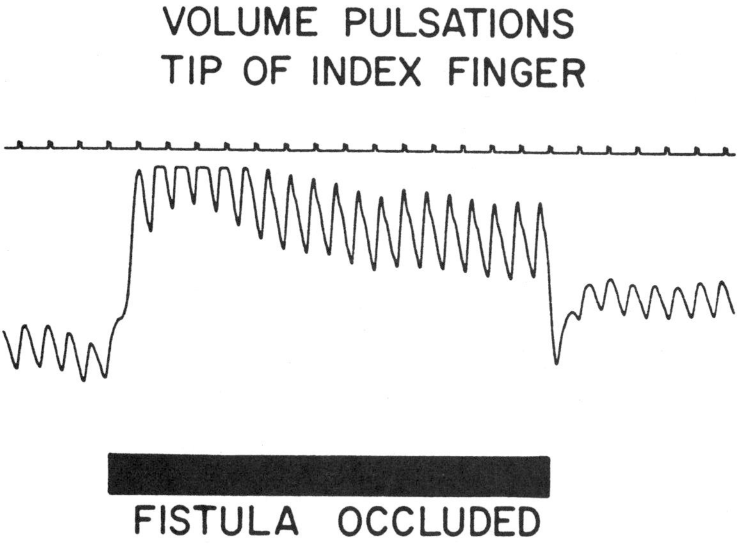

VOLUME PULSATIONS
TIP OF INDEX FINGER

FISTULA OCCLUDED

Figure 16. Effect of manual compression of a radial artery-cephalic vein fistula on pulse volume and distal phalangeal volume of the ipsilateral index finger. From Strandness DE Jr, Sumner DS: *Hemodynamics for Surgeons*, Grune and Stratton, New York, 1975.

peripheral pressure, sometimes returning it to normal levels. When the collaterals are small and the involved artery continues to serve as the major source of peripheral blood flow, compression of the fistula and the involved artery will decrease the peripheral pressure.

Digital plethysmographic pulses may be normal (when the fistula is small) but are frequently reduced in volume and may have an abnormal contour. Compression of the fistula may increase the pulse volume and restore the contour to a normal configuration (Figure 16).

Of course, when other arterial lesions exist in conjunction with the arteriovenous fistula, the observations discussed above will be modified. However, the basic changes will remain the same.

Patients with functioning side-to-side or side-to-end radial artery-cephalic vein fistulas occasionally complain of ischemic pain on the radial side of their hand—the so-called radial steal syndrome.[101,103] In these cases, flow in the distal radial artery will be reversed. Blood pressure in the thumb and index finger will be decreased but will return to normal (or near normal) when the distal artery is manually compressed. By ligating the distal radial artery, the surgeon can alleviate the symptoms and increase the digital blood pressure.

The findings in patients with congenital fistulas are similar but generally more complex.[9] Even with large lesions, the increase in proximal blood flow is seldom as marked as it is with acquired fistulas; and due to the multiple and diffuse communications, it is unusual to demonstrate improved distal perfusion with compression of the fistula. Peripheral flow, blood pressure, and pulses may be markedly reduced, especially in conjunction with diffuse arteriovenous malformations of the hand, but more proximally located fistulas seldom result in marked flow deprivation. Because of the diffuse nature of the arteriovenous communications, volume pulses, obtained by applying the plethysmograph to the site of the fistula, are often markedly increased.[102] Since this phenomenon occurs with no other lesion, it is diagnostic of congenital arteriovenous malformation.

Congenital fistulas can be visualized with the duplex scanner, which also permits the diameter and morphology of the feeding artery to be examined.[49] Imaging has been shown to be valuable in the follow-up of surgically constructed arteriovenous fistulas used for vascular access.[104] Constrictions of the distal vein, the venous anastomosis, and of the graft itself may be evident on the B-mode scan, and are confirmed by increased frequencies and by alterations in the Doppler spectrum.

Microvascular Injuries

Certain injuries, such as frostbite or the intra-arterial injection of toxic substances, can obstruct the microvasculature while leaving the major arteries and veins open, at least initially. In frostbite, flow may continue via arteriovenous shunts even though nutritional (capillary) blood flow is absent. Similar changes are sometimes seen in patients who have been in shock. These changes presumably reflect the effect of profound adrenergic stimuli, which divert blood flow away from the periphery. The hands and fingers may be cold, swollen, and have a grayish color.

Early in the course of these poorly understood conditions, weak Doppler signals may be present even in the distal portions of the involved digits. Plethysmographic pulses are absent or reduced and, when present, usually have an abnormal contour. Blood pressure at the base of the digits may be normal. With time, the arterial signals disappear, the pressures drop to unobtainable levels, and the fingers become gangrenous.

When Doppler signals are good and the distal digital pressures are normal, the prognosis is better. In some of these cases, I have observed complete recovery.

Revascularization and Replantation

The remarkable advances in microvascular surgery now permit the restoration of flow to many completely severed or partially severed fingers, hands, and arms. Although survival of the severed part implies the successful restoration of blood flow through at least some of the anastomoses, it does not necessarily indicate that the blood supply has been returned to normal levels. Noninvasive measurement of digit pulses, digital blood flow, and digital pressures permits the surgeon to objectively assess the adequacy of the reconstruction.[29,105,106] Imaging with the duplex scanner has also proved to be helpful.[48]

In a study of 33 digital replants and revascularizations, 80% of the operated fingers demonstrated a statistically significant reduction in blood pressure and blood flow when compared with the same finger on the opposite hand.[29] However, 75% of the blood pressures and all of the blood flows fell within the 95% confidence limits of control normal values. In other words, the perfusion of tissues surviving replantation or revascularization is usually within normal limits but is often reduced when compared to that of normal tissues of the same individual.

References

1. McNamara MF, Takaki HS, Yao JST, Bergan JJ: A systematic approach to severe hand ischemia. *Surgery* 83:1–11, 1978.
2. Porter JM, Rivers SP, Anderson CJ, Baur GM: Evaluation and management of patients with Raynaud's syndrome. *Am J Surg* 142:183–189, 1981.
3. Erlandson EE, Forrest ME, Shields JJ, et al: Discriminant arteriographic criteria in the management of forearm and hand ischemia. *Surgery* 90:1025–1036, 1981.
4. Sumner DS: Noninvasive assessment of upper extremity ischemia. In: Bergan JJ, Yao JST (eds): *Evaluation and Treatment of Upper and Lower Extremity Circulatory Disorders.* Orlando: Grune & Stratton, Inc; 1984, pp. 75–95.
5. Yao JST: Preoperative assessment of upper extremity ischemia. In: Greenhalgh RM (ed): *Diagnostic Techniques and Assessment Procedures in Vascular Surgery.* London: Grune & Stratton, Inc; 1985, pp. 359–378.
6. Berger AC, Kleinert JM: Noninvasive vascular studies: A comparison with arteriography and surgical findings in the upper extremity. *J Hand Surg* 17A: 206–210, 1992.
7. Mendlowitz M, Naftchi N: The digital circulation in Raynaud's disease. *Am J Cardiol* 4:580–584, 1959.
8. Hirai M: Cold sensitivity of the hand in arterial occlusive disease. *Surgery* 85:140–146, 1979.
9. Strandness DE, Jr, Sumner DS: Raynaud's disease and Raynaud's phenomenon. In: *Hemodynamics for Surgeons,* New York: Grune and Stratton; 1975, pp. 543–581.
10. Lewis T: Experiments relating to the peripheral mechanism involved in spastic arrest of the circulation in the fingers: A variety of Raynaud's disease. *Heart* 15:7–101, 1929.
11. Rösch J, Porter JM, Gralino BJ: Cryodynamic hand angiography in the diagnosis and management of Raynaud's syndrome. *Circulation* 55:807–814, 1977.

12. Edwards JM, Phinney ES, Taylor LM, et al: α_2 Adrenergic receptor levels in obstructive and spastic Raynaud's syndrome. *J Vasc Surg* 5:38–45, 1987.
13. Carter SA, Dean E, Kroeger EA: Apparent finger systolic pressures during cooling in patients with Raynaud's syndrome. *Circulation* 77:988–996, 1988.
14. Jamieson GG, Ludbrook J, Wilson A: Cold hypersensitivity in Raynaud's phenomenon. *Circulation* 44:254–264, 1971.
15. Krähenbühl B, Nielsen SL, Lassen NA: Closure of digital arteries in high vascular tone states as demonstrated by measurement of systolic blood pressure in the fingers. *Scand J Clin Lab Invest* 37:71–76, 1977.
16. Ohgi S, Moore DJ, Miles RD, et al: The effect of cold on circulation in normal and cold sensitive fingers. *Bruit* 9:9–15, 1985.
17. Lynn RB, Steiner RE, Van Wyk FAK: Arteriographic appearances of the digital arteries of the hands in Raynaud's disease. *Lancet* 1:471–474, 1955.
18. Pyykkö I, Kolari P, Fäkkilä M, et al. Finger peripheral resistance during local cold provocation in vasospastic disease. *Scand J Work Environ Health* 12: 395–399, 1986.
19. Singh S, de Trafford JC, Baskerville PA, Roberts VC: Digital artery calibre measurement—A new technique of assessing Raynaud's phenomenon. *Eur J Vasc Surg* 5:199–203, 1991.
20. Sumner DS, Lambeth A, Russell JB: Diagnosis of upper extremity obstructive and vasospastic syndromes by Doppler ultrasound, plethysmography, and temperature profiles. In: Puel P, Boccalon H, Enjalbert A (eds): *Hemodynamics of the Limbs*, Toulouse, France; GEPESC, 1979, pp. 365–373.
21. Yao JST, Gourmos C, Pathanasiou K, Irvine WT: A method for assessing ischemia of the hands and fingers. *Surg Gynecol Obstet* 135:373–378, 1972.
22. Gross WS, Flanigan P, Kraft RO, Stanley JC: Chronic upper extremity arterial insufficiency. *Arch Surg* 113:419–423, 1978.
23. Barnes RW, Peterson JL, Krugmire RB, Strandness DE Jr: Complications of brachial artery catheterization: Prospective evaluation with the Doppler velocity detector. *Chest* 66:363–367, 1974.
24. Gunderson J: Segmental measurement of systolic blood pressure in the extremities including the thumb and the great toe. *Acta Chir Scand (Suppl)* 426: 1–90, 1972.
25. Nielsen PE, Bell G, Lassen NA: The measurement of digital systolic blood pressure by strain gauge technique. *Scand J Clin Lab Invest* 29:371–379, 1972.
26. Downs AR, Gaskell P, Morrow I, Munson RN: Assessment of arterial obstruction in vessels supplying the fingers by measurement of local blood pressures and the skin temperature response test-correlation with angiographic evidence. *Surgery* 77:530–539, 1975.
27. Hirai M: Arterial insufficiency of the hand evaluated by digital blood pressure and arteriographic findings. *Circulation* 58:902–908, 1978.
28. Salem ME-S, El-Girby AH, El-Moneim NAA, Khalil SA: Value of finger arterial blood pressure in diagnosis of vascular changes in some connective tissue diseases. *Angiology* 44:183–187, 1993.
29. Manke DA, Sumner DS, Van Beek AL, Lambeth A: Hemodynamic studies of digital and extremity replants or revascularizations. *Surgery* 88:445–452, 1980.

30. Hirai M, Ohta T, Shionoya S: Development of a bladder-free cuff for measuring the blood pressure of the fingers and toes. *Circulation* 61:704–709, 1980.
31. Sumner DS: Mercury strain-gauge plethysmography. In: Bernstein EF (ed): *Vascular Diagnosis*, 4th ed. St. Louis: Mosby; 1993, pp. 205–223.
32. Sumner DS, Strandness DE, Jr: An abnormal finger pulse associated with cold sensitivity. *Ann Surg* 175:294–298, 1972.
33. Thulesius O: Methods for the evaluation of peripheral vascular function in the upper extremities. *Acta Chir Scand (Suppl)* 465:53–54, 1975.
34. Ohgi S, Moore DJ, Miles RD, et al: Physiology of the peaked finger pulse in normal and cold-sensitive subjects. *J Vasc Surg* 3:516–522, 1986.
35. Hertzman AB, Roth LW: The reactions of the digital artery and minute pad arteries to local cold. *Am J Physiol* 136:680–691, 1942.
36. Huff SE: Observations on peripheral circulation in various dermatoses. *Arch Dermatol* 71:575–578, 1955.
37. Alexander S, Cummings C, Figg-Hoblyn L, et al: Usefulness of digital peaked pulse for diagnosis of Raynaud's syndrome. *J Vasc Technol* 12:71–75, 1988.
38. Peller JS, Gabor GT, Porter JM, Bennett RM: Angiographic findings in mixed connective tissue disease. Correlation with fingernail capillary photomicroscopy and digital photoplethysmography findings. *Arthritis Rheum* 28: 768–774, 1985.
39. Holmgren K, Bauer GM, Porter JM: Vascular laboratory evaluation of Raynaud's syndrome. *Bruit* 5:19–22, 1981.
40. Pistorius M-A, Planchon B, de Faucal P: Plethysmographic cold test for diagnosis and evaluation of the severity of Raynaud's phenomenon. *Int Angiol* 13:10–14, 1994.
41. McLafferty RB, Edwards JM, Taylor LM Jr, Porter JM: Diagnosis and long-term clinical outcome in patients diagnosed with hand ischemia. *J Vasc Surg* 22:361–369, 1995.
42. Burch GE: *Digital Plethysmography*. New York, Grune and Stratton, 1954.
43. Honda N: The periodicity in volume fluctuations and blood flow in the human finger. *Angiology* 21:442–446, 1970.
44. Browse NL, Hardwick PJ: The deep breath-venoconstriction reflex. *Clin Sci* 37:125–135, 1969.
45. Delius W, Kellerova E: Reactions of arterial and venous vessels in the human forearm and hand to deep breath or mental strain. *Clin Sci* 40:271–282, 1971.
46. Balas P, Katsogiannis A, Katsiotis P, Karaitianos J: Comparative study of evaluation of digital arterial circulation by Doppler ultrasonic tracing and hand arteriography. *J Cardiovasc Surg* 21:455–462, 1980.
47. Mozersky DJ, Buckley CJ, Hagood CO Jr, et al. Ultrasonic evaluation of the palmar circulation. A useful adjunct to radial artery cannulation. *Am J Surg* 126:810–, 1973.
48. Koman LA, Bond MG, Carter RE, Poehling GG: Evaluation of upper extremity vasculature with high resolution ultrasound. *J Hand Surg* 10:249–255, 1985.
49. Payne MP, Blackburn DR, Peterson LK, et al: B-Mode imaging of the hand and upper extremity. *Bruit* 10:168–176, 1986.
50. Trager S, Pignatoro M, Anderson J, Kleinert JM: Color flow Doppler: Imaging the upper extremity. *J Hand Surg* 18A:621–625, 1993.

51. Hutchison DT: Color duplex imaging: Applications to upper extremity and microvascular surgery. *Hand Clin* 9:47–57, 1993.
52. Langholz J, Ladleif M, Blank B, et al: Colour coded duplex sonography in ischemic finger artery disease—A comparison with hand arteriography. *Vasa* 26:85–90, 1997.
53. Porter JM, Snider RL, Bardana EJ, et al: The diagnosis and treatment of Raynaud's phenomenon. *Surgery* 77:11–23, 1975.
54. Peacock JH: The effect of changes in local temperature on the blood flows of the normal hand, primary Raynaud's disease and primary acrocyanosis. *Clin Sci* 19:505-512, 1960.
55. Nielsen SL, Lassen NA: Measurement of digital blood pressure after local cooling. *J Appl Physiol* 43:907–910, 1977.
56. Hoare M, Miles C, Girvan R, et al: The effect of local cooling on digital systolic pressure in patients with Raynaud's syndrome. *Br J Surg* 69(Suppl):527–528, 1982.
57. Nobin BA, Nielsen SL, Eklov B, Lassen NA: Reserpine treatment of Raynaud's disease. *Ann Surg* 87:12–16, 1978.
58. Corbin DOC, Wood DA, Housley E: An evaluation of finger systolic-pressure response to local cooling in the diagnosis of primary Raynaud's phenomenon. *Clin Physiol* 5:383–392, 1985.
59. Maricq HR, Weinrich MC, Valter I, et al: Digital vascular responses to cooling in subjects with cold sensitivity, primary Raynaud's phenomenon, or scleroderma spectrum disorders. *J Rheumatol* 23:2068–2078, 1996.
60. Naidu S, Baskerville PA, Goss DE, Roberts VC: Raynaud's phenomenon and cold stress testing: A new approach. *Eur J Vasc Surg* 8:567–573, 1994.
61. Maricq HR, Spencer-Green G, LeRoy EC: Skin capillary abnormalities as indicators of organ involvement in scleroderma (systemic sclerosis), Raynaud's syndrome and dermatomyositis. *Am J Med* 61:862–870, 1976.
62. Blockmans D, Beyens G, Verhaeghe R: Predictive value of nailfold capillaroscopy in the diagnosis of connective tissue diseases. *Clin Rheumatol* 15:148–153, 1996.
63. Priollet P, Vayssairat M, Housset E: How to classify Raynaud's phenomenon. Long-term follow-up study of 73 cases. *Am J Med* 83:494–498, 1987.
64. Fitzgerald O, Hess EV, O'Connor GT, Spencer-Green G: Prospective study of the evolution of Raynaud's phenomenon. *Am J Med* 84:718–726, 1988.
65. Konan LA, Smith BP, Smith TL: Stress testing in the evaluation of upper-extremity perfusion. *Hand Clin* 9:59–83, 1993.
66. Allen JA, Devlin MA, McGrann S, Doherty CC: An objective test for the diagnosis and grading of vasospasm in patients with Raynaud's syndrome. *Clin Sci* 82:529–534, 1992.
67. Binaghi F, Cannas F, Mathieu A, Pitzus F: Correlations among capillaroscopic abnormalities, digital flow and immunologic findings in patients with isolated Raynaud's phenomenon. Can laser Doppler flowmetry help identify a secondary Raynaud phenomenon? *Int Angiol* 11:186–194, 1992.
68. Lütolf O, Chen D, Zehnder Th, Mahler F: Influence of local finger cooling on laser Doppler flux and nailfold capillary blood flow velocity in normal subjects and in patients with Raynaud's phenomenon. *Micovasc Res* 46:374–382, 1993.

69. Wollersheim H, Reyenga J, Thien Th: Postocclusive reactive hyperemia of fingertips, monitored by laser Doppler velocimetry in the diagnosis of Raynaud's Phenomenon. *Microvasc Res* 38:286–295, 1989.
70. Sumner DS: Noninvasive assessment of upper extremity and hand ischemia. *J Vasc Surg* 3:560–564, 1986.
71. Mozersky DJ, Barnes RW, Sumner DS, Strandness DE Jr: Hemodynamics of innominate artery occlusion. *Ann Surg* 178:123–127, 1973.
72. Corson JD, Menzoian JO, LoGerfo FW: Reversal of vertebral artery blood flow demonstrated by Doppler ultrasound. *Arch Surg* 112:715–719, 1977.
73. Berguer R, Higgins R, Nelson R: Noninvasive diagnosis of reversal of vertebral-artery blood flow. *N Engl J Med* 302:1349–1351, 1980.
74. Machleder HI, Sweeney JP, Barker WF: Pulseless arm after brachial artery catheterization. *Lancet* 1:407–409, 1972.
75. Hirai M: Digital blood pressure and arteriographic findings under selective compression of the radial and ulnar arteries. *Angiology* 31:21–31, 1980.
76. Koman LA, Urbaniak JR: Ulnar artery insufficiency: A guide to treatment. *J Hand Surg* 6:16–24, 1981.
77. Bartel P, Blackburn D, Peterson L, et al: The value of non-invasive tests in occupational trauma of the hands and fingers. *Bruit* 8(March):15–18, 1984.
78. Silcott GR, Polich VL: Palmar arch arterial reconstruction for the salvage of ischemic fingers. *Am J Surg* 142:219–225, 1981.
79. Zweifler AJ, Trinkaus P: Occlusive digital artery disease in patients with Raynaud's phenomenon. *Am J Med* 77:995–1001, 1984.
80. Dabich L, Bookstein JJ, Zweifler A, Zarofonetis CJD: Digital arteries in patients with scleroderma. Arteriographic and plethysmographic study. *Arch Intern Med* 130:708–714, 1972.
81. Mills JL, Friedman EI, Taylor LM Jr, Porter JM: Upper extremity ischemia caused by small artery disease. *Ann Surg* 206:521–528, 1987.
82. Maricq HR, Weinrich MC, Keil JE, LeRoy EC: Prevalence of Raynaud phenomenon in the general population. A preliminary study by questionnaire. *J Chron Dis* 39:423–427, 1986.
83. Balas P, Tripolitis AJ, Kaklamanis P, et al: Raynaud's phenomenon. Primary and secondary causes. *Arch Surg* 114:1174–1177, 1979.
84. Jacobs MJHM, Breslau PJ, Slaaf DW, et al: Nomenclature of Raynaud's phenomenon: A capillary microscopic and hemorheologic study. *Surgery* 101:136–145, 1987.
85. Tordoir JHM, Haeck LB, Winterkamp H, Dekkers W: Multifinger photoplethysmography and digital blood pressure measurement in patients with Raynaud's phenomenon of the hand. *J Vasc Surg* 3:456–461, 1986.
86. Porter JM, Bardana EJ, Baur GM, et al: The clinical significance of Raynaud's syndrome. *Surgery* 80:756–764, 1976.
87. Pardy BJ, Hoare MC, Eastcott HHG, et al: Prostaglandin E$_1$ in severe Raynaud's phenomenon. *Surgery* 92:953–965, 1982.
88. Rodeheffer RJ, Rommer JA, Wigley F, Smith CR: Controlled double-blind trial of nifedipine in the treatment of Raynaud's phenomenon. *N Engl J Med* 308:880–883, 1983.
89. Roald OK, Seem E: Treatment of Raynaud's phenomenon with ketanserin in patients with connective tissue disorders. *Br Med J* 289:577–579, 1984.

90. Creager MA, Pariser KM, Winston EM, et al: Nifedipine-induced fingertip vasodilation in patients with Raynaud's phenomenon. *Am Heart J* 108: 370–373, 1984.
91. Mohrland JS, Porter JM, Smith EA, et al: A multiclinic, placebo-controlled, double-blind study of prostaglandin E_1 in Raynaud's syndrome. *Ann Rheum Dis* 44:754–760, 1985.
92. Sanders RJ, Monsour JW, Baer SB: Transaxillary first rib resection for the thoracic outlet syndrome. *Arch Surg* 97:1014–1023, 1968.
93. Gelabert HA, Machleder HI: Diagnosis and management of arterial compression at the thoracic outlet. *Ann Vasc Surg* 11:359–366, 1997.
94. Towner KM, McDonnell AE, Turcotte JK, Zarins CK: Noninvasive assessment of upper extremity deep venous obstructions. *Bruit* 5:21–22, 1981.
95. Gray B, Williams LR, Flanigan DP, et al: Upper extremity deep venous thrombosis: diagnosis by Doppler ultrasound and impedance plethysmography. *Bruit* 7:30–34, 1983.
96. Knudson GJ, Wiedmeyer DA, Erickson SJ, et al: Color Doppler sonographic imaging in the assessment of upper-extremity deep venous thrombosis. *AJR* 154:399–403, 1990.
97. Baxter GM, Kincaid W, Jeffrey RF, et al: Comparison of colour Doppler ultrasound with venography in the diagnosis of axillary and subclavian vein thrombosis. *Br J Radiol* 64:777–781, 1991.
98. Grassi CJ, Polak JF: Axillary and subclavian venous thrombosis: Follow-up evaluation with color Doppler flow US and venography. *Radiology* 175: 651–654, 1990.
99. Salles-Cunha S, Beebe HG, Andros G: Preoperative assessment of alternate veins. *Semin Vasc Surg* 8:172–178, 1995.
100. Patwardhan NA, Anderson FA Jr, Cutler BS, Wheeler HB: Noninvasive detection of axillary and subclavian venous thrombosis by impedance plethysmography. *J Cardiovasc Surg* 24:250–255, 1983.
101. Summer DS: Hemodynamics and pathophysiology of arteriovenous fistulae. In: Rutherford RB (ed), *Vascular Surgery*, 4th edition, Philadelphia: WB Saunders Co; 1995, pp. 1166–1191.
102. Rutherford RB, Sumner DS: Diagnostic evaluation of arteriovenous fistulae. In: Rutherford RB (ed), *Vascular Surgery*, 4th edition, Philadelphia: WB Saunders Co; 1995, pp. 1192–1207.
103. Bussell JA, Abbott JA, Lim RC: A radial steal syndrome with arteriovenous fistula for hemodialysis. *Ann Intern Med* 75:387–394, 1971.
104. Glickman MH, Clark S, Goodrich V: Determination of outflow stenosis of arteriovenous fistulas for hemodialysis. *Bruit* 9:16–19, 1985.
105. Balas P, Giannikas AC, Harto-Garofalides G, Plessas S: The present status of replantation of amputated extremities. Indications and technical considerations. *Vasc Surg* 4:190–209, 1970.
106. Matsuda M, Shibahara H, Kato N: Long-term results of replantation of 10 upper extremities. *World J Surg* 2:603–612, 1978.

3

Angiography in the Diagnosis and Management of Vascular Disorders of the Upper Extremity

Antoinette S. Gomes, MD

Angiography has a major role in the diagnosis of vascular lesions of the upper extremities. Recently, with the development of interventional angiographic technique, arteriography now also has a therapeutic role.

Techniques

Arteriography of the upper extremity is performed using the modified Seldinger technique, with either a transfemoral or high brachial artery approach. When the axilla and entire arm are to be visualized, the femoral route is usually used. When visualization of the hand or forearm is desired, a direct brachial or axillary approach may be used. Patients should be given adequate premedication analgesic. Low osmolar contrast agents are preferred. Although these agents cost more than conventional ionic contrast material, the newer agents produce less pain and discomfort. When conventional ionic agents are used, 60% (w/v) contrast medium is adequate for most studies. The contrast may be mixed with 1% lidocaine

From Machleder HI, (ed): *Vascular Disorders of the Upper Extremity*. Third Revised Edition. Futura Publishing Company, Inc., Armonk, NY, © 1998.

(10 mL per 100 mL of contrast). This has been shown to decrease the pain of injection.[1] Lidocaine should not be used when the catheter tip is in a position that will permit reflux into the cerebral circulation.[2] Vasodilators such as priscoline or papaverine should be used when visualization of the small vessels of the hand is desired or when characterization of tumor vascularity is desired.[3,4] Wrapping the extremity in warm towels will also result in vasodilatation and improve visualization.[5] Reactive hyperemia may also be induced by the application of tourniquets.[6,7]

Venography of the upper extremity is accomplished by injection of 30 to 40 cc of contrast medium through a butterfly infusion set or Intracath placed in the basilic vein. Unlike arteriography where contrast injection is typically by power injection, venography is performed by hand injection of contrast. When the patient is being evaluated for superior vena cava obstruction, bilateral injections are performed to avoid errors in interpretation due to wash-in of unopacified blood. Digital subtraction angiographic techniques and utilization of large field of view image intensifiers are recommended for arterial and venous studies because subtraction techniques allow removal of soft tissues and confusing overlying bony shadows in the thoracic outlet.

Arterial Trauma

Arterial trauma may occur from numerous causes including penetrating or blunt trauma, fractures, dislocations, repeated small trauma, and thermal injuries. The arteriographic changes seen may be arterial spasm, segments of tapered narrowings or occlusions, arterial intimal tears, dissections, transections, displacement of the artery by hematoma, or bleeding with extravasation of contrast into the soft tissues (Figure 1). Arteriography is the single most useful diagnostic procedure in suspected arterial injury, and is frequently used when the wound is in close proximity to a major vessel. Although patients with normal physical findings, with the exception of the wound site itself, usually have negative arteriograms,[8] arteriography is often requested because the state of the peripheral pulses distal to the trauma is not always a reliable indicator of the extent of the vascular injury. The pulse may be palpable in the presence of severe arterial trauma with inadequate flow, and similarly, the pulses may be absent or diminished secondary to arterial spasm in the absence of significant arterial damage.[9]

Aneurysms

Although aneurysms are uncommon in the upper extremity,[10] they are usually due to trauma.[11] Other less common causes of aneurysm in-

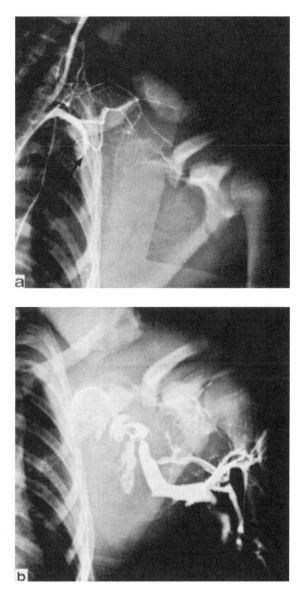

Figure 1. Traumatic avulsion of the left subclavian artery and axillary vein. This trauma victim sustained multiple fractures of the scapula and clavicle. **a:** The subclavian artery injection shows traumatic laceration of the left subclavian artery with abrupt occlusion of the artery proximally (arrow). **b:** Left axillary venogram shows active venous bleeding from a transected left axillary vein. Thrombosis is seen in a segment of the cephalic vein.

clude cystic medial necrosis, syphilis, polyarteritis nodosa, Takayasu's disease, and fibromuscular hyperplasia and atherosclerosis (Figure 2). The radiographic appearance of aneurysms varies. They may be fusiform and appear as a diffuse uniform dilatation of the vessel. The saccular type present as a localized outpouching of a vessel. Dissecting aneurysms in DeBakey type I and type II can extend into the brachiocephalic vessels. Radiographically, a linear lucency representing the border of the false lumen can be seen extending into the innominate or subclavian arteries. The false lumen may produce compression and occlusion of the subclavian artery. False aneurysms representing a rent in the arterial wall may appear similar to saccular aneurysms. The true size of the aneurysm may be difficult to ascertain and a false-negative arteriogram obtained if there is laminated thrombus in the wall of the aneurysm partially filling the aneurysm sac. Aneurysms also occur in the ulnar artery as a result of repetitive blunt trauma. Repetitive injury to the palmar and digital arteries of the hand results in thrombosis and occlusion of these vessels, and in the larger vessels pseudoaneurysms, the hypothenar hammer syndrome. The aneurysms typically occur in the ulnar artery where the artery crosses the hamate bone and is compressed by the hook of the hamate. This is usually the result of occupational trauma, and is seen most often in the dominant hand of manual laborers whose work involves repetitive use of the hand.[12]

Embolism

Emboli to the upper extremity usually are of cardiac origin.[13,14] They usually impact at an arterial bifurcation and in the upper extremity they most frequently lodge at the bifurcation of the brachial artery.[15] Radiographically, they are seen as filling defects with convex margins. Filling of the artery distally is usually not seen because of poor collateral formation or propagation of the thrombus (Figure 3).

Atherosclerosis

Atherosclerosis of the upper extremity usually involves the subclavian arteries and does not usually extend beyond them.[16] The radiographic picture of the atherosclerotic changes varies with the extent and duration of the disease. Plaques that may be concentric, eccentric, or ulcerated are seen and may be localized or diffuse. Varying degrees of stenosis or dilatation may occur. Lesions in the subclavian arteries are best visualized with a large bolus injection made with the catheter positioned in the ascending aorta.

When complete occlusion of the subclavian artery occurs proximal to the vertebral artery, a subclavian steal syndrome may occur in which there is preferential flow of blood retrograde down the vertebral artery on the affected side into the low-pressure subclavian artery distal to the

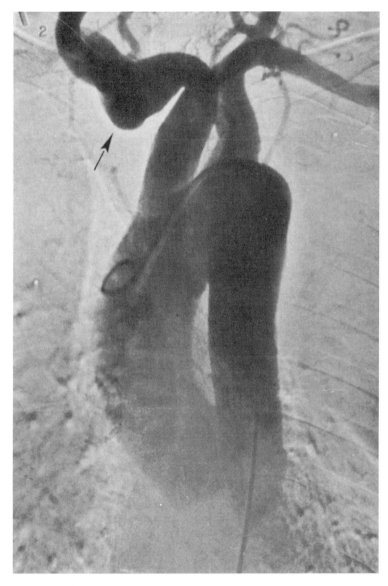

Figure 2. Arteriosclerotic aneurysm. A fusiform aneurysm is seen in the proximal right subclavian artery (arrow).

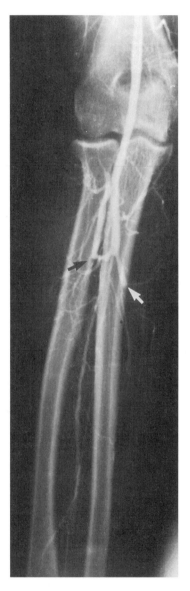

Figure 3. Occlusion of the radial and ulnar arteries. This patient had a recently repaired subclavian artery aneurysm. Following the repair, multiple emboli occurred resulting in occlusion of the radial (black arrow) and ulnar arteries (white arrow). Collaterals reconstitute the common interosseus artery.

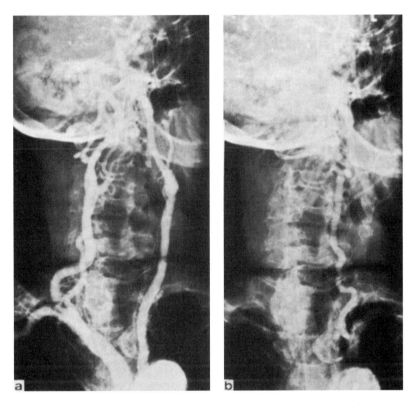

Figure 4. Subclavian steal syndrome. **a**: The aortic arch injection in the RPO projection shows opacification of the right innominate, common carotid, and right subclavian arteries. The left common carotid artery is also identified. There is no filling of the left subclavian artery on the left vertebral vein. **b**: Late in the injection, there is retrograde filling of the left vertebral artery down to the left subclavian artery with antegrade filling of the left subclavian artery. The area of stenosis at the origin of the left subclavian artery is identified.

stenosis.[17] The pattern of flow in the steal syndrome is best seen on an arch injection with a delayed filming sequence (Figure 4).

Thoracic Outlet Syndromes

The subclavian and axillary arteries and nerves of the brachial plexus are subject to compression at various sites in their passage through the supraclavicular triangle into the axillary fossa. The subclavian artery and plexus may be compressed against the scalenus anticus tendon or first rib by the scalenus medius tendon at the point of its traverse through the scalene tunnel and ascent onto the first rib. The presence of a cervical rib with associated fibrous band attaching to the under surface of the first rib produces further compromise of this space. Compression may occur at the costoclavicular space due to a prominent subclavius muscle or following healing of clavicular fractures with associated callus formation. With the arm in hyperabduction, compression of the axillary artery may occur at the site of insertion of the pectoralis minor tendon onto the coracoid process (Figures 5 through 7). Compression may also occur in the quadrilateral space. In this condition the posterior humeral circumflex artery and axillary nerve may be compressed as they pass through a space

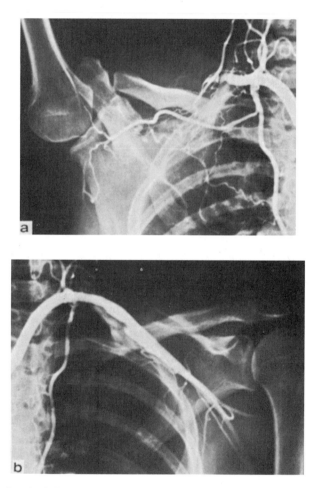

Figure 5. Cervical rib syndrome. **a:** Injection at the origin of the right subclavian artery with complete occlusion of right subclavian artery at the level of the right cervical rib. Note multiple collaterals distal to the level of occlusion. **b:** On the left, there is marked irregularity with thrombus formation in the distal left subclavian artery at the level of the cervical rib.

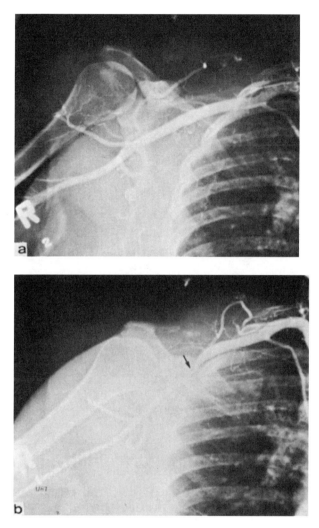

Figure 6. Thoracic outlet syndromes. **a**: The right subclavian artery injection in neutral position shows no evidence of structural abnormality to the right subclavian artery. **b**: With the shoulder depressed, narrowing of the right subclavian artery (arrow) at the site of insertion of the pectoralis minor muscle is shown. Similar findings were seen on the left side.

formed between the triceps head laterally and the teres major and teres minor muscles above and below.

Symptoms of thoracic outlet syndromes (TOS) are usually neurological due to compression of the brachial plexus and not due to compression of the subclavian artery in the thoracic outlet. Arteriography should

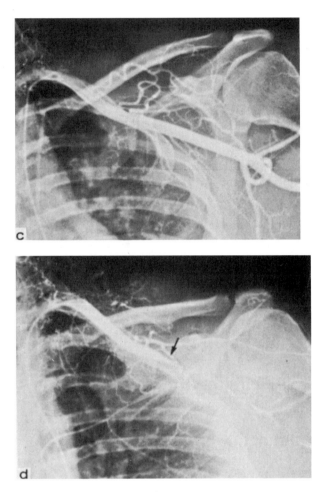

Figure 6. c: In neutral position, no abnormality of the left subclavian artery is identified. **d:** With the shoulder pulled back, however, there is evidence of severe obstruction to flow in the left subclavian artery (arrow).

be interpreted cautiously in patients with TOS. The intermittent arterial compression may be difficult to demonstrate, and the patient should be studied with the arms in a position that reproduces symptoms. Many patients with TOS have no arterial compression. Many normal patients without TOS can have their subclavian artery compressed in arm elevation, or shoulder bracing positions.[18] Arteriography is recommended in patients with arm symptoms who have a weak pulse or a significantly lower blood pressure in the symptomatic arm as compared to the normal side. It should be performed in patients with a subclavian

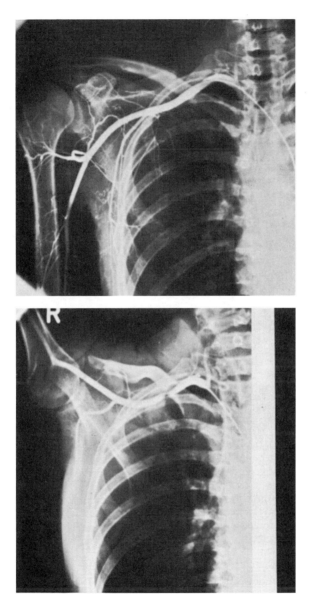

Figure 7. Thoracic outlet syndromes. **Top**: Subclavian arteriogram in neutral position shows no abnormality. **Bottom:** Extension of the arm with Adson's maneuver shows extrinsic compression of the right subclavian artery in the costoclavicular tunnel.

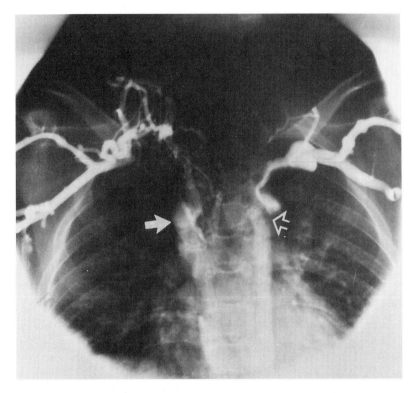

Figure 8. Superior vena cavagram. Bilateral subclavian vein occlusion. On the **right**, there is abrupt termination of the right subclavian vein with an abundant collateral network. The collaterals communicate with the azygous vein (arrow) which drains into the proximal superior vena cava. On the **left**, occlusion of the left subclavian vein is noted and collaterals communicate with the left hemiazygous vein (arrowhead).

artery bruit and suspected subclavian artery stenosis, and in patients suspected of having a subclavian artery aneurysm, or in those in whom a source for peripheral emboli is sought. Patients who manifest venous symptoms of TOS characterized by intermittent venous compression with edema or sudden thrombotic occlusion of the axillary or subclavian vein should have venography. Cut film or digital subtraction images are obtained and examined for evidence of thrombus or the presence of collateral vessels indicating obstruction to flow in the major venous channels (Figure 8).

Arteritis

Arteriography is useful in the diagnosis of arteritis.

Buerger's Disease

Buerger's disease (thromboangiitis obliterans) is a panangiitis affecting Caucasian and Asiatic men in their third or fourth decade. It is a segmental, inflammatory, and occlusive disease of medium and small arteries of young adult male smokers affecting mainly the distal upper and lower extremities.[19-21] There is often a history of recurrent migratory thrombophlebitis. The exact etiology is unknown. Certain HLA haplotypes may be involved in susceptibility to the disease.[22] The mechanism of the relationship of exacerbations to smoking and remissions to abstinence is striking. The acute lesion is a panangiitis involving all layers of the vessel wall, but the architecture of the vessel wall is preserved. The occluding thrombus is very vascular and contains nuclei of many fibroblasts. The histopathologic changes in the involved superficial arteries and veins are similar.[22] In the subacute phase there is less cellularity, and recanalizaion of the thrombi is apparent. In the late phase of the disease there is often organized and recanalized thrombus and perivascular and perineural fibrosis.[22] The arteriographic findings in Buerger's disease, while not pathognomonic, are usually typical to permit diagnosis.[21] There is a high frequency of involvement of the upper extremities and the lesions are frequently bilateral. No calcium is seen in the lesions, and there is an absence of arteriosclerotic changes. The arterial lumen is smoothly narrowed with a smooth reduction in caliber of the vessel above the thrombosed segment. The lesions may be totally occlusive, or have a stringlike appearance. Multiple segmental occlusive lesions occur predominantly in the forearm and hand, with the majority of the lesions occurring in the cubital arch, palmar arch, and digital arteries. Affected vessels may have normal segments. The collateral circulation is generally less well developed than in arteriosclerotic vascular disease, and is primarily through the vasa vasorum of the thrombosed segment, giving a winding corkscrew appearance of the fine vessels accompanying the occluded segment. In distal lesions the artery may terminate with a series of small branches having a tree-root or spider-leg appearance.[21]

Takayasu's Disease

Takayasu's disease is a panarteritis believed to be autoimmune in origin.[23] High levels of γ-globulins, circulating immune complexes, and rheumatoid factor provide evidence of a humoral-mediated pathogenesis. It is more common in females with peak incidence between 15 and 25 years of age.[24] There may be hormonal modulation of the immune response. The disease has an early systemic phase that may be undetected and a late occlusive phase. Arteriography is usually performed in patients with the occlusive or pulseless phase, at which time the patient presents with is-chemic manifestations secondary to arterial occlusion. In the early stages, the adventitia and media are infiltrated by lymphocytes and plasma cells.[25] Marked thickening of the intima due to accumulation of mucopoly-saccharides produces longitudinal irregularity of the inner luminal vessel surface. A mixed cellular infiltrate with giant cells and granuloma forma-tion involves the media and adventitia.[26] Later, degeneration of the inter-nal elastic lamina of the media occurs with progressive replacement of the adventitia and media by fibrous tissue.[27] Obliteration of the nutrient arteries occurs and adventitial neovascularization. The aortitis frequently affects the thoracic and abdominal aorta and its branches.[28] The lesions are most often solitary or segmental rat-tailed narrowings affecting the aorta and visceral vessels at their aortic origin. The common carotid arter-ies are more often affected than the vertebral arteries. The subclavian arteries are frequently involved with the tapered narrowings and occlu-sions typically occurring just beyond the thyrocervical trunk (Figure 9).[27] Aneurysms may be present and affect the aorta rather than its branches and linear vascular calcification seen.[25] Because of good collateral circula-tion, occlusion of the subclavian arteries usually is asymptomatic and claudication is rare.[27] The changes seen are often indistinct from giant cell arteritis. Cardiac involvement with vessel occlusion or stenosis or myocardial involvement occurs in 6% to 16% of patients.[29] Pulmonary artery inflammation may occur.[30,31]

Giant Cell (Temporal) Arteritis

Giant cell arteritis is a granulomatous arteritis of uncertain etiology with characteristic giant cells in the media and intimal thickening. The localization of inflammatory cells and giant cells around fragmented inter-nal elastic lamina suggested an autoimmune reaction. Immunohistochem-ical studies have revealed that monocyte derived macrophages and CD4$^+$ T lymphocytes dominate the lesions.[32,33] Typically, tissue infiltrating cells, primarily T lymphocytes and macrophages form granulomas in the arte-rial media. Multinucleated giant cells may be part of the disease process, but are not always present. Destruction of the smooth muscle layer and fragmentation of the internal elastic lamina of the vessel occur. Calcifica-tion may occur. Intimal proliferation and thrombosis occur and damage of medial smooth muscle cells is followed by fibrosis. The disease has a predilection for medium-sized vessels of the carotid system, especially the temporal arteries, but also can involve major branches of the aortic arch producing symptoms in the upper extremity.[34-36] It is a disease of the elderly, rare in patients under 60 years of age,[37] and is more common in females. It is frequently associated with the symptom complex polymy-

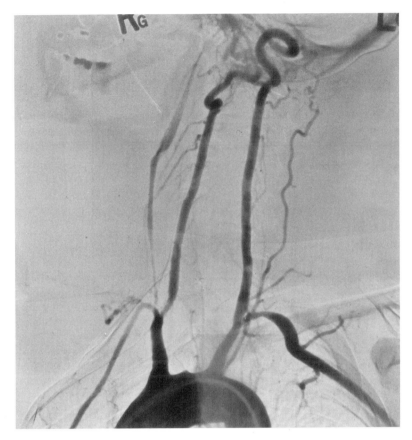

Figure 9. Takayasu's disease. Aortic arch injection in the RPO projection shows occlusion of the right subclavian artery. A long segment of tapered narrowing is seen in the right common carotid artery. The left common carotid artery is occluded at its origin. A short segment of narrowing is seen in the proximal left subclavian artery.

algia rheumatica.[34] Patients with upper extremity involvement may manifest bruits, absent pulses and claudication.[34–36]

The angiographic features are long segments of smooth arterial stenoses alternating with areas of normal or increased caliber and smooth tapered occlusions of affected large arteries. There is absence of irregular plaques and ulceration. Aneurysms of the subclavian and axillary arteries have been described,[38,39] and more recently, aortic aneurysms have been described as a late complication.[40]

The angiographic appearance in the upper extremity is similar to Takayasu's disease and may be indistinguishable (Figure 10).

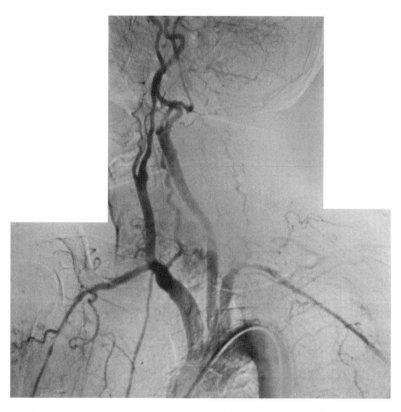

Figure 10. Giant cell arteritis. The aortic root injection in the RPO projection shows a long segment of smooth arterial narrowing in the right axillary artery. No plaques of ulcerations are identified. Similar changes are seen in a localized segment of the proximal left subclavian artery.

Raynaud's Syndrome and Vasospastic Disorders of the Upper Extremity

Raynaud's syndrome is defined as episodic attacks of vasoconstriction of the arteries and arterioles of the extremity in response to cold or emotional stimuli. Clinically there are sequential color changes in the extremity consisting of pallor, cyanosis, and rubor with associated paresthesias. When the attacks occur in a patient who has evidence of other local or systemic diseases such as a collagen disease, it is referred to as Raynaud's phenomenon. The attacks are limited to the upper extremity but rarely involve the feet and toes as well. Primary Raynaud's disease usually follows a benign clinical course. The diagnostic criteria of Allen and Brown[41] allow 95% diagnostic accuracy. These include:

- Intermittent attacks of discoloration of the extremities;
- Absence of evidence of organic arterial occlusion;
- Symmetrical bilateral distribution;
- Absence of gangrene or cutaneous changes;
- Occurrence in young females;
- History of symptoms for 2 years, during which time no manifestations of conditions associated with Raynaud's phenomenon have occurred.

A wide variety of diseases may be associated with Raynaud's phenomenon.

Arteriography is best performed by the femoral approach with the catheter tip positioned in the midbrachial artery.[42] Arteriography is useful to determine the distribution of arterial obstructive lesions and the presence of resting vasospasm. Arteriography may be performed after immersion of the hand in cold water for 20 to 30 seconds. The study can then be repeated after warming the hand and administering a vasodilator. The vasospastic changes are most evident in the digital arteries. The palmar arteries and arteries of the forearm are usually involved. Patients with Raynaud's phenomenon have extensive luminal obstruction in addition to vasospasm.

Recurrent arterial vasospasm may also occur after cold injury. These patients manifest cold hypersensitivity in the area of previous frostbite. Arteriography reveals vasospasm of the large and small arteries of the affected area.

Arterial vasospasm can also be induced by ergotamine and its derivatives. Ergotamine stimulates smooth muscle and has a toxic effect on the endothelium predisposing to thrombus. Arteriographically, there is markedly delayed flow; the arteries are threadlike in appearance with tapered occlusions. The findings are usually reversible with drugs.[43,44]

Medium and Small Vessel Occlusive Disease

Medium and small vessel occlusive disease may be the end result of a wide number of diseases. In some instances, there may be distinct morphological changes in the vessel indicating the etiology, but frequently the diagnosis must be based on clinical and laboratory findings. Arteriography can define the site and extent of the lesions. Conditions involving the upper extremity that should be considered are the collagen diseases, most frequently scleroderma. Other entities that may produce medium- and small-sized vessel occlusions are chronic recurrent trauma, disproteinemias, polycythemia vera, adverse reaction to warfarin or other drugs, pseudoxanthoma elasticum, and excess circulatory catecholamines (Figure 11).

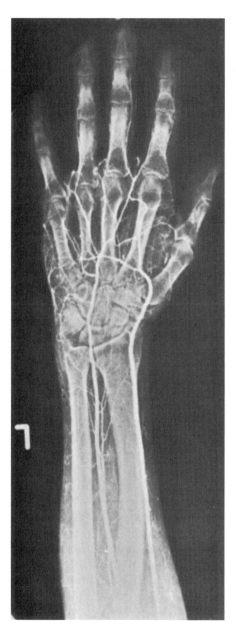

Figure 11. Vasospastic disorder, unknown etiology. This patient presented with cyanosis, numbness and coldness of the hands and feet, developing over a period of 1 month. There was a prior history of heavy smoking and coronary heart disease. The arteriogram shows occlusion of the digital arteries of the left thumb, radial and ulnar digital vessels of the left second digit, the ulnar digital artery of the third digit, the radial digital artery of the fourth digit, and the radial and ulnar digital artery of the fifth digit. The biopsy was nonrevealing. The findings seen are consistent with vasculitis of the vasospastic type.

Surgical Arteriovenous Fistulas

Chronic hemodialysis requires long-term access to the vascular tree. In most patients the upper extremity is the preferred site of fistula construction or graft placement. The surgically created fistulas are usually between the radial artery and cephalic vein. The direct arteriovenous (DAV) Brescia-Cimino fistula constructed between the radial artery (preferably distal) and the cephalic vein is still the best access for long-term hemodialysis and has the highest patency rate and lowest incidence of complications.[45–48] For patients with no suitable vessel for a forearm or antecubital DAV fistula, a straight (radial artery/antecubital vein) or looped (brachial artery antecubital vein) forearm bridge graft can be used. Currently, expanded polytetrafluoroethylene (E-PTFE) is the preferred graft material[47–50] with the longest shunt survival and fewer complications compared with saphenous vein or bovine carotid artery.

The most common complication of dialysis vascular access is thrombosis of the fistula or graft. The likelihood of thrombosis depends on the type of fistula or shunt constructed, site of the arteriovenous anastomosis, selection of prosthetic material, and adequacy of the patient's vessels. Graft thrombosis may occur at any time. Technical factors or lack of adequate runoff is the primary cause of early failure. Later thrombosis may be due to repeated trauma from needle punctures with subsequent fibrosis and narrowing, hypotensive episodes during dialysis and venous intimal hyperplasia.

Angiography plays an important role in the demonstration of graft abnormalities and in the management of graft malfunction. It has been recommended the subclavian vein be imaged with venography before placement of a vascular graft in all patients with a previous history of subclavian catheters.[51] Contrast injection into the fistula or graft is the best way to assess the lumen of the access device and the status of the venous outflow.[52–54]

Direct graft injection is used to evaluate graft hypertension and extremity edema. Graft hypertension is a common indication for graft angiography, and is determined by an increase in measured pressure in the dialysis outflow line and by abnormal graft pulsation. Normally, palpable graft pulse amplitude diminishes progressively toward the venous end of the graft. A forceful pulse palpable throughout the graft length and a loud bruit at the venous end is indicative of inadequate graft or venous runoff. Direct graft injection of the graft permits evaluation of the graft, graft venous anastomosis, and regional draining veins.[54]

Direct graft injection is performed by graft puncture, using a thin wall disposable scalp vein needle, Intracath, micropuncture catheter or with a dialysis needle left in place postdialysis. The direction of graft puncture should be in line with the direction of graft flow. In patients with a direct arteriovenous fistula, the scalp vein is inserted into the proximal or distal venous limb of the anastomosis so the tip lies 1 cm from the anastomosis. Twenty to 30 mL of 60% methylglucamine diatrizoate diluted to 30% is attached by a connecting tube. A blood pressure cuff is positioned proximal to the area of interest and inflated to at least 250 mm Hg to occlude all flow in the arm. Once the tourniquets are inflated, a closed system is created and material injected will cross from the vein to the artery permitting visualization. Filming is started with the injection of contrast. Midway through the injection the tourniquets are released and arterial blood flow washes the contrast agent out, permitting visualization of remote veins.[52] Several views may be necessary to remove overlap of vessels.

The arterial injection technique is used to investigate reduced dialysis line inflow or to evaluate symptoms of extremity ischemia. Arterial graft anastomosis, regional arterial status and runoff are principally evaluated with this technique. Lidocaine should be added to the contrast to reduce patient discomfort. When evaluating symptoms of peripheral arterial runoff, the study is performed with temporary compression occlusion of the graft. This results in improved filling of the arterial system distal to the graft. The graft is compressed by the patient. Arteriography is then repeated without graft compression and is used to evaluate the degree of graft steal.

As a normal fistula matures, the involved artery becomes longer and more tortuous.[52] Similar, more prominent changes affect the anastomotic vein and, to a lesser degree, other veins in the extremity. Stenosis may result from angulation of the artery as it elongates (Figure 12).

Graft thrombosis with occlusion is characterized by abrupt occlusion of a short segment. Intrinsic narrowing can occur anywhere along the course of the graft. The stenosis may be focal or involve a long segment of the graft. Anastomotic narrowing is seen almost exclusively at the graft venous junction and is the most common anatomic lesion leading to graft hypertension and ultimate graft thrombosis. With the Cimino-Brescia fistula occlusions or narrowings may involve the connecting artery, the anastomosis, and the main or collateral vessels.[52]

Venous outflow stenosis or occlusion leads to extremity edema and graft malfunction. Venous stenoses may arise a considerable distance from the fistula or graft, and the entire arm and innominate vessels should be examined in cases of resistance to venous return. With grafts, the lesions are localized a short distance beyond the level of the graft venous anastomosis. Stenosis or occlusion of the arterial limb is usually the result of regional atherosclerosis. Aneurysmal dilatation or multiple outpouchings develop at venipuncture sites, and are common in bovine grafts (Figure 13). False aneurysms, large bulbous vascular outpouchings, form most

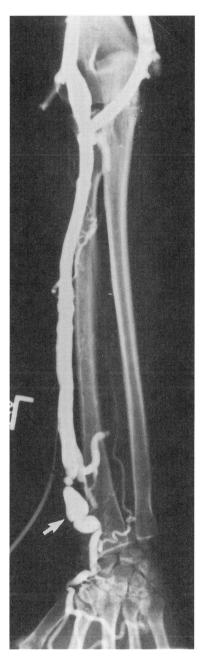

Figure 12. Hemodialysis arteriovenous fistula. The fistula has been created between the radial artery and cephalic vein. Just distal to the needle is an area of stenosis in the vein followed by a segment with aneurysmal dilatation (arrow) and an area of mild narrowing of the anastomosis to the radial artery. The adjacent radial artery is dilated.

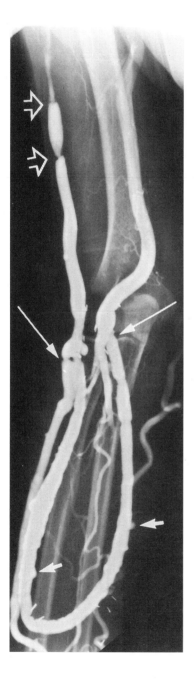

Figure 13. Bovine hemodialysis graft. The graft (arrows) has been placed between the cephalic vein and the brachial artery. Note the dilatation of the brachial artery. The graft itself shows multiple small false aneurysms at the site of repeated venipunctures (short arrows). Minimal narrowing is seen at the site of the graft anastomosis to the venous limb. The venous limb is dilated and shows changes consistent with arterialization. Anastomotic narrowing is seen almost exclusively at the graft venous junction and is the most common anatomic lesion leading to graft hypertension. Venous stenosis, however, may also arise a considerable distance from the fistula as in this case (arrowheads).

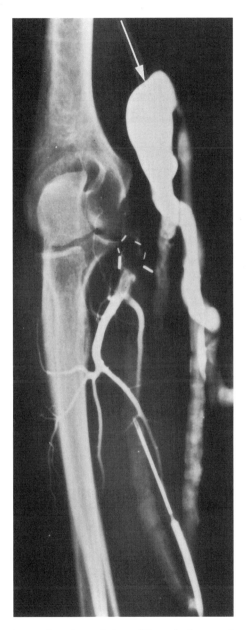

Figure 14. Bovine hemodialysis graft. Late filling of a forearm bovine hemodialysis graft showing an aneurysm in the proximal portion of the graft (arrow).

often at venipuncture sites.[52] Large aneurysms may be saccular or fusiform (Figure 14). Perigraft infection usually associated with an infected false aneurysm can occur.

Soft Tissue and Bone Tumors of the Upper Extremity

Multiple musculoskeletal tumors arise in the upper extremities.

Soft Tissue Tumors

The soft tissue tumors that occur include benign lipomas, malignant fibrosarcomas, liposarcomas, synoviomas, and rhabdomyosarcomas. The primary use of angiography is in the determination of the true extent of the lesions, their blood supply and degree of vascularity. Both benign and malignant soft tissue lesions may be hypervascular.[55] Certain findings are suggestive of malignancy. Tumor vessels have an erratic course and lack progressive diminution in caliber as is seen in normal or inflammatory vessels. They often end in an area of pooling called a tumor lake.[55,56] Nonhomogeneous staining is seen during the capillary phase, and arteriovenous shunting may be present. Failure to see abnormal vascularity, however, does not rule out malignancy.[4]

Inflammatory lesions may be hypervascular but show a more systematic branching and orderliness of the vascular pattern. The involved vessels are smooth and fine and diminish in caliber as they traverse the mass. The capillary stain may be inhomogeneous. Vascular lakes and AV shunting are usually not present. Sharp delineation of the margin of the mass from the surrounding soft tissue favors the diagnosis of neoplasm. Masses that are poorly circumscribed may be either neoplastic or inflammatory in origin.[57] Masses that produce only displacement of arteries, but which themselves are entirely avascular on optimal studies using vasodilators, can be considered benign and non inflammatory in the majority of cases (Figure 15).[55]

Angiography is frequently used to determine recurrence of tumor after previous resection. Although post-surgical changes in vessels may produce difficulty, arteriography can provide information as to the area to be re-explored, and sometimes can be of assistance in determining the site for repeat biopsy.

Bone Tumors

The more frequently occurring bone tumors are osteosarcomas, chondrosarcomas, giant cell tumors, and fibrous histiocytomas. Several limita-

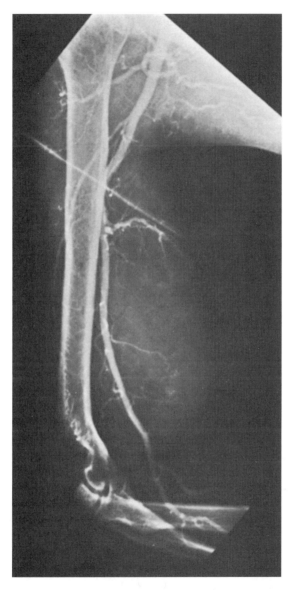

Figure 15. Sarcoma of the right forearm. Subclavian artery injection reveals marked draping of vessels around a hypovascular soft tissue mass lesion in the right arm. No clear-cut tumor stain is identified. Several of the draped arteries show increased tortousity and disorganization in their terminal portions.

tions exist in the use of arteriography in the evaluation of bone tumors. Although most benign neoplasms are hypovascular and show vascular displacement,[58] malignancy cannot be excluded completely when the arteriogram shows avascularity. The abundant intra-osseous vascular network of bone tumors is not visualized in arteriograms. Centrally located, even well vascularized tumors, are rarely demonstrated angiographically until the lesion has broken through the cortex.[58] Differential diagnostic difficulties often arise in hypervascular lesions because hypervascularity per se is not a specific sign of malignancy. Hypervascularity may be present in giant cell tumors, aneurysmal bone cysts, osteoid-osteomas, and inflammatory lesions. Tumor vessels, however, are usually not present, and the angiographic differentiation between benign and malignant disease is again based on the presence or absence of tumor vascularity.

The appearance of malignant tumor vascularity in bone is similar to that in other parts of the body and is characterized by vessels with an erratic course, the presence of puddling in tumor lakes, and AV shunting. Another finding reported in malignant bone tumors is the presence of

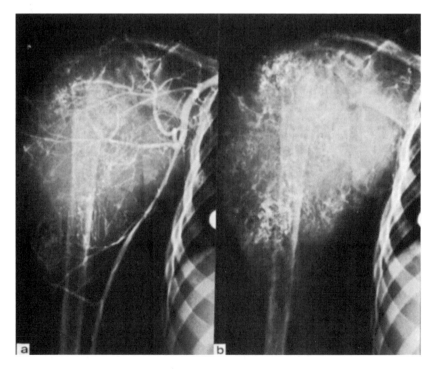

Figure 16. a: Osteogenic sarcoma. There is extensive involvement of the humerus with an associated soft tissue mass. The arterial phase of the angiogram shows extensive tumor vascularity. **b**: Osteogenic sarcoma. In the parenchymal phase, a dense tumor stain with areas of puddling of contrast is seen.

straight veins coursing at right angles to the normal flow of venous blood (Figure 16).[59]

Arteriovenous Malformations

Arteriovenous malformations (AVMs) are abnormal communications between arteries and veins. They may be congenital or acquired.

Congenital Arteriovenous Malformations

AVMs are developmental abnormalities present from birth. They assume a wide variety of appearances ranging from cavernous hemangiomas to large, multi-feeder AVMs. The malformation may be predominantly arterial, venous, or mixed. They may be diffuse or circumscribed. The abnormal communications may be microfistulous or macrofistulous.[60,61] Woollard[62] has described the embryological basis for these lesions. The lesions and their appearance appear to be determined by the point at which developmental arrest occurs in the differentiation of the vascular network. The primitive vasculature first appears as a diffuse network of blood spaces in the mesenchyme. Arrest at this time may give rise to hemangiomas. Embryonic arrest occurring after varying degrees of differentiation into arteries and veins has occurred may explain the varied appearances seen. Although more common in the lower extremity, AVMs occur in the upper extremity (Figure 17).

Magnetic resonance imaging (MRI) of vascular malformations is recommended. It will demonstrate the extent of the subcutaneous tissue and muscle involvement. All patients with high-flow congenital AVMs or suspected mixed lesions should undergo arteriography to determine the nature and extent of the malformation. Large volumes of contrast injected at rapid rates are usually necessary to opacify the AVM. Selective injections are usually necessary also.

Upper extremity venous involvement can usually be determined on the late phase of the arteriogram; however, in selected cases with a dominant venous component, upper extremity venography may be necessary. Only then can a reasonable approach to management be determined.

Acquired Arteriovenous Fistulas

Acquired AV fistulas in the extremities are usually the result of penetrating trauma. They may occur post-surgically, and rarely are seen in association with neoplasms, infection, or atherosclerotic aneurysms. They are frequently associated with false aneurysms.[63] High-volume rapid injection arteriography may or may not opacity the fistula itself, but there is immediate filling of the vein. Depending on the age and size of the AV fistula, the proximal artery may be dilated tortuous and show atherosclerosis.[64] Proximal veins are usually dilated.

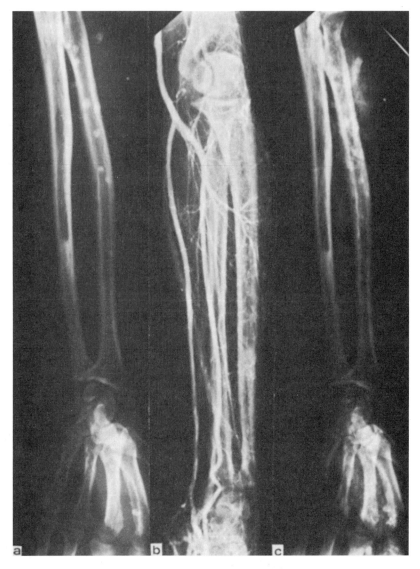

Figure 17. Cavernous hemangioma in the left forearm. **a**: The plain films show multiple phleboliths in the forearm with an area of increased density mid shaft of ulna. **b**: Arterial phase of angiogram is typically normal. **c**: Venous phase of the injection reveals an intense tissue stain indicating pooling of blood in the hemangioma.

Superior Vena Cava Syndrome

Superior vena cava (SVC) syndrome is caused by partial or complete obstruction of the SVC and its major venous tributaries. The most common etiology is thoracic neoplasm. SVC syndrome may occur in the course of other mediastinal processes such as mediastinal fibrosis, idiopathic thrombosis, and secondary to long-term central venous catheters. Symptoms consist of venous congestion and edema in the upper half of the body. Shortness of breath, hoarseness from laryngeal edema, headache, visual disturbances, and other neurological manifestations from cerebral edema may occur. Radiation therapy and chemotherapy have been the initial traditional treatments of choice. Surgical palliation by means of a venous bypass graft has been used, but is a major intervention that is difficult to justify in pre-terminal cancer patients because success is not guaranteed.[65] More recently transcatheter thrombolytic therapy and in appropriate cases placement of stents have been found to be useful means of relieving the obstruction.

Interventional Angiography

In addition to providing diagnostic information, angiography may be utilized therapeutically. Selective transcatheter arterial embolization or dilatation techniques (percutaneous transluminal angioplasty [PTA]) may be used.

Transcatheter Arterial Embolization

Transcatheter arterial embolization is useful in the control of post-traumatic bleeding and is a useful therapeutic alternative in the management of traumatic and congenital AVMs.

With transcatheter embolization the catheter is positioned selectively or subselectively in the vessel to be occluded and the embolic agent introduced through a catheter. Embolization therapy may be performed by direct injection. A variety of embolic agents are available. The selection of an agent used is determined by the permanence of occlusion required. For control of bleeding, nonpermanent agents such as Gelfoam[66] or autogenous clot[67] are suitable. When permanent occlusion is necessary, as in the management of congenital AVMs, permanent agents such as Gianturco-Wallace coils[68] or Ivalon (polyvinyl alcohol) particles are used.[69] Other permanent agents that have been used include detachable balloons,[70] silicone microspheres,[71] liquid silicone,[72] and bucrylate adhesive.[73] Sclerosing agents such as dehydrated alcohol, hot contrast material, and sotradechol have been used.

In the management of congenital AVMs it is important that the embolic agent reach and occlude the interstices of the AVM. Simple occlusion of the feeding vessel alone is inadequate and equivalent to simple surgical ligation of feeders that have been found to be ineffective due to regrowth of new collateral feeders.[74,75] Embolization techniques require careful sub-selective arteriography. Complications of the procedure include inadvertent reflux of the embolic agent with occlusion·of normal structures. Patients undergoing therapeutic embolization of congenital AVMs manifest a systemic response to the procedure characterized by pain, fever, and elevated muscle enzymes. Fibrin split products may be transiently elevated. The symptoms usually resolve within the first week postembolization, however, pain may be protracted and low-grade fever may persist for several weeks. With large AVMs it is usually necessary to perform the embolization in stages. The technique is an effective palliative therapy for large lesions, may be curative in small lesions especially hemangiomas or may be an adjunct to surgery (Figure 18).

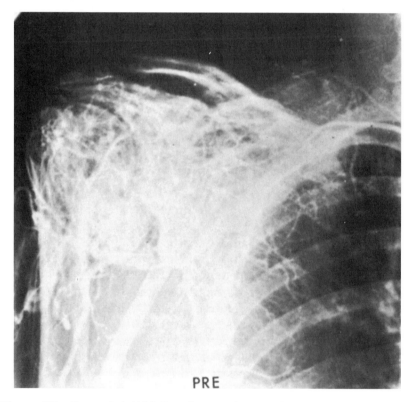

Figure 18A. Congenital AVM. Baseline arteriogram shows an AVM of the right shoulder.

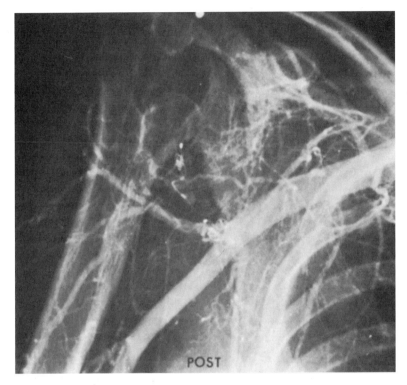

Figure 18B. Congenital AVM. Arteriogram following embolization of AVM using Ivalon particles and Gianturco coils shows marked reduction in AVM.

Percutaneous Transluminal Angioplasty

Areas of vascular stenosis in the arteries of the upper extremity are also amenable to dilatation using PTA.[76,77] PTA has been shown to be a safe, efficacious treatment of focal stenosis in the subclavian artery.[78] It has been used to treat subclavian steal syndrome[79] and in the treatment of coronary subclavian steal syndrome.[80] Caution is advised in dilating lesions originating proximal to the origin of the vertebral arteries as the potential for cerebral embolization of fragmented plaques exists. Either the femoral or brachial approach may be used. Using a guidewire to cross the stenosis, the balloon portion of the catheter is positioned at the area of stenosis and inflated several times. Immediately, postdilatation patients are given intra-arterial heparin, and most are discharged on antiplatelet drugs for varying intervals. PTA can also be used in the treatment of venous stenoses. It has been used successfully to dilate the venous stenoses that often occur proximal to dialysis shunt anastomoses and has been used with less success to dilate anastomotic stenoses in the shunts themselves.[81]

Thrombolytic Therapy

Thrombolytic therapy is used routinely in the treatment of upper extremity axillosubclavian vein thrombosis, and thromboembolic disease of the arteries of the arm and hand.

Lytic therapy can be delivered locally via a catheter placed in the thrombus or in close proximity to the clot. The thrombolytic agent is then infused in local low- or high-dose infusions.[82] Urokinase is generally preferred because it is associated with a lower incidence of bleeding and allergic complications. Recombinant tissue type plasminogen activator (rt-PA) may be used. Streptokinase is associated with a high incidence of bleeding and therefore is no longer frequently used. Good results have been reported with lytic therapy infusion into the brachial artery in patients with acute and sub acute hand ischemia from thromboembolic disease.[84,85]

Localized thrombolytic therapy is used routinely in the treatment of proximal venous thrombosis of the upper extremity with good results.[86] The catheter is embedded in the thrombus. The success of thrombolytic therapy is influenced by the age of the thrombus, with fresh thrombus being more likely to lyse. Nonetheless, successful lysis has been accomplished in thrombi older than 6 weeks and it is therefore worthwhile to attempt thrombolysis in patients with arterial or venous thrombosis (Figure 19). With older thrombi, infusions may be several days duration. Thrombolytic therapy is also used in the management of occluded central lines and in the treatment of SVC obstruction.

Interventional Radiological Salvage of Dialysis Access

Urokinase in conjunction with PTA is widely used to re-establish flow and function of thrombosed dialysis grafts. The graft is punctured using a single wall needle and an infusion catheter inserted with the puncture performed close to the arterial inflow directed toward the venous outflow. A variety of methods have been used. Urokinase may be imbedded into the thrombus followed by an infusion. A more widely used technique in patients with PTFE grafts is the pulsed spray crossed catheter technique. Single-wall needle puncture of the graft is again performed close to the arterial inflow directed toward the venous outflow. A guidewire is passed and the wire manipulated to the venous outflow and into the venous outflow if possible. A second puncture in the opposite direction is then performed. A pulse spray multiside hole catheter is introduced at each puncture site and pulsed spray of urokinase performed. Typically a 250,000 U of urokinase vial is reconstituted with 9 mL saline and 1 mL of 5000 U/mL of heparin. Aliquots (0.2 mL) of the mixture are forcefully injected. After 250,000 U of urokinase have been injected, angiography is done and angioplasty of the obstructing lesions performed.[87] With this

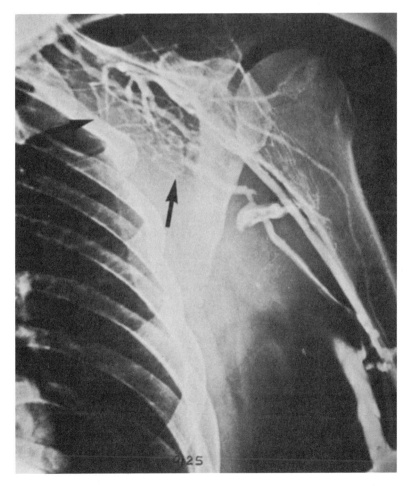

Figure 19. Thrombolytic therapy of venous thrombosis. **A**: Upper extremity venogram shows no flow in the basilic, axillary or subclavian veins. The cephalic vein fills. Extensive collaterals are seen in the axilla (arrows). The patient was treated with intermediate dose urokinase infusion via a catheter placed in the basilic vein.

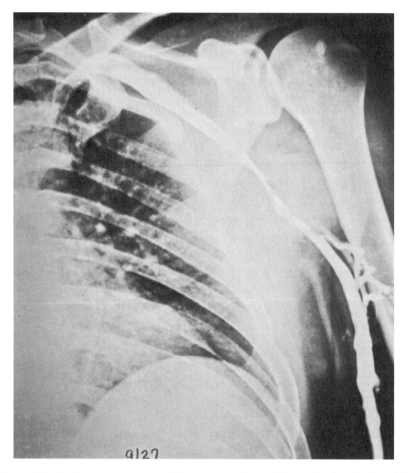

Figure 19. B: Repeat venogram 48 hours later shows filling of the basilic, brachial axillary and subclavian veins with cessation of collateral flow.

technique, patency is established in 98.5% of grafts. Additional urokinase may be administered if needed. Other techniques under evaluation include the use of mechanical devices for thrombolysis. Their efficacy is under evaluation. Dialysis access stenoses are usually due to scarring at the surgical anastomosis or intimal hyperplasia and may require high balloon pressures for dilation. Stenoses secondary to scarring may recur following balloon deflation. Restenosis is a frequent occurrence after angioplasty and a 1-year patency rate of 45% has been reported in postangioplasty dialysis shunt stenosis.[88] Intimal hyperplasia is a major problem. Complications of access angioplasty include intimal shearing, vein rupture or dissection, thrombosis, and late development of pseudoaneurysm

at the catheterization site. Complications of thrombolysis include embolization of partially lysed clot, extravasation, and septicemia.[89] These complications however, are infrequent and interventional techniques do pro-
long the life of the dialysis shunt.

Vascular stents have been placed most commonly in the efferent vein
and subclavian vein. Intimal hyperplasia limits the utility of current stents,
although it responds in the short term to angioplasty or atherectomy. In
patients in whom the central veins have all occluded secondary to previous catheter placements, recanalization followed by PTA or stent placement is an alternative to maintain patency of venous access.

Vascular Stents

The role of vascular stents in the treatment of upper extremity disease
is controversial primarily because of lack of long-term follow-up. Major
considerations in the placement of stents in the upper extremity relate to
the size of the stent, location of intended placement, and the type of stent
used. Although a variety of stents have been developed, the Palmaz balloon-expandable stent, the self-expanding Wallstent (Medinvent SA, Lau-
sanne, Switzerland, Schneider Corp, Minneapolis, MN) and the Gianturco
Z stent (Cook, Inc, Bloomington, IN) are the most frequently used in peripheral vessels in the United States. The Palmaz balloon-expandable stent
is the only device currently approved by the Food and Drug Administration (FDA) for use in the peripheral arterial system.

All three stents have been used in treatment of SVC syndrome. The
largest early experience has been with the Gianturco Z stent.[91-94] The
Wallstent has the advantage of being flexible and is useful in vessels of
curvature. It is easy to deploy and is available in a variety of sizes and
lengths. Clinical success is high.[95-97] Prompt and complete relief of SVC
syndrome is usually obtained with resolution of facial cyanosis and edema
within 24 hours. The diameter of the stent must be larger than the SVC
to prevent migration and its length sufficient to cover the area of stenosis;
larger stents (eg, ≥14 mm diameter) are preferred. The stents may be
placed prior to radiation therapy as the SVC syndrome may progress after
radiation. The stainless steel stent is thrombogenic and anticoagulation is
usually required after placement. Patency of the stent can be monitored
with helical computed tomography (CT). Restenosis or occlusion of the
stent is usually due to tumor in growth and/or secondary thrombosis.
Thrombosis can be managed with thrombolysis or clot aspiration and
tumor in growth can be managed by PTA and placement of a second stent
within the first. The use of vascular stents in treatment of SVC syndrome
due to nonmalignant causes presents the problem of maintaining stent
patency with normal life expectancy.

Vascular stents have been used in treatment of occluded dialysis fistulas, however as noted earlier, recurrent occlusion of the stent is a problem. It is generally accepted that vascular stents should not be used in TOS (Paget-Schroetter) prior to surgical release and there is controversy whether their use is justified in the thoracic outlet because of the high incidence of stent thrombosis. As noted earlier (see section on dialysis grafts) vascular stents have been used in the management of recurrent dialysis graft occlusion, but rethrombosis is frequent.[90] In the arterial system, vascular stents, usually the Palmaz or the Wallstent have been used with success in the treatment of subclavian artery stenoses that are refractory to traditional angioplasty.[98–100]

Arterial Infusion Therapy

Percutaneously placed indwelling arterial catheters are frequently used for the administration of chemotherapy. Using a high brachial artery puncture the catheter can be passed from the brachial artery down into the hepatic artery or other branches for infusion chemotherapy. The technique is frequently used in the management of liver tumors. The arterial lines may be left in place for extended periods up to 13 months.[101] Patients who require repeated short-term infusions may have the lines removed and replaced several times. The left brachial artery approach is preferred. When not available, the right side may be used, however, the increased tortuosity of the arch vessels in older patients makes this approach difficult.

For the management of lesions involving the arm or forearm, the catheter is usually introduced transfemorally with the tip positioned distal to the vertebral artery. Although some angiographers perform arteriography of upper extremity lesions using a retrograde axillary puncture with subsequent manipulation of the catheter to direct the tip downstream in the direction of flow, this technique has not been widely used for long-term infusions because of the risk of brachial artery spasm and damage during manipulation.

Small catheters 4F or 5F, are usually used for long-term infusions. Flow is maintained using an infusion pump. A small amount of heparin (1000 U in 500 mL D5W) is used to prevent catheter occlusion. The distribution of the arterial infusate in extremities can be determined by intra-arterial injection of flourescein and visualization using a Wood's light.

In Wirtanen's series[102] of more than 1000 cases of infusion therapy via the standard retrograde brachial artery approach, the radial pulse was lost in 20% due to thrombus at the puncture site. Because of the distal position of the puncture site, however, sufficient flow occurred through the deep brachial artery and thrombectomy was not required. Infection

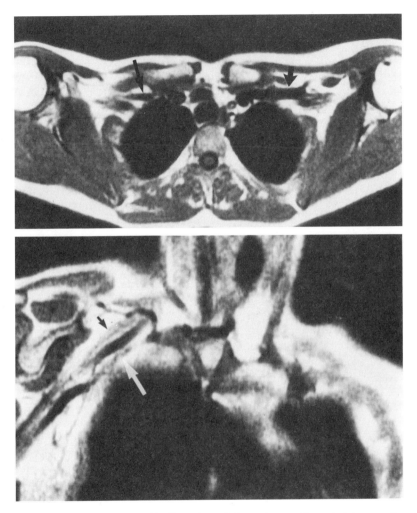

Figure 20. MRI of patient with thoracic outlet syndrome. **Top**: Axial scan shows right subclavian vein (long arrow) is smaller than the left (short arrow). A focal area of narrowing is seen in the right subclavian vein behind the clavicle at the junction of the right subclavian and brachiocephalic vein. **Bottom**: Coronal oblique scan showing the axillary and basilic veins (white arrow). The axillary artery is seen superior to the vein (black arrow).

at the puncture site occurred in less than 5% of the patients. Five had peripheral septic emboli and visual field problems occurred in 2, presumably secondary to vertebral artery embolization.

Magnetic Resonance Imaging

MRI is a new imaging technique that does not require the use of ionizing radiation. Images are constructed using magnetic fields and radiofrequency pulses. MRI is particularly suited to imaging the vascular system because of the high contrast it affords between flowing blood and soft tissues. Depending on the pulse sequence used, flowing blood shows up as signal void while slow flowing blood and thrombus have intermediate to bright signal. MRI has been used successfully to delineate soft tissue masses in the upper extremity[103] (Figure 20) and to define the size and extent of AVMs before and after treatment.[104] It has also been used in patients with Takayasu's disease and often demonstrates wall thickening and aneurysm formation. MRI is used frequently to evaluate patency of the SVC, and has shown encouraging results in the evaluation of the arteries and veins in patients with suspected TOS. Magnetic resonance angiography using gadolinium injection is currently utilized in the evaluation of the vessels of the upper extremities. New, rapid pulse sequences allow visualization of the vessels of the upper thorax in a manner that often obviates conventional angiography.

References

1. Guthaner DF, Silverman JF, Hayden WG, et al: Intra-arterial analgesia in peripheral arteriography. *Am J Roentgenol* 128:737–739, 1977.
2. Chuang VP, Widrich WC: Complications from intra-arterial lidocaine in upper extremity arteriography. *Am J Roentgenol* 131:906, 1978.
3. Jacobs BJ, Hanafee WN: The use of Priscoline in peripheral arteriography. *Radiology* 88:957–960, 1967.
4. Hawkins IF, Hudson T: Priscoline in bone and soft tissue angiography. *Radiology* 110:541–546, 1974.
5. Rosch J, Antonovic R, Porter JM: The importance of temperature in angiography of the hand. *Radiology* 123:323–326, 1977.
6. Hishida Y: Peripheral arteriography using the reactive hyperemia. *Jpn Circ J* 27:349–358, 1963.
7. Kahn PC, Boyer DN, Moran JM, et al: Reactive hyperemia in lower extremity arteriography: An evaluation. *Radiology* 90:975–980, 1968.
8. McDonald EJ, Goodman PC, Winestock DP: The clinical indications for arteriography in trauma to the extremity. *Radiology* 116:45–47, 1975.
9. Perry MO, Thal ER, Shires GT: Management of arterial injuries. *Ann Surg* 173:403–408, 1971.

10. Dent TL, Lindenauer M, Ernst CB, et al: Multiple arteriosclerotic arterial aneurysms. *Arch Surg* 105: 338–344, 1962.
11. Louis DS, Simon MA: Traumatic false aneurysms of the upper extremity. *J Bone J Surg* 56-A:176–179, 1974.
12. Latshaw RF, Weidner WA: Ulnar artery aneurysms: Angiographic considerations in two cases. *Am J Roentgenol* 131:1093–1095, 1978.
13. Darling CR, Austen WG, Linton RR: Arterial embolism. *Surg Gynecol Obstet* 124:106–114, 1967.
14. Levy JR, Butcher HR: Arterial emboli: An analysis of 125 patients. *Surgery* 68:968–973, 1970.
15. Champion HR, Gill W: Arterial embolus to the upper limb. *Br J Surg* 60: 505–508, 1973.
16. Crawford ES, DeBakey ME, Morris GC, et al: Thrombo-obliterative disease of the great vessels arising from the aortic arch. *J Thorac Cardiovasc Surg* 43: 38–53, 1962.
17. New vascular syndrome—The subclavian steal (editorial). *N Engl J Med* 265: 912, 1961.
18. Roos DB: Thoracic outlet and carpal tunnel syndromes. In: Rutherford RB, ed. *Vascular Surgery*. Philadelphia, PA: W.B. Saunders Co, 1977; p. 605.
19. McKusick VA, Harris WS, Otteson OE, et al: Buerger's disease: A distinct clinical and pathological entity. *JAMA* 181:5–12, 1962.
20. Lambeth J, Yong NK: Arteriographic findings in thromboangiitis obliterans. *Am J Roentgenol* 109:553–562, 1970.
21. Rivera R: Roentgenographic diagnosis of Buerger's disease. *J Cardiovasc Surg* 14:40–46, 1973.
22. Olin JW: Thromboangiitis obliterans. *Curr Opin Rheumatol* 6:44–49, 1994.
23. Hirsch MS, Aikat BK, Basu AK: Takayasu's arteritis: report of five cases with immunologic studies. *Bull Johns Hopkins Hosp* 115:29–64, 1964.
24. Onat T, Zeren E: Coarctation of the abdominal aorta. *Cardiologia* 54:140–157, 1969.
25. Lande A, Gross A: Total aortography in the diagnosis of Takayasu's arteritis. *Am J Roentgenol* 116:165–178, 1972.
26. Kerr GS: Takayasu's arteritis. *Rheum Dis Clin North Am* 21:1041–1058, 1995.
27. Lande A, Rossi P: The value of total aortography in the diagnosis of Takayasu's arteritis. *Radiology* 114:287–297, 1975.
28. Nasa T: Pathology of pulseless disease. *Angiology* 11:225–242, 1963.
29. Cipriano PR, Silverman JF, Perlroth MG, et al: Coronary arterial narrowing in Takayasu's aortitis. *Am J Cardiol* 39:744–750, 1977.
30. Sharma S, Kamalakar T, Rajani R, et al: The incidence and patterns of pulmonary artery involvement in Takayasu's arteritis. *Clin Radiol* 42:177–181, 1990.
31. Yamada I, Shibuya H, Matsubara O, et al: Pulmonary artery disease in Takayasu's arteritis: Angiographic findings. *Am J Roentgenol* 159:263, 1992.
32. Nordborg E, Nordborg C, Malmvall B, et al: Giant cell arteritis. *Rheum Dis Clin North Am* 21:1013–1026, 1995.
33. Calamia KT, Moore SB, Elveback LR, et al: HLA-DR locus antigens in polymyalgia rheumatica and giant cell arteritis. *J Rheumatol* 8:993–996, 1981.
34. Hamrin B, Jonsson N, Landberg: Involvement of large vessels in polymyalgia arteritica. *Lancet* 1:1193–1196, 1965.

35. Hunder GG, Ward LE, Burbank MK: Giant cell arteritis producing an aortic arch syndrome. *Ann Intern Med* 66:578–592, 1967.
36. Klein RB, Hunder GG, Stanson AW, et al: Large artery involvement in giant cell (temporal) arteritis. *Ann Intern Med* 83:806–812, 1975.
37. Hauser WA, Ferguson RH, Holley KE, et al: Temporal arteritis in Rochester, Minnesota, 1951–1967. *Mayo Clin Proc* 46:597–602, 1971.
38. Gilmor JR: Giant cell chronic arteritis. *J Pathol Bacteriol* 53:263–277, 1941.
39. Harrison RJ, Harrison CU, Kopelman H: Giant cell arteritis with aneurysms: Effects of hormone therapy. *Br Med J* 2:1593–1595, 1955.
40. Evans HM, O'Fallon WM, Hunder GG: Increased incidence of aortic aneurysmal disease in patient with giant cell arthritis: A population-based study (abstract). *Arthritis Rheum* 36(suppl 9):342, 1993.
41. Allen VE, Brown GE: Raynaud's disease: A critical review of minimal requisites for diagnosis. *Am J Med Sci* 183:187, 1932.
42. Porter JM, Snider RL, Bardana EJ, et al: The diagnosis and treatment of Raynaud's phenomenon. *Surgery* 77:11–23, 1975.
43. Johnsson KA: Angiography in two cases of Ergotism. *Acta Radiol (Stockh)* 57:280, 1962.
44. Fagerberg S, Jorulf H, Sandberg CG: Ergotism, arteriospastic disease and recovery studied angiographically. *Acta Med Scand* 182:769–772, 1967.
45. Zeit RM, So SKS, Ferral H: The problems and management of hemodialysis accesses. In: Castaneda-Zuniga W, Tadavarthy SM, Qian Z, et al, eds. *Interventional Radiology.* Vol 1. Philadelphia: Williams & Wilkins; 1997, pp. 566–598.
46. Hirschman GH, Wolfson M, Mosimann JE, et al: Complications of dialysis. *Clin Nephrol* 15:66–74, 1981.
47. So SKS: Access for dialysis. In: Simmons RL, Finch ME, Ascher NL, et al, eds. *Manual of Vascular Access, Organ Donation and Transplantation.* New York: Springer-Verlag; 1984, pp. 3–87.
48. Brescia MJ, Cimino JE, Appel K, et al: Chronic hemodialysis using venipuncture and a surgically created arteriovenous fistula. *N Engl J Med* 275:1089–1092, 1966.
49. Sabanayagam P, Schwartz AB, Soricelli RR, et al: A comparative study of 402 bovine heterografts and 225 reinforced expanded PTFE grafts as AVF in the ESRD patient. *Trans Am Soc Artif Intern Organs* 26:88–92, 1980.
50. Akhondzadeh L, Wilson SE, Williams R, et al: Infection of materials used in vascular access surgery: An evaluation of Dacron, bovine heterograft, Teflon, and human umbilical vein grafts. *Dial Transplant* 9:697, 1980.
51. Surratt RS, Picus D, Hicks ME, et al: The importance of preoperative evaluation of the subclavian vein in dialysis access planning. *Am J Roentgenol* 156:623–625, 1991.
52. Gilula LA, Staple TW, Anderson CB, et al: Venous angiography of hemodialysis fistulas. *Radiology* 115: 555–562, 1975.
53. Gothlin J, Linstedt E: Angiographic features of ciminobrescia fistulas. *Am J Roentgenol* 125:582–590, 1975.
54. O'Reilly RJ, Hansen CC, Rosental JJ: Angiography of chronic hemodialysis arteriovenous grafts. *Am J Roentgenol* 130:1105–1113, 1978.
55. Levin DC, Watson RC, Baltaxe HA: Arteriography in diagnosis and management of acquired peripheral soft-tissue masses. *Radiology* 103:53–58, 1972.

56. Herzberg DL, Schreier MH: Angiography in mass lesions of the extremities. *Am J Roentgenol* 111:541–546, 1971.
57. Lagergren C, Lindbom A, Soderberg G: Vascularization of fibromatous and fibrosarcomatous tumors. *Acta Radiol* 53:1–16, 1960.
58. Voegeli E, Uehlinger E: Arteriography in bone tumors. *Br J Radiol* 49:407–415, 1976.
59. Strickland B: The value of arteriography in bone tumors. *Skeletal Radiol* 1: 3–14, 1976.
60. Malan E, Puglionisi A: Cognital angiodysplasias of the extemities. (Note I: Generalities and classification; Venous dysplasia). *J Cardiovasc Surg* 5:87, 1964.
61. Malan E, Puglionisi A: Congenital angiodysplasias of the extremities. (Note II: Arterial, arterial and venous, and hemolymphatic dysplasias). *J Cardiovasc Surg* 6:255, 1965.
62. Woollard HH: The development of the principal arterial stems in the forelimb of the pig. *Contrib Embryol* 14: 139, 1922.
63. Elken DC, Schumacker HB Jr: Arterial aneurysms and arteriovenous fistula. In: Elkin DC, DeBakey ME, eds. *Surgery in World War II, Vascular Surgery.* Office of the Surgeon General, Dept of the Army, 1955.
64. Lindenauer SM, Thompson NW, Draft RO, et al: Late complications of traumatic arteriovenous fistulas. *Surg Gynecol Obstet* 129:525–532, 1969.
65. Perez CA, Presant CA, Van Amburg AL: Management of superior vena cava syndrome. *Semin Oncol* 5:123–134, 1978.
66. Carey LS, Grace DM: The brisk bleed: Control by arterial catheterization and Gelfoam plug. *J Can Assoc Radiol* 25:113–115, 1974.
67. Ring EJ, Athanasoulis C, Waltman AC, et al: Arteriographic management of hemorrhage following pelvic fracture. *Radiology* 109:65–70, 1973.
68. Gianturco C, Anderson JH, Wallace S: Mechanical devices for arterial occlusion. *Am J Roentgenol* 124:428–435, 1975.
69. Tadavarthy SM, Moller JH, Amplatz K: Polyvinyl alcohol (Ivalon) anew embolic material. *Am J Roentgenol* 125:609–616, 1975.
70. Kaufman SL, Kumar AA, Roland JA, et al: Transcatheter embolization in the management of congenital arteriovenous malformations. *Radiology* 137: 21–29, 1980.
71. Hilal SK, Michelson WJ: Therapeutic percutaneous embolization for extra-axial vascular lesions of the head, neck and spine. *J Neurosurg* 43:275–287, 1975.
72. Hilal SK, Sane P, Michelson WJ, et al: The embolization of vascular malformations of the spinal cord with low viscosity silicone rubber. *Neuroradiology* 16: 430–433, 1978.
73. Pevsner PH, Doppman SL: Therapeutic embolization with a microballoon catheter system. *Am J Roentgenol* 134:949–958, 1980.
74. Szilagyi DE, Elliott JP, DeRusso FJ, et al: Peripheral congenital arteriovenous fistulas. *Surgery* 57:61–81, 1965.
75. Gomes MMR, Bernatz PE: Arteriovenous fistulas. A review and ten years experience at the Mayo Clinic. *Mayo Clin Proc* 45:81–102, 1970.
76. Gruntzig A, Kumpe D: Technique of percutaneous transluminal angioplasty with the Grutzig balloon catheter. *Am J Roentgenol* 132:547–552, 1979.

77. Zeitler E, Gruntzig A, Shoop W: *Percutaneous Vascular Recanalization*. New York: Springer Verlag; 1979.
78. Burke DR, Gordon RL, Mishkin JD, et al: Percutaneous transluminal angioplasty of subclavian arteries. *Radiology* 164:699–704, 1987.
79. Motarjeme A, Keifer JW, Zuska AJ, et al: Percutaneous transluminal angioplasty for treatment of subclavian steal. *Radiology* 155:611–613, 1985.
80. Hallisey MJ, Rees JH, Meranze SG, et al: Use of angioplasty in the prevention and treatment of coronary subclavian steal syndrome. *J Vasc Interv Radiol* 6: 125–129, 1995.
81. Saeed M, Newman GE, McCann RI, et al: Stenoses in dialysis fistulas: Treatment with percutaneous angioplasty. *Radiology* 164:693, 1987.
82. McNamara TO, Fischer JR: Thrombolysis of peripheral arterial and graft occlusions: Improved results using high dose urokinase. *Am J Roentgenol* 144: 769–775, 1985.
83. Risius B, Graor RA, Geisinger MA, et al: Recombinant human tissue-t type plasminogen activator for thrombolysis in peripheral arteries and bypass grafts. *Radiology* 160:183–188, 1986.
84. Tisnado J, Cho S, Beachley MC, et al: Low dose fibrinolytic therapy in hand ischemia. *Semin Intervent Radiol* 2:367–380, 1985.
85. Lambiase RE, Paolella LP, Haas RA, et al: Extensive thromboembolic disease of the hand and forearm: Treatment with thrombolytic therapy. *J Vasc Interv Radiol* 2:201–208, 1991.
86. Becker GJ, Holden RW, Mail JT, et al: Local thrombolytic therapy for "thoracic inlet syndrome." *Semin Intervent Radiol* 2:349–353, 1985.
87. Roberts AC, Valji K, Bookslein JJ, et al: Pulsed spray pharmacomechanical thrombolysis for treatment of thrombosed dialysis access grafts. *Am J Surg* 166:221–226, 1993.
88. Glanz S, Bashist B, Gordon DH, et al: Angiography of upper extremity access fistulae for dialysis. *Radiology* 143:45–52, 1982.
89. Graor RA, Risius B, Young JR et al: Low dose streptokinase for selective thrombolysis: Systemic effects and complications. *Radiology* 152:35–39, 1984.
90. Vorwerk D, Guenther RW, Mann H, et al: Venous stenosis and occlusion in hemodialysis shunts: Follow-up results of stent placement in 65 patients. *Radiology* 195:140–146, 1995.
91. Putnam JS, Uchida BT, Antonovic R, et al: Superior vena cava syndrome associated with massive thrombosis: Treatment with expandable wire stents. *Radiology* 167:727–728, 1988.
92. Charnsangavej C, Carrasco CH, Wallace S, et al: Stenosis of the vena cava: Preliminary assessment of treatment with expandable metallic stents. *Radiology* 161:295–298, 1986.
93. Rosch J, Uchida BT, Hall LD, et al: Gianturco-Rosch expandable Z stents in the treatment of superior vena cava syndrome. *Cardiovasc Intervent Radiol* 15: 319–327, 1992.
94. Irving JD, Dondelinger RF, Reidy JF, et al: Gianturco self-expanding stents: Clinical experience in the vena cava and large veins. *Cardiovasc Intervent Radiol* 15:328–333, 1992.
95. Hennequin LM, Fade O, Fays JG, et al: Superior vena cava stent placement: Results with the Wallstent Endoprosthesis. *Radiology* 196:353–361, 1995.

96. Dondelinger RF, Goffette P, Kurdziel JC, et al: Expandable metal stents for stenoses of the venae cavae and large veins. *Semin Intervent Radiol* 8:252–263, 1991.

97. Watkinson AF, Hansell DM: Expandable Wallstent for the treatment of obstruction of the superior vena cava. *Thorax* 48:915–920, 1993.

98. Duber C, Klose KJ, Kopp H, et al: Percutaneous transluminal angioplasty for occlusion of the subclavian artery: Short and long term results. *Cardiovasc Intervent Radiol* 15:205–210, 1982.

99. Mufti SI, Young KR, Schulthes T: Restenosis following subclavian artery angioplasty for treatment of coronary subclavian steal syndrome: Definitive treatment with Palmaz stent placement. *Cathet Cardiovasc Diagn* 33:172–174, 1994.

100. Sueoka BL: Percutaneous transluminal stent placement to treat subclavian steal syndrome. *J Vasc Interv Radiol* 7:351–356, 1996.

101. Clouse ME, Ahmed R, Ryan RB, et al: Complications of long term transbrachial hepatic arterial infusion chemotherapy. *Am J Roentgenol* 129:799–803, 1977.

102. Wirtanen GW: Percutaneous transbrachial artery infusion catheter techniques. *Am J Roentgenol* 117:696–700, 1973.

103. Pettersson H, Gillespy T, Hamlin DJ, et al: Primary musculoskeletal tumors: Examination with MR imaging compared with conventional modalities. *Radiology* 164:237–241, 1987.

104. Cohen JM, Weinreb JC, Redman HC: Arteriovenous malformations of the extremities: MR imaging. *Radiology* 158:475–479, 1986.

Part II

The Cumulative Trauma Disorders

4

Introduction to Neurovascular Compression Syndromes at the Thoracic Outlet

Herbert I. Machleder, MD

The region generally referred to as the thoracic outlet is characterized by a number of unique embryological and developmental characteristics that have particular and often dramatic effects on the neurovascular structures. The boundaries of clavicle above and first rib below form an unyielding yet mobile passage for axillosubclavian artery, vein, and brachial plexus as they traverse the area from neck and chest to upper arm. The scalenus anticus and scalenus medius muscles form the interscalene triangle, an additional anatomic passage for artery and nerve not encountered elsewhere in the body (Figures 1 and 2). An understanding of neurovascular compression at the thoracic outlet is perhaps best developed in the context of the historical evolution of etiologic concepts, and the unique anatomic characteristics that underlie the varied clinical manifestations.[1]

In 1986 the neurologist W.S. Fields[2] wrote:

All shoulder girdle compression syndromes have one common feature, namely, compression of the brachial plexus, the subclavian artery, and subclavian vein, usually between the first rib and the clavicle. With elevation of the upper limb, there is a scissorlike approximation of the clavicle superiorly and the first rib inferiorly. Grouping the various conditions under the single heading of thoracic outlet syndrome has resulted in

From Machleder HI, (ed): *Vascular Disorders of the Upper Extremity*. Third Revised Edition. Futura Publishing Company, Inc., Armonk, NY, © 1998.

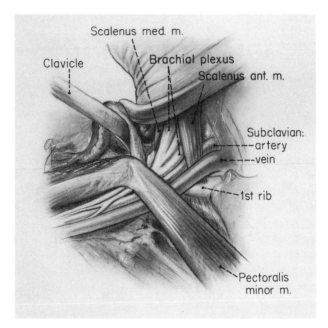

Figure 1. Anatomic dissection showing the anatomy at the thoracic outlet. Cadaver head is turned to the left and clavicle is reflected laterally.

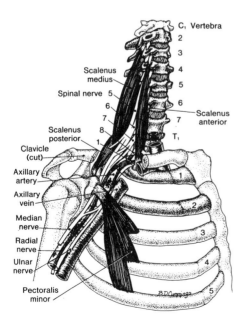

Figure 2. Diagram of interscalene triangle showing passage of brachial plexus and axillosubclavian artery. (Reproduced with permission from Travell JG, Simons DG: *Myofascial Pain and Dysfunction*. Baltimore: William and Wilkins; 1983.)

more correct diagnoses and improved therapy. This syndrome should be considered in all neurologic and vascular complaints of the arm previously reported as scalenus anticus, hyperabduction, costoclavicular, cervical rib, fractured clavicle, cervicobrachial compression, pneumatic hammer, effort vein thrombosis, subcoracoid pectoralis minor, and first thoracic rib syndromes.

Development of Anatomic Concepts

The Cervical Rib

In the spring of 1861, a 26-year-old servant woman was admitted to St. Bartholomew's hospital in London, England with a painful, dysesthetic, and somewhat ischemic left arm. It was noted on examination that she had a walnut-sized pulsation above the left clavicle and a clinical diagnosis was made of cervical rib displacing the subclavian artery and brachial plexus. It was noted that the patient had pain in her arm, particularly the elbow, and decreased sensation in her fingers. She dropped objects from her left hand. On March 30th (8 days after admission) Mr. Holmes Coote proceeded with surgery to remove the cervical rib. His operative comments as recorded in *The Lancet* remain instructive, and reiterate some of the anatomic features.

> The region was not a pleasant one for any proceeding demanding the use of the knife. The subclavian artery and vein were in front; the axillary plexus of nerves lay spread out above; below, the apex of the lung, covered by the pleura, rose up in dangerous proximity; on the scalenus was the phrenic nerve; while towards the mesial line were the important vessels and nerves passing to the head, together with the vertebral vessels and thoracic duct. You can understand, therefore, why I was cautious in what I did.

Despite the technical challenge, the patient had return of the radial pulse and was discharged improved, with an optimistic prognosis.[3]

At the time of this report it was recalled by the writer that a similar case was seen in Charing Cross Hospital several months previously. Mary O, a 21-year-old girl, had been admitted to Dr. Willshire's service and a pulsatile supraclavicular mass was noted and cervical rib diagnosed. The striking difference was that this young woman had been admitted for the treatment of anemia, her arms presumably asymptomatic, and the pulsatile mass and cervical rib were of no demonstrable clinical significance.[4]

As with other diseases, it is perhaps axiomatic that an underlying anomaly is only a predisposing factor in a complex interaction of events that lead to the manifestations of a clinical disorder.

The First Rib

After Coote's successful case, cervical rib and its syndrome were increasingly encountered, particularly after 1900, when recognition was facilitated by the growing use of roentgen diagnosis. A number of subsequent surgical reports appeared in the literature, and cervical rib excision became an accepted therapeutic approach for upper extremity radicular neurovascular symptoms.

Paradoxically, patients were increasingly recognized with seemingly identical symptoms but without a demonstrable cervical rib. Some of these were found to have a rudimentary cervical rib manifest by an enlarged C7 transverse process and a radiologically undetected fibrocartilagenous band that compressed the brachial plexus (Figures 3 through 5).[5] However, there were other patients with no discernible bony abnormality. Particularly in the industrial regions of England and Australia, physicians reported patients with neurogenic and vasomotor symptoms of the cervical rib syndrome without radiological evidence of a cervical rib or enlarged C7 transverse process.

These reports proved to be an important milestone in the development of a more generalized concept of upper extremity neurovascular

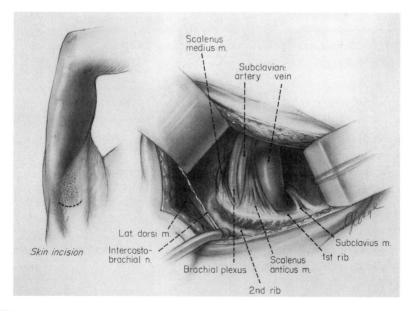

Figure 3.   Thoracic outlet anatomy as seen from the transaxillary surgical approach.

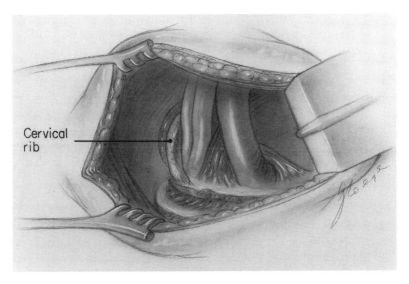

Figure 4. Appearance of cervical rib from the transaxillary approach. (Reproduced with permisson from Reference 32.)

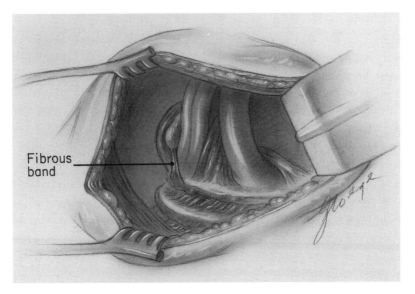

Figure 5. Fibrocartilagenous band as described as Gilliat. This lesion has been implicated in the "wasted hand." (Reproduced with permisson from Reference 32.)

compression. In a landmark clinical and anatomic study of a large number of men, women, and children, T. Wingate Todd[6] concluded in 1912 that "symptoms of 'cervical rib' may be caused by an apparently normal first dorsal rib, and may be cured by its removal." He concluded from his studies that, "in consequence of the action of these forces, pressure symptoms on the lowest brachial trunk are most likely to occur in women at the commencement of adult age." These observations, derived from anatomic measurements of postnatal shoulder development, would foretell the actual clinical prevalence reported over the next 80 years.

Todd expanded his observations by noting that the upper limb develops at the level of the seventh cervical segment, and consequently the first and second thoracic nerves must travel upward until they have crossed the uppermost rib and then angulate downward to enter the arm. Because of this configuration any elevation of the rib or depression of the shoulder must stretch these lower connections with the brachial plexus. He had shown additionally that in the course of normal skeletal development there is a gradual descent of the shoulder with advancing years. This tendency, he noted, is exaggerated when the individual carries a heavy weight, and is reduced when the weight is taken off the arm by supporting the elbow in a sling or on the arm of a chair. "It is just these maneuvers which frequently result in exacerbation or relief of symptoms."

In 1920, Stopford and Telford[7] reported a group of clinical cases seen in Manchester where the lower trunk of the brachial plexus was compressed by the first thoracic rib rather than a supernumerary cervical rib. They described the essential characteristics of these cases of neurovascular compression.

As Todd had predicted, the symptoms were predominantly in the sensory and motor distribution of the lower trunk of the brachial plexus. These patients complained of loss of grip strength, fatigue of the hand with exercise, weakness of the intrinsic muscles, loss of sensation in the distribution of the lower trunk (of brachial plexus), and vasomotor instability with episodes of cyanosis and coolness. They noted that after removal of the impinging portion of the first rib there was rapid resolution of the vasomotor and sensory changes and slow resolution of atrophic and motor changes.

In succeeding years abnormalities in development of the first thoracic rib would be recognized and, as with cervical rib, be associated with radicular neurovascular symptoms.[8,9]

The Anterior Scalene Muscle

At about the time of Stopford and Telford's report, the large neurosurgical clinics in the United States were encountering similar perplexing cases of "cervical rib syndrome without cervical rib." At the Mayo Clinic, Adson and Coffey[10] had begun to treat cervical rib patients by scalenectomy alone. Their work, emphasizing the compressive role of the anterior scalene muscle, directed attention in the United States to soft tissue abnormalities, whereas in Great Britain research and treatment continued to focus on the normal and abnormal first rib.

It is not surprising that in the United States, scalenectomy would be applied to this new group of patients with cervical rib-type symptoms of radicular neurovascular compression. Adson and Coffey's discovery inaugurated a remarkable intensity of clinical work involving university departments and large private clinics in all parts of the United States.

Naffziger,[11,12] Chief of Neurosurgery at the University of California, considered the anterior scalene muscle to be the key to the neurovascular compressive abnormalities, and used the term scalenus syndrome. Ochsner and colleagues[13] first published the term in a landmark article entitled, "Scalenus anticus (Naffziger) syndrome," giving credit to Naffziger although their paper antedated his by 3 years. The concept began to flourish with dramatic cures and failures.

In this period of time, before the widespread recognition of patients with carpal tunnel syndrome, cervical disk disease, and neuroforaminal compression, the application of scalenotomy was certain to lead to failures, particularly when applied to patients with predominantly upper plexus or median nerve distribution symptoms.

Despite considerable interest in scalenotomy in the United States it was likely applied too broadly. There were failures, partly due to diagnostic imprecision during the gradual recognition of other overlapping neurogenic syndromes, and partly due to incomplete decompression of the neurovascular structures. As a consequence, scalenotomy did not entirely live up to expectations.

Thoracic Outlet Compression Syndrome

It seems evident that sometime in the 1950s the term thoracic outlet syndrome (TOS) crept into general usage as well as first appearing in the medical and surgical literature. The term was used to describe both the arterial and neurogenic presentations, recognizing the commonality of etiology and frequent overlap of vascular and neurogenic symptoms.[14,15] The "Mayo Clinic Number" of the 1946 *Surgical Clinics of North America* was devoted to a symposium on pain in the shoulder and arm.[16] Eaton,[17] the consultant in neurology described what he would regularly refer to 10 years later (in 1956) as the "thoracic outlet syndrome."

Almost always the patient seeks relief from pain and paresthesia of the upper extremity. The patient most often complains of a dragging sensation through the shoulders and pain distributed over the deltoid area to the elbow. When the condition is more severe, pain and paresthesia occur in the ulnar aspect of the forearm and hand, and in the fourth and fifth digits. At times, it spreads to the radial aspect of the forearm, hand and digits, and to the neck, scapular and pectoral regions. Sometimes, the patient may complain of pain in the head and face on the same side. There is a decided tendency for the symptoms to become worse at night while the patient is lying down. At this time paresthesia may be particularly intense and may involve the whole upper extremity. The patient may be awakened several times and find relief by lying prone and swinging the arm over the side of the bed. However, when the syndrome is well developed, symptoms also occur at other times. They may be aggravated by the use of the arms and particularly by use which depresses the shoulder girdle, such as the carrying of heavy objects or the maintenance for long periods of the position of the arms required in holding a book to be read.

The Decline of Scalenotomy

O.T. Clagett,[18] chief of the section of thoracic surgery at the Mayo Clinic, became interested in the new syndrome of thoracic outlet compression. He noted the very frequent cases of residual and recurrent symptoms from the scalenotomy era of his surgical predecessor Adson, and drawing from his experience with thoracoplasty and a rediscovery of the English literature he inaugurated the new era of first rib removal.

Clagett described a posterior approach to first rib removal that for most surgeons was a difficult operation devised primarily for the treatment of tuberculosis by thoracoplasty. Although Clagett's article had considerable impact, delivered as the Presidential Address to the American Thoracic Society, there was relatively limited further clinical application.

Present Concepts

A major milestone appeared in 1966 when Roos[19,20] reported a series of 15 patients treated by removal of the first thoracic rib from a transaxillary approach. The dramatic superiority of this technique was readily appreciated and became widely accepted. The combination of the improved ability to identify patients with carpal tunnel syndrome and cervical disk disease, and a very effective operative approach to TOS led to renewed interest in the treatment of thoracic outlet compression syndrome. Roos' superb ability in communicating the critical elements in the clinical work-up as well as the operative details proved to be one of the keys to acceptance in every country with modern surgical practice. The transaxillary procedure became the standard operation for removal of the first thoracic rib.

Recognition that cumulative trauma disorders (due to performance of repetitive tasks) account for extensive upper extremity disability has been increasing in all industrialized countries.[21] These musculoskeletal disorders make up more than 50% of all occupational illnesses in the United States today.[22] In emerging industrial countries the same experience is being reported. On a large hand service in Shanghai China, for example, 20% of cases of upper extremity neurovascular symptoms were attributed to compression at the thoracic outlet.[23]

In many regards, the acceptance of soft tissue abnormalities in thoracic outlet compression syndromes parallels the evolution of thinking about carpal tunnel syndrome. In reviewing the history of this entity at the Mayo Clinic, Amadio[24] had the following to say: "initially, treatment was limited to those patients with the most severe neuropathies and derangement of wrist anatomy. As confidence with the diagnosis and therapy increased, progressively less severe anatomic deformities and then progressively less severe neurologic impairments were considered for surgical management." In the early years, during the 1920s, many centers began experimenting with decompression of the median nerve by removing bony deformity. There was a progressive building on previous operations that eventually led to the understanding of the soft tissue abnormality. Until the late 1940s the condition was known by a variety of names. Diagnosis was entertained only "when a severe and obvious distal median neuropathy was present." In 1947, the eminent British neurologist, Sir Russell Brain proposed that less severe neuropathies characterized by intermittent paresthesias, pain, and weakness might be part of the same spectrum and might, in fact, be fairly common.[25]

Pathological Anatomy

Anatomic variation at the region of the thoracic outlet has intrigued surgical anatomists from the early descriptions of supernumerary ribs to modern studies of ultrastructural changes in the scalene muscles.[26,27] During transaxillary resections of the first rib for arterial, venous, or brachial plexus compression at the thoracic outlet, a spectrum of changes representing intermediate developmental variation can be recognized in addition to the discrete abnormalities such as cervical ribs, cervical fibrocartilagenous bands, and supernumerary scalene muscles.[28,29]

Working in Paris, Milliez[30] emphasized that anomalies at the thoracic outlet rarely exist in isolation as there is interaction in development of the different elements. The anatomist White and his colleagues[31] clarified this concept in describing cervical ribs and congenital malformations of

first thoracic ribs as linked to errors of bodily segmentation in early embryonic development, where variation in the formation of the brachial plexus
appears before bony skeleton development. Cervical rib development, for
example, is determined by the formation of the spinal nerve roots. The
regression of the C5 through C7 ribs is occasioned by the rapid development of the enlarging roots of the brachial plexus in the region of the limb
bud. In cases of a cervical C7 rib there is generally a pre-fixed plexus with
only a small neural contribution from the T1 nerve root. The inhibition
to rib development at that level is lost or reduced, and the size of the
cervical rib is then related to the extent of contribution of this T1 root to
the brachial plexus. As a corollary, in the postfixed plexus where there is
a contribution of the T2 root to the brachial plexus, the first thoracic rib
is often rudimentary, having been inhibited in its development by the
unusual nerve growth.[31] This embryologically determined morphological
interdependence is evident with other structural relationships at the thoracic outlet.

A series of 200 consecutive cases reported from UCLA gives an idea
of the relative frequency of the three forms of TOS as well as the anatomic
variations that can be seen from the transaxillary exposure.[32]

Forty cases (20%) in this series presented with problems related to
venous obstruction, or arterial insufficiency and embolization. Twenty-
six cases (65%) of this vascular subgroup had additional neurogenic symptoms associated with abnormal sensory evoked responses in the affected
extremity. In the entire group, of 200 symptomatic extremities, 153 (76.5%)
exhibited signs of arterial compression in stress positions on clinical examination or with digital photoplethysmography.

In 68 cases (34%) there was no structural abnormality discernible
from the transaxillary surgical approach. Seventeen cases (8.5%) had a
cervical rib articulating with the first rib directly or by fibrocartilagenous
extension. Twenty (10%) had a scalenus minimus muscle inserting either
on the first rib or Sibsons fascia. Thirty-nine patients (19.5%) had an anomaly of the subclavius tendon or its insertion tubercle. Eighty-six cases
(43%) had an anomaly of scalene muscle development or insertion. In 15
cases (7.5%) there were other categories of anomalies that could not be
related to specific developmental characteristics. These included ligamen-
tous or fibrous structures that did not correspond to regression residua
of recognized embryological structures. More than one abnormality was
recognized in 22.5% of the cases, and 32% of 25 patients undergoing bilateral procedures had similar anomalies on both sides.

There was only one clinical setting that could be correlated with a
characteristic anatomic abnormality. Of 33 patients presenting with spontaneous axillosubclavian vein thrombosis (Paget-Schroetter's syndrome),
18 (55%) had hypertrophy of the subclavius tendon associated with enlargement of the insertion tubercle. Among male patients with Paget-
Schroetter syndrome 14 of 20 (70%) had this anomaly.[33]

Embryological Development

The abdominal, thoracic, and cervical musculature develops from the hypomeric portion of the paraxial and epaxial mesoderm, with the scalene and prevertebral muscles in the neck corresponding to the intercostal and ventrolateral abdominal muscles in the thorax and abdomen, respectively.[34] In the embryo, plates of axially running muscle segments differentiate into the discrete muscle groups seen in the adult.

The subclavian artery, which is the artery of the seventh cervical segment, as well as the spinal nerves from C5 to T1 pierce the muscle plates in the cervical segment much the same as the intercostal nerve and artery do in the thoracic segments. The growth of the limb bud and development of the pectoral girdle then lead to the particular structural changes seen in this region, specifically the segmentation of the scalenic muscle mass into discrete muscles.

First Rib and Cervical Rib Anomalies

During development, the C7 rib forms and then regresses to the C7 transverse process. Various stages in this evolution range from a complete C7 rib to rudimentary forms associated with a fibrocartilagenous band.[35,36] The only radiological indication of this residual band may be an enlarged C7 transverse process (Figures 4 and 5).

Anomalies of the first or cervical rib are encountered in about 10% of modern series of patients with TOS. The incidence of these autosomal dominant abnormalities in the general population can be estimated from the medical literature. Adson and Coffee[37] report that Galen and Vesalius both described cervical ribs in their anatomical dissections.[38]

In a study of 40,000 consecutive chest x-rays in American army recruits, Etter[39] encountered 68 complete articulated cervical ribs (0.17%), 31 anomalous first ribs and 67 rudimentary first ribs (0.25%). Additionally, 77 synostoses of first and second ribs and 16 bifid first ribs were recognized. In 1947, Adson[40] reviewed his experience with cervical ribs citing a Mayo Clinic radiological study prior to 1927 that identified an incidence of 0.563% or 5.6 patients per 1000 with cervical rib. Twenty-eight percent were males, 72% were females, and 47% of the cervical ribs were bilateral. The right side was involved in 23% and the left side in 30%. Forty-five percent of the group were symptomatic. Adson[41] quotes a review by Haven of 5000 routine roentgenograms of the thorax in which he found 38 first rib abnormalities and 37 cervical ribs, an incidence of 0.74% or 7.4 persons per 1000. Adson[41] subscribed to the concept linking formation of cervical ribs to a failure of rudimentary rib regression as the nerve roots form.

Firsov[42] in the Soviet Union reported fluorographic examination of 510,893 people, observing 1379 cervical ribs for an incidence of 0.27%. Women accounted for 76.8% and men 23.2%; 33.3% were bilateral. A cervical rib or C7 rib is most often associated with a pre-fixed type of brachial plexus where there is a minor contribution to the brachial plexus from the T1 nerve root and a major contribution from C4. When the C7 rib is incomplete, there is often a rudimentary band in place of the regressed portion of the rib.

Cervical rib clearly represents one of the predisposing abnormalities for development of thoracic outlet compression syndrome. The significantly higher incidence of these recognized congenital abnormalities in women compared with men may also be reflected in the higher incidence of thoracic outlet nerve compression symptoms in women.

The symptom characteristics associated with the presence of cervical ribs have been addressed by several authors. In 205 patients treated for cervical rib or TOS at Montefiore Medical Center (Bronx, NY), 12 patients had arterial lesions (5.9%).[43] Halsted[44] indicated that in 716 cases of cervical rib he had reviewed, there were 27 cases of subclavian artery dilatation (3.7%). He indicates that of 360 symptomatic clinical cases 235 or 65.3% had nerve symptoms alone, 106 or 29.4% had nerve and vascular symptoms and 19 or 5.3% had vascular symptoms alone.

Charlesworth and Brown[45] performed 23 cervical rib excisions and indicated that 15 (65%) had predominantly neurological symptoms, and 8 (35%) had vascular symptoms.

Telford and Mottershead[46] encountered anomalous fibrous bands from rudimentary cervical ribs in 12 and complete cervical ribs in 70 of 105 surgical cases. Telford, writing with Stopford,[47] attributed the vascular complications of cervical rib to stimulation of the sympathetic innervation through the lowest two nerve roots, a view that prevailed for many years. In their otherwise excellent discussion, they seem to have neglected the possibility of arterial embolism.

Fibrocartilagenous bands extending from the end of incompletely formed cervical ribs are best thought of as an anomaly of cervical rib formation. These abnormalities have been referred to as type 1 and type 2 bands by Roos (Figures 1, 3, and 5).

Scalene Muscle Anomalies

Milliez,[30] in his studies of scalene muscle in a 2.5-cm embryo has emphasized the influence of neurovascular structure development on the ultimate configuration of the scalene muscle mass. He recognized a confluent scalene muscle distinguished only by a groove at the site of anterior and middle scalene differentiation. Actual separation into two muscles occurred at the points where the muscle mass was traversed by the roots of the brachial plexus. Rather than the scalenus minimus forming as a separate muscle entity it represents one form of segmentation of the scalenic mass. Milliez quotes Poitevin's studies of 1988 indicating that the scalenic mass is only differentiated into specific muscle groups by the traversing of the neurovascular bundle. The persistence of certain muscle inclusions in the brachial plexus, as well as muscle groups that traverse various elements of the brachial plexus, is related to the original mass of the scalene variously segmented by the passage of these advancing structures as the limb bud develops. However, he acknowledges an alternate opinion that accessory scalene muscles may be representations of phylogenetic recapitulation wherein muscles persist that ordinarily would regress either completely or to a small tendon.

This separation of muscle bundles interdigitating between the neurovascular structures accounts for the muscular bridges seen between the middle and anterior scalene that often penetrate the brachial plexus. Sanders and Roos[48] demonstrated in their recent anatomical dissections that these abnormalities of scalene segmentation are seen quite frequently in the adult. Although not pathological in their own right, these fibers may result in neurogenic symptoms as a consequence of later abnormal growth, peculiarities of occupational or recreational use, or post-traumatic changes (Figure 6). Adson, Ochsner, Naffziger and their coworkers made

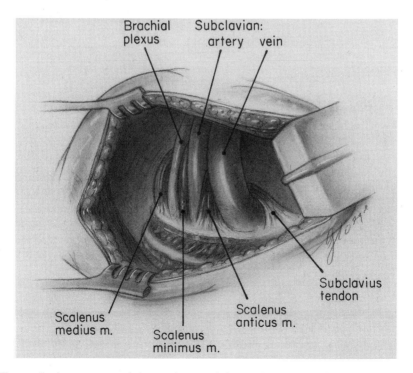

Figure 6. Appearance of the scalenus minimus abnormality. (Reproduced with permisson from Reference 32.)

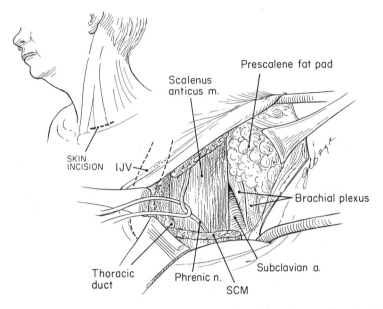

Figure 7. Transcervical approach to thoracic outlet and neurovascular structures.

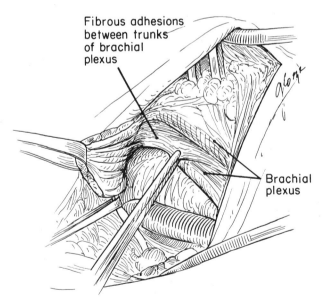

Figure 8. A: Drawing of fibrous bands or muscle, traversing area between trunks of the brachial plexus.

the initial observations of scalene muscle involvement in neurovascular compression at the thoracic outlet.[13,14] Recent ultrastructural studies have helped to clarify the fiber type and hypertrophic changes that underlie the gross morphological observations.[27]

In addition to metabolic changes and the discrete anomalies previously described, there is wide variation in normal scalene muscle anatomy. These variations may well explain differing sequelae in individual patients after comparable trauma or in comparable work situations. In a series of methodical dissections, Lang[49] described the range of scalene muscle insertions and configurations of the interscalene triangle. These variations govern the available passage space for artery and brachial plexus through the interscalene triangle (Figures 7, 8A, 8B, and 9).

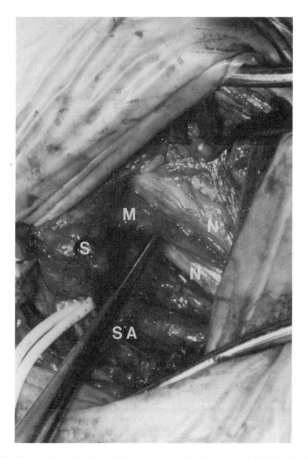

Figure 8. B: Operative view from the transcervical approach. SA indicates subclavian artery; S, scalene muscle stump being lifted from its bed; N, divisions and trunks of brachial plexus; M, fibrotic or muscular band.

Telford and Mottershead[46] found the ventral attachment of the anterior scalene to vary from 2.4 to 6.0 cm from the chondrosternal junction, and the width of the anterior scalene insertion to vary from 0.4 to 2.5 cm with the interscalene interval varying from 0 to 2.4 cm. They encountered crossing of the insertions of the anterior and middle scalene muscles in 8 of 105 operative cases and in 15% (15) of 102 cadaver dissections. Sunderland and Bedbrook encountered this crossing of the scalene insertions in 15% of 35 cadaver dissections.[50]

This abnormality (which in the extreme is a sling-like crossing of the scalene muscles described by some as a V-shaped deformity) traps the subclavian artery and brachial plexus. It corresponds to the type 4 band

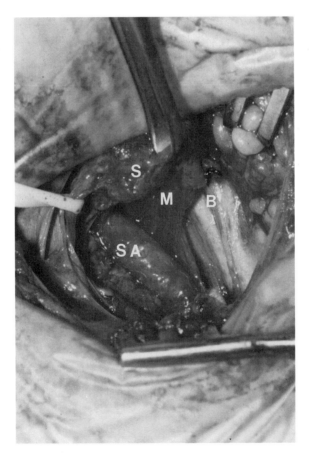

Figure 9. Supernumerary scalene muscle slip going between subclavian artery and brachial plexus. SA indicates subclavian artery; S, stump of scalene muscle being elevated by a Babcock clamp; M, extra muscle slip; B, brachial plexus trunks.

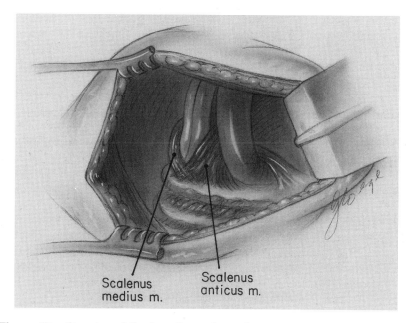

Scalenus
medius m.

Scalenus
anticus m.

Figure 10. Crossing of the insertions of anterior and middle scalene muscles. (Reproduced with permisson from Reference 32.)

described by Roos and has been called intercostalization by Makhoul and Machleder,[32] to reflect the embryonic derivation of these muscles (first recognized by Todd[51]) (Figure 10).

Roos[52] subdivided these crossing bands into an eighth and ninth abnormality in 1980; the type 8 representing a band from the middle scalene to the costochondral junction and type 9 a fascial band in the concave curve of the first rib.

Unique configurations of scalene muscle insertion, that tend to compress the neurovascular structures in the interscalene triangle, accounted for 43% of the congenital variations seen in the series reported from UCLA.[30]

The scalenus minimus muscle, present in 20 of the UCLA cases (10%) can be represented by a residual ligament which has variously been called the costovertebral, or pleurospinal ligament when the muscle has regressed. Roos[52] described these as type 5 or type 6 bands depending on the site of insertion to rib or apical pleura (Figures 6 and 9).

Sanders and Roos[48] studying the anatomy of the interscalene triangle found interdigitating fibers between the scalene muscles through the brachial plexus in 75% of dissections in TOS patients and in 40% of 60 cadaver dissections. In 45% of cadaver dissections the C5, C6 nerve roots emerged between fibers of the anterior scalene muscle rather than between the anterior and middle scalene muscles.

Subclavius Anomalies

Telford and Mottershead[46] noted in anatomic dissections that during movements of abduction or retraction of the shoulder, the tendon of the subclavius muscle compressed the subclavian vein against the first rib. In the Paget-Schroetter type deformity Sampson[53] emphasized the striking hypertrophy of the subclavius tendon, with these observations later corroborated by Aziz et al[54] and Kunkel and Machleder.[33]

This particular manifestation of compression at the thoracic outlet is related to progressive enlargement of the subclavius muscle system with repetitive compressive trauma to the subclavian vein followed by fibrosis, stricture, and thrombosis. An abnormality in this system was found in 19.5% of the UCLA cases with 15.5% having an exostosis at the subclavius tubercle (Figure 11).

Despite the congenital nature of these deformities, the onset of symptoms in early to mid adult life has been recorded by virtually all physicians

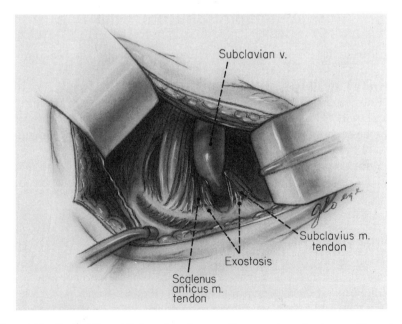

Figure 11. Typical Paget-Schroetter abnormality, seen from the transaxillary view. Note compression of the axillosubclavian vein. (Reproduced with permisson from Reference 33.)

treating the clinical disorders. This delay in onset is most likely related to postnatal development. The chest widens and the clavicle continues its growth to approximately age 22 or 25 after which the pectoral girdle begins to descend. Still later, with loss of strength or tone in the supporting musculature of the thoracic girdle, there is further traction on the neurovascular structures at the thoracic outlet.

Summary

In their most obvious manifestations, the congenital and acquired abnormalities recognized in association with the thoracic outlet compression syndrome are considered discrete anomalies. However, they should more properly be viewed as part of a continuum of developmental variation. The particular spectrum of developmental variations seen may be significant as predisposing elements when complicated by either increased functional requirements or a change in muscle fiber type (or isoforms of myosin) consequent to trauma.[55]

Greater resilience of the arterial and venous system seems to result in relatively innocuous symptoms until compression reaches levels of hemodynamic significance or structural damage. It is evident that the threshold for neurogenic symptoms from the brachial plexus is lower than that of the vascular system. Coincident with the range and continuum of developmental abnormalities, there is a range and continuum of compression of the normal structures that traverse the thoracic outlet area. Symptoms associated with the extremes of the compressive abnormalities are easy to distinguish since they represent the "classic" cases:

(1) Paget-Schroetter axillosubclavian vein occlusion;
(2) hand ischemia from thrombosis or embolization from the compressed or aneurysmal subclavian artery;
(3) the "wasted hand" of cervical band compression of the brachial plexus.

In addition to these end-stage conditions, it is important to recognize the full spectrum of symptoms that can arise from neurovascular compression at the thoracic outlet. The lessor degrees of compression will often be disabling, in settings of specific physical or occupational requirements.

References

1. Machleder HI: Thoracic outlet syndromes: New concepts fiom a century of discovery. *Cardiovasc Surg* 2:137–145, 1994.
2. Fields WS, Lemak NA, Ben-Menachem Y: Thoracic outlet syndrome: Review and reference to stroke in a major league pitcher. *AJNR* 7:73–78, 1986.

3. Coote H: Exostosis of the left transverse process of the seventh cervical verte-brae, surrounded by blood vessels and nerves, successful removal. *Lancet* 1: 360–361, 1861.
4. Wilshire WH: Supernumerary first rib: Clinical records. *Lancet* 2:633, 1860.
5. Gilliat RW, LeQuesne PM, Logue V, Sumner AJ: Wasting of the hand associ-ated with a cervical rib or band. *J Neurol Neurosurg Psychiatry* 33:615–624, 1970.
6. Todd TW. The descent of the shoulder after birth. Its significance in the pro-duction of pressure-symptoms on the lowest brachial trunk. *Anat Anz Bd* 41: 385–395, 1912.
7. Stopford JSB, Telford ED: Compression of the lower trunk of the brachial plexus by a first dorsal rib. *Br J Surg* 7:168–77, 1919.
8. White JC, Poppel N, Adams R: Congenital malformations of the first thoracic rib. *Surg Gynecol Obstet* 81:643–59, 1945.
9. Edwards PR, Moody AP, Harris PL: First rib abnormalities in association with cervical ribs: A cause for postoperative failure in the thoracic outlet syndrome. *Eur J Vasc Surg* 6:677–681, 1992.
10. Adson AW, Coffey JR: Cervical rib: A method of anterior approach for relief of symptoms by division of the scalenus anticus. *Ann Surg* 85:839–53, 1927.
11. Naffziger HC: The scalenus syndrome. *Surg Gynecol Obstet* 64:119–20, 1937.
12. Naffziger HC, Grant WT: Neuritis of the brachial plexus, mechanical in origin: The scalenus syndrome. *Surg Gynecol Obstet* 67:722–30, 1938.
13. Ochsner A, Gage M, DeBakey M: Scalenus anticus (Naffziger) syndrome. *Am J Surg* 28:669–95, 1935.
14. Peet RM, Henriksen JD, Anderson TP, Martin GM: Thoracic-outlet syndrome: Evaluation of a therapeutic exercise program. *Proc Mayo Clinic* 31:281–87, 1956.
15. Rob CG, Standeven A: Arterial occlusion complicating thoracic outlet compression syndrome. *Br Med J* 2:709–19, 1958.
16. Eaton LM: Neurologic causes of pain in the upper extremities; with particular reference to syndromes of protruded intervertebral disk in the cervical region and mechanical compression of the brachial plexus. *Surg Clin North Am* 4–6: 810–832, 1946.
17. Eaton LM: in discussion of Peet et. al. *Proc Mayo Clinic* 312:81–87, 1956.
18. Clagett OT: Research and prosearch. *J Thorac Cardiovasc Surg* 44:153–66, 1962.
19. Roos DB: Transaxillary approach for first rib resection to relieve thoracic outlet syndrome. *Ann Surg* 163:354–58, 1966.
20. Roos DB: Experience with first rib resection for thoracic outlet syndrome. *Ann Surg* 173:429–42, 1971.
21. Dawson DM. Entrapment neuropathies of the upper extremities. *N Engl J Med* 329:2013–2018, 1993.
22. Rempel DM, Harrison RJ, Barnhard S: Work-related cumulative trauma disor-ders of the upper extremity. *JAMA* 267:838–842, 1992.
23. Gu YD, Yan JG, Shang GM, et al: Thoracic outlet syndrome. *Chin Med J* 101: 689–694, 1988.
24. Amadio PC: The Mayo Clinic and carpal tunnel syndrome. *Mayo Clin Proc* 67: 42–48, 1992.
25. Brain WR, Wright AD, Wilkinson M: Spontaneous compression of both median nerves in the carpal tunnel: Six cases treated surgically. *Lancet* 1:277–82, 1947.

26. Machleder HI, Moll F, Verity A. The anterior scalene muscle in thoracic outlet compression syndrome: Histochemical and morphometric studies. *Arch Surg* 121:1141–1144, 1986.

27. Sanders RJ, Jackson CGR, Banchero N, Pearce WH: Scalene muscle abnormalities in traumatic thoracic outlet syndrome. *Am J Surg* 159:231–236, 1990.

28. Law AA: Adventitious ligaments simulating cervical ribs. *Ann Surg* 72: 497–499, 1920.

29. Roos DB: Congenital anomalies associated with thoracic outlet syndrome. *Am J Surg* 132:771–778, 1976.

30. Milliez PY: Contribution A L'Etude De L'Ontogenese Des Muscles Scalenes (Reconstruction D'Un Embryon De 2.5 cm). June 28, 1991 Universite Paris 1 Pantheon-Sorbonne Musee De L'Homme, Museum D, Histoire Naturelle.

31. White JC, Poppel N, Adams R: Congenital malformations of the first thoracic rib: A cause of brachial neuralgia which simulates the cervical rib syndrome. *Surg Gynecol Obstet* 81:643–659, 1945.

32. Makhoul RG, Machleder HI: Developmental anomalies at the thoracic outlet: An analysis of 200 consecutive cases. *J Vasc Surg* 16:534–545, 1992.

33. Kunkel JM, Machleder HI: Treatment of Paget-Schroetter syndrome: A staged multidisciplinary approach. *Arch Surg* 124:1153–1158, 1989.

34. Hamilton, Boyd, Massman: *Human Embryology.* Third edition. Cambridge: 1952, pp. 548–559.

35. Todd TW: The relations of the thoracic operculum considered in reference to the anatomy of cervical ribs of surgical importance. *J Anat Physiol* 45:293–304, 1911.

36. Gruber W: Uber die Halsrippen des Menschen mit vergleichend-anatomischen Bemerkungen. *Mem Acad Imper Sci St Petersburg* 7(ser 13), No 2, 1869.

37. Adson AW, Coffee JR: Cervical rib. *Ann Surg* 85:839–857, 1927.

38. Schapera J: Autosomal dominant inheritance of cervical ribs. *Clin Genet* 31: 386–388, 1987.

39. Etter LE: Osseous abnormalities of the thoracic cage seen in forty thousand consecutive chest photoroentgenograms. *AJR* 51:359–363, 1944.

40. Adson WA: Surgical treatment for symptoms produced by cervical ribs and the scalenus anticus muscle. *Surg Gynecol Obstet* 85:687–700, 1947.

41. Adson AW: Cervical ribs: Symptoms, differential diagnosis and indication for section of the insertion of scalenous anticus muscle. *J Int Coll Surg* 16:546–559, 1951.

42. Firsov GI: Cervical ribs and their distinction from under-developed first ribs. *Arkhiv Anatomii Gistologii I Embriologii* 67:101–103, 1974.

43. Scher LA, Veith FJ, Haimovici H, et al: Staging of arterial complications of cervical rib: Guidelines for surgical management. *Surgery* 95:644–649, 1984.

44. Halsted WS: An experimental study of circumscribed dilation of an artery immediately distal to a partially occluding band and its bearing on the dilation of the subclavian artery observed in certain cases of cervical rib. *J Exp Med* 24:271–279, 1916.

45. Charlesworth D, Brown SCW: Results of excision of a cervical rib in patients with the thoracic outlet syndrome. *Br J Surg* 75:431–433, 1988.

46. Telford ED, Mottershead S: Pressure at the cervico-brachial junction (an operative and anatomical study). *J Bone Joint Surg* 308:249–263, 1948.

47. Telford EC, Stopford JSB: The vascular complications of cervical rib. *Br J Surg* 18:557–564, 1931.
48. Sanders RJ, Roos DB: The surgical anatomy of the scalene triangle. *Contemp Surg* 35:11–16, 1989.
49. Lang J: *Topographische Anatomie des Plexus brachialis und Thoracic-Outlet Syndrom.* Berlin: Walter de Gruyter; 1985.
50. Sunderland S, Bedbrook GM: Narrowing of the second part of the subclavian artery. *Anat Rec* 104:299–307, 1949.
51. Todd TW: Cervical rib: Factors controlling its presence and its size, its bearing on the morphology of the shoulder, with four cases. *J Anat Physiol* 45:293–304, 1911–1912.
52. Roos DB: Pathophysiology of congenital anomalies in thoracic outlet syndrome. *Acta Chir Belgica* 79:353–361, 1980.
53. Sampson JJ: In: *Medico-Surgical Tribute to Harold Brunn.* Berkeley: University of California Press; 1942, pp. 453–471.
54. Aziz S, Straehley CJ, Whelan TJ: Effort-related axillosubclavian vein thrombosis: A new theory of pathogenesis and a plea for direct surgical intervention. *Am J Surg* 152:57–61, 1986.
55. Juvonen T, Satta J, Laitala P, et al: Anomalies at the thoracic outlet are frequent in the general population. *Am J Surg* 170:33–37, 1995.

—————— 5 ——————

Neurogenic Thoracic Outlet Compression Syndrome

Herbert I. Machleder, MD

Initial Assessment

Predominantly neurogenic symptoms may affect up to 75% of patients presenting with neurovascular compression at the thoracic outlet. These patients often incur symptoms in the overhead position (abduction and external rotation [AER]) typically developing numbness of the fourth and fifth fingers and ulnar aspect of the forearm. They rapidly note impairment in strength and endurance with exercise in AER. When fatigue occurs in this position, a bruit can often be auscultated inferior to the lateral third of the clavicle over the axillary artery. This positional neurovascular compression will affect mechanics, painters, stone masons, electricians, and others who work with arms in abduction. The symptom characteristics can be replicated on physical examination by having the patient clench and unclench the fingers with arms elevated. The so-called elevated arm stress test (EAST). The EAST or AER maneuver has been studied in industrial workers in Sweden and found to correlate both with symptoms at work and with the presence of nocturnal dysesthesias.[1] During elevated arm exercise the hand will often become pale and show reactive hyperemia upon resuming the neutral position.

Characteristically there is tenderness over the anterior scalene muscle and hypersensitivity to clavicular percussion on the affected side. This hypersensitivity is very often associated with a positive Tinnel's sign at the brachial plexus. In addition, fine finger movement and grip strength

From Machleder HI, (ed): *Vascular Disorders of the Upper Extremity*. Third Revised Edition. Futura Publishing Company, Inc., Armonk, NY, © 1998.

becomes progressively impaired as patients develop difficulty performing tasks in both the AER position and with their arms in neutral positions. This accounts for the disabilities seen in many patients from industrial and white collar repetitive-motion occupations.

The loss of tactile ability and fine motor coordination is a consequence of impairment in the C8-T1 nerve root contribution to both median and ulnar nerves. Median nerve innervated muscles such as the opponens pollicis, and lumbricalis-interossei on the radial side are supplied completely by the C8-T1 roots. The flexor pollicis longus and brevis as well as the abductor pollicis brevis derive substantial innervation from C8-T1 as does flexor digitorum profundus and sublimis.

Most of the ulnar innervated muscles derive their entire innervation from C8-T1. These include the flexor digitorum profundus (fingers 3 and 4), adductor pollicis, dorsal interossei, palmar interossei, and abductor digiti quinti. The motor innervation of the fifth finger; opponens digiti quinti and flexor digiti quinti is predominantly from inferior trunk of brachial plexus (C8-T1).

It is essential to evaluate the patient for the possibility of cervical disk or neuroforaminal disease, as well as for peripheral nerve entrapment. In this regard the motor and sensory examination augments the clinical history in establishing the diagnosis. Additionally the deep tendon reflexes have characteristic patterns in the different disorders.

These sensory and motor changes in neurogenic thoracic outlet compression explain the various complaints and disabilities described by patients in a variety of occupational and daily life situations. They also emphasize the necessity for differentiating compression of the inferior trunk of brachial plexus from isolated median nerve compression at the wrist and ulnar nerve compression at the cubital tunnel or Guyon's tunnel. In this regard the clinical evaluation is enhanced by careful electrophysiological assessment.

Particular care must be exercised in patients who may have the "double crush" syndrome of multiple sites of peripheral nerve compression. Compression at the thoracic outlet can often be seen concurrently with carpal tunnel syndrome and tardy ulnar palsy.[2]

Patients who fail to achieve symptomatic relief after median nerve decompression or ulnar nerve translocation often have an unrecognized site of brachial plexus compression at the thoracic outlet. The converse can also be seen with residual focal neuropathic symptoms after otherwise successful correction of thoracic outlet compression.

Electrophysiological Examination

When advanced, the neurogenic symptom complexes of the thoracic outlet syndrome can be associated with characteristic electrophysiological changes. At the outset it is important to recognize the limitations of electrophysiological evaluation. Pain and dysesthesias are the predominant early symptoms of patients presenting with brachial plexus compression at the thoracic outlet, particularly when these symptoms are positionally enhanced. This pain is considered to be mediated by the smaller myelinated or unmyelinated nerve fibers. The integrity or function of these fibers is not tested by the standard electrophysiological techniques. In advanced cases of brachial plexus compression (similar to the findings with carpal tunnel compression of the median nerve) where weakness and atrophy are evident on clinical examination there will generally be concomitant abnormalities on electromyography and nerve conduction studies.

A more sensitive method for determining abnormalities in these larger fibers would be by the use of electrical tests in the symptomatic positions. Although this is feasible for carpal tunnel compression of the median nerve the parameters have not been established for the brachial plexus. It is likewise important to recognize that there are substantial variations in normal nerve conduction that tend to limit sensitivity and specificity. Consequently, the electrophysiological findings must frequently be interpreted in light of the presenting signs and symptoms.

Nerve conduction, electromyography, and F-wave determinations are often normal in patients with neurogenic thoracic outlet compression. In more advanced stages of compression there may be evidence of denervation in the distribution of the inferior trunk of the brachial plexus. In these cases the ulnar nerve F-wave response may likewise be abnormal. A more sensitive evaluation of the brachial plexus may be accomplished by measuring somatosensory evoked responses for median and ulnar nerves in neutral and stress positions. In neurogenic thoracic outlet compression there may be a characteristic loss of amplitude at the brachial plexus (or Erb's point) potential. Occasionally there will be an increase in latency. These changes have been documented in the literature with pre- and postoperative studies.[3–5]

Radiological Studies

Chest and cervical spine x-rays are obtained regularly, particularly in patients in the third decade of life and older. Neither the computed tomographic (CT) nor magnetic resonance imaging (MRI) scan has demonstrated any particular usefulness in evaluating the thoracic outlet compression syndromes. Their current application is confined to research protocols. The three-dimensional MRI reconstructions, as done by Collins, appear to be the most promising of the new imaging studies. Helical CT has been applied to the study of the thoracic outlet area.[6]

Arteriography and venography are used in the particular settings where arterial insufficiency or venous obstruction are prominent components of the clinical picture. These tests should be performed with the arms in neutral position (at the sides) and again with the arm abducted (humerus at right angles to the chest). It has been demonstrated additionally that arteriography should be done in the erect position to be most useful in documenting positional, nonocclusive compression.[7]

Conservative Management

From the initial physiotherapy management program described by Peet at the Mayo Clinic, there have been additions and modifications.[13] In France, Aligne and Barral[8] reviewed the general principles of physical therapy as improving and strengthening the muscle groups which they consider "openers" of the thoracic outlet area. These are the middle and superior segments of the trapezius, the levator scapulae, and the sternocleidomastoid muscles. This is done concomitantly with relaxation of the muscle group called "closers" anterior and middle scalene, subclavius, pectoralis minor, and pectoralis major. They recognized that moderate to severe cases should be referred for surgical treatment but reported a 70% success rate with physical therapy when the following criteria were met:

(1) early entrance into the physical therapy program;
(2) absence of bony abnormalities;
(3) symptoms are neurological only, without vascular compromise;
(4) physical therapy is combined with exercises done at home.

They recognized poor outcomes in cases where there was antecedent cervical trauma, and with what they termed "moderate-to-average severity, combining vascular and neurological involvement."[8] These observations have been confirmed by others, and seem to hold true for cases treated surgically.[9,10]

References

1. Toomingas A, Hagberg M, Jorulf L, et al: Outcome of the abduction external rotation test among manual and office workers. *Am J Indust Med* 19:215–227, 1991.
2. Wood VE, Biondi J: Double-crush nerve compression in thoracic outlet syndrome. *J Bone Joint Surg* 72:85–87, 1990.
3. Siivola J, Sulg I, Pokela R: Somatosensory evoked responses as diagnostic aid in thoracic outlet syndrome. *Acta Chir Scand* 148:647–652, 1982.
4. Yiannikas C, Walsh JC: Somatosensory evoked responses in the diagnosis of thoracic outlet syndrome. *J Neurol Neurosurg Psychiatry* 46:234–240, 1983
5. Machleder HI, Moll F, Nuwer M, Jordan S: Somatosensory evoked potentials

in the assessment of thoracic outlet compression syndrome. *J Vasc Surg* 6: 177–184, 1987.

6. Matsumura JS, Rilling WS, Pearce WH, et al: Helical computed tomography of the normal thoracic outlet. *J Vasc Surg* 26:776–783, 1997.

7. Benzian SR, Mainzer F: Erect arteriography: Its use in the thoracic outlet syndrome. *Radiology* 111:275–277, 1974.

8. Aligne C, Barral X: Rehabilitation of patients with thoracic outlet syndrome. *Ann Vasc Surg* 6:381–384, 1992.

9. Green R, McNamara J, Ouriel K: Long-term follow-up after thoracic outlet decompression: An analysis of factors determining outcome. *J Vasc Surg* 14: 739–746, 1991.

10. Poole GV, Thomas KR: Thoracic outlet syndrome reconsidered. *Am Surg* 62: 287–291, 1996.

6

Electrodiagnostic Evaluation of Patients with Painful Syndromes Affecting the Upper Extremity

*Sheldon E. Jordan, MD and
Herbert I. Machleder, MD*

Based on observations from the history and physical examination alone, establishing a diagnosis of thoracic outlet syndrome may be difficult. In certain cases, the difficulty arises from the lack of objective findings with too much reliance placed on the patient's subjective reports and responses to bedside stress maneuvers. Even with objective findings, specificity may be limited; for example, normal individuals may show pulse changes or supraclavicular bruits with arm positioning maneuvers.[1–4] In addition, thoracic outlet syndrome is uncommon and must be differentiated from other, more common, causes of upper extremity pain and numbness including cervical radiculopathy, carpal tunnel syndrome, and ulnar compression neuropathy. To complicate matters even further, in cumulative trauma disorders, multiple sources of neurogenic and musculoskeletal pain coexist, which makes it difficult to sort out which problem needs the most aggressive management.

The role of electrophysiological testing is twofold: (1) to help confirm and objectify the diagnosis of thoracic outlet syndrome and (2) to exclude other neuropathic conditions that may occur in patients presenting with painful syndromes affecting the upper limb.

From Machleder HI, (ed): *Vascular Disorders of the Upper Extremity*. Third Revised Edition. Futura Publishing Company, Inc., Armonk, NY, © 1998.

General Considerations

Electrophysiological testing has its own limitations; the sensitivity is low for the majority of patients who present with a possible thoracic outlet syndrome. Pain in the upper limb is the complaint that most often brings the patient with thoracic outlet to the doctor; the pain is probably mediated by smaller myelinated or unmyelinated nerve fibers. However, standard electrophysiological techniques do not test integrity or function of these small nerve fibers. Abnormalities found with electromyography (EMG) and nerve conduction tests generally reflect damage to larger myelinated nerve fibers found in the more severe cases of thoracic outlet syndrome with patients exhibiting atrophy on bedside examination. In contrast, most patients do not have atrophic muscles and only develop weakness and sensory loss with certain stressful positions. Therefore, with the arms at rest, the typical patient with possible thoracic outlet syndrome will be expected to have normal EMG and nerve conduction tests.

It would seem that stress-positioning electrical tests would play a role in these patients. Stress positioning nerve conduction tests have been available for carpal tunnel syndrome[5,6] and ulnar compression neuropathy[7]; however, similar testing for motor pathways is not yet available for thoracic outlet syndrome. The stress position testing of sensory pathways is available for thoracic outlet syndrome patients using evoked potential techniques; this approach is reviewed in this book in Chapter 7.

Specificity is also limited with electrophysiological testing; potentially misleading information can be obtained with tests designed to detect median or ulnar compression neuropathies. For example, in asymptomatic normal individuals, there may be up to a 46% false-positive rate using standard electrodiagnostic test batteries for carpal tunnel syndrome.[8] The explanations for false-positives are partly statistical and partly biological. From a statistical view, assuming a normal distribution of test results, the expected false-positive rate for each variable may be a small percent; however, if multiple tests are performed in a given individual, the chances become much greater that at least one of the tests will be abnormal.[8] From a biological standpoint, it is possible that everyday wear and tear may be responsible for subclinical electrophysiological abnormalities in asymptomatic individuals. From a practical view, consider the example of a manual laborer who may demonstrate slowing of median conduction across the wrist without actually having a carpal tunnel syndrome; if surgery on his wrist had been based solely on electrophysiological criteria, then an optimal outcome would not have been expected if the actual cause of symptoms had been a more proximal compression. Note that "normal" laboratory values used to interpret median nerve and ulnar nerve conduction tests do not typically take the person's occupation into account. In comparison to the general population, manual laborers may, in fact, have slowed nerve conductions across the wrist or elbow due to habitual occupational trauma; this potentially important factor needs to be considered. In our experience, it is not unusual for a worker with symptoms of proximal brachial plexus compressions at the thoracic outlet to have had unsuccessful carpal tunnel release based on a median nerve conduction abnormality at the wrist.

The sensitivity of EMG and nerve conduction tests for cervical radiculopathy and peripheral entrapments is substantially less than perfect. Therefore, a negative test does not exclude whatever diagnosis may be otherwise considered on the basis of clinical data.

A standard admonition is to correlate the electrophysiological test results with the clinical examination; unfortunately, as in the case of thoracic outlet syndrome, the signs elicited at the bedside examination in patients with peripheral entrapment may, in some cases, be neither sensitive nor specific.[9,10]

Electromyography

Appreciation of the role of EMG in confirming a case of thoracic outlet syndrome depends on a general understanding of anatomy and pathophysiology of motor units. Each motor unit is made up of a single neuron, its branching axon, and all the scattered muscle fibers that it innervates within a given muscle (Figure 1). When a normal motor unit is activated, most or all of its muscle fibers become simultaneously excited, producing a summated electrical potential that can be detected by an electromyography electrode placed nearby. With slight voluntary muscular contraction, a few motor units are detected by the EMG electrode and subsequently displayed on the oscilloscope screen. With maximum voluntary effort, so many motor units are recruited that the potentials fill up the oscilloscope screen. With a normal muscle at rest, no motor unit potentials are detected.

After nerve injury, some axons may degenerate immediately; their muscle fibers will become orphans. The orphaned muscle fibers begin to atrophy; this can be detected clinically as gross muscle atrophy. The orphaned fibers spontaneously depolarize, producing the electrical signs of acute denervation, positive sharp waves, and fibrillation potentials detectable in muscles at rest (Figures 2 and 3). In the typical patient with chronic thoracic outlet, such electrical signs of acute denervation are rarely seen.[11,12]

Over the course of months, peripheral axon sprouts growing from nearby intact motor units will reinnervate some of the orphaned muscle fibers. The sprouts may conduct a motor impulse slowly and irregularly so that the newly reinnervated fibers are activated later and more asyn-

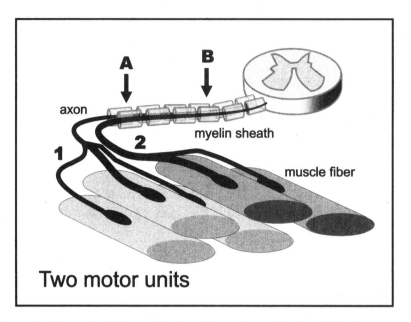

Figure 1. Two motor units number 1 and 2, are shown. Each unit includes a parent spinal motor neuron and its myelinated axon branching and innervating many muscle fibers. With standard nerve conduction studies recording electrodes are placed over a distal muscle in order to detect surface electrical activity generated by contracting muscle fibers. Nerve stimulation is applied to a distal location (site A) and then a more proximal site (site B).

chronously than other muscle fibers in the same motor unit. As a consequence of this, it will take a longer time period to activate all of the muscle fibers within the motor unit. Therefore, after reinnervation, motor units will demonstrate prolonged durations of their electrical potentials and the units may appear irregular in configuration (polyphasic) (Figures 4 and 5).

In patients with thoracic outlet syndrome, there may be chronic muscular atrophy; in these patients, careful electromyographic examinations may reveal excessively prolonged and polyphasic motor unit potentials characteristic of chronic denervation with subsequent reinnervation in the affected C8 and T1 myotomes.[11,12] The abductor pollicis, opponens pollicis, first dorsal interosseous, and abductor digiti minimi muscles would be key muscles to examine by EMG in order to localize the site of injury to the lower trunk of the brachial plexus. As expected, in patients without muscular atrophy of the intrinsic hand muscles, the EMG is characteristically normal.[11,13]

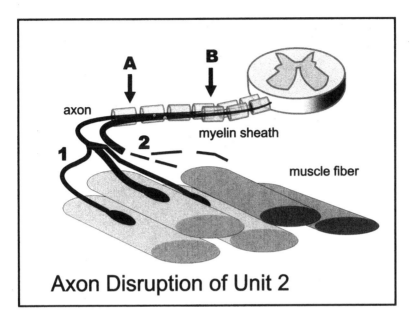

Figure 2. Motor unit 2 has been disrupted, its muscle fibers become orphans and begin to atrophy. Nerve stimulation at either site A or B will only excite the remaining motor unit 1.

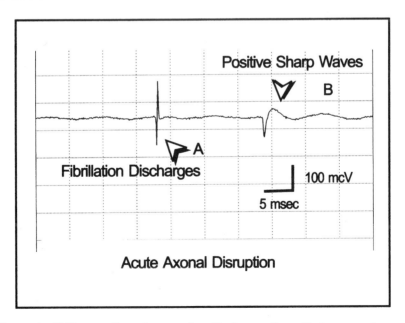

Figure 3. EMG recording of a muscle with denervation will show spontaneous discharges with the muscle at rest.

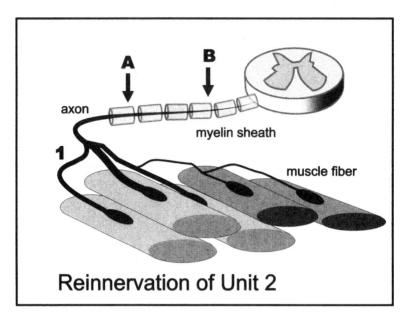

Figure 4. Orphan muscle fibers remaining from unit 2 have become reinnervated by peripheral axon sprouts from unit 1. Each time that unit 1 becomes activated, a larger number of motor units will be excited as compared with the initial state as seen in Figure 1.

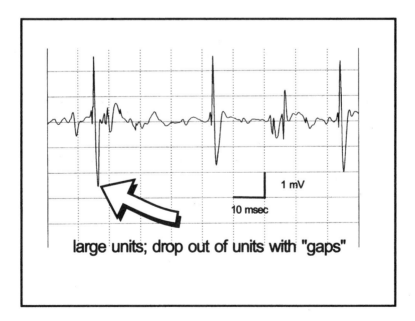

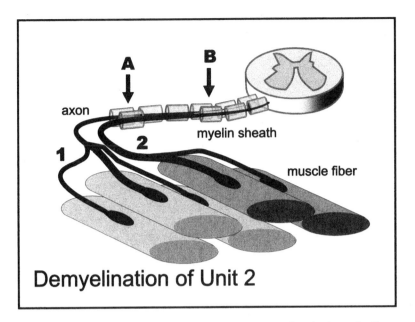

Demyelination of Unit 2

Figure 6. Unit 2 has a length of demyelinated axon; electrical conduction over this segment may result in complete failure (conduction block) or slowing of impulse transmission (conduction slowing).

Nerve Conduction Studies

The type of abnormality observed with nerve conduction testing would depend on whether the nerve is stimulated proximal or distal to a site of nerve compression and upon the severity of nerve injury. Fast nerve impulse conduction velocity from a proximal stimulus to a distal recording site depends largely on the health of nerve axons as well as on the integrity of their respective myelin sheaths. Damage to a myelin sheath due to a mild nerve compression injury produces either conduction slowing or complete conduction block of a nerve impulse traveling distally through a single nerve fiber (Figure 6).[14,15] If the myelin sheaths of many fibers are damaged in a given nerve, then many impulses become blocked

---

Figure 5. After reinnervation, motor units consist of a greater number of muscle fibers which tends to make EMG amplitudes larger than the normally expected 3–5 mV; durations tend to be longer than 10 to 15 ms and many polyphasic units are seen (normal units have three phases). Because fewer motor units are available for maximal voluntary contraction, large empty gaps between remaining units are seen during EMG recording.

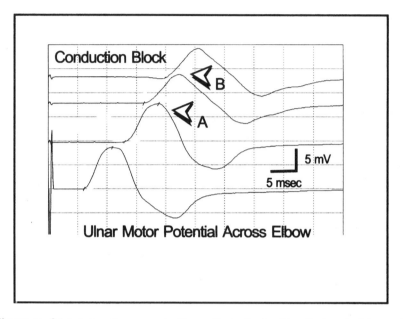

Figure 7. Stimulating the nerve in Figure 6 at site A will activate all of the units normally; however, when stimulating at a proximal site B, conduction block will occur for unit 2 so that a smaller compound motor potential is recorded from the muscle.

or slowed (Figures 7 and 8). As a consequence, stimulating a nerve proximal to a site of compression will produce less than the expected electrical potential recorded distally. The distal response may also be delayed. If only myelin is damaged, then all of the nerve fibers can be successfully stimulated distal to the site of injury. However, in severe nerve injury, some nerve fibers are completely disrupted and axon degeneration ensues. In the latter case, stimulating the nerve distal to the site of injury will produce a diminutive potential due to a reduced number of excitable nerve fibers (Figure 9).

Initially, it was thought that measuring nerve conduction velocity from Erb's point to the upper arm for the ulnar nerve would be an accurate test for Thoracic outlet syndrome.[16–18] The reliability and accuracy of these tests have been questioned.[19–21] There are many technical problems with this approach; most importantly, percutaneous stimulation at Erb's point often results in nerve activation distal to the actual site of anatomical compression. As noted in the discussion above, a proximal stimulation site would be needed in order to detect conduction block or conduction delay in milder cases of nerve compression. More recent techniques have been devised in order to stimulate proximally at the C8 or T1 roots[22];

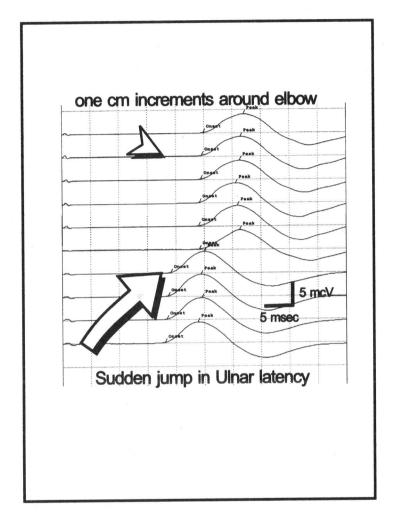

Figure 8. Conduction slowing can be demonstrated by performing an "inching technique." Stimulation is performed for the ulnar nerve at 1-cm increments around the elbow; when a segment with demyelination is under the stimulation site, there will be a sudden delay resulting in a step off of the sequential waveforms. See the potentials at and immediately above the arrow. Note that in this particular case, the amplitudes are relatively constant above and below the demyelinated segment, so that there is only conduction slowing without conduction block.

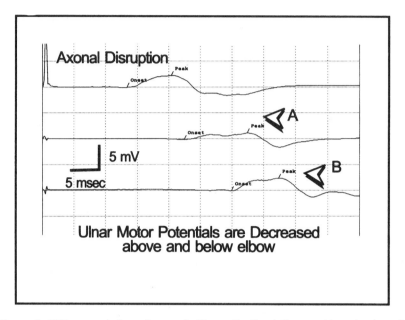

Figure 9. With axonal disruption, as in Figure 2, stimulating at either site A or site B will activate only unit 1 resulting in a constant low amplitude motor potential as seen in this figure.

however, it is not established whether these techniques will be more accurate in diagnosing thoracic outlet syndrome. In the occasional patient with severe neurogenic thoracic outlet syndrome, there may be sufficient axonal degeneration so that the sensory nerve action potential is reduced in size all along the course of the ulnar nerve. This type of abnormality can be detected with measurement of ulnar sensory nerve action potentials generated and recorded distally.[23] By contrast, median sensory fibers travel in the uppermost trunks of the brachial plexus and are not as commonly affected as the ulnar sensory fibers.[11]

F-Wave Studies

Percutaneous stimulation of the median or ulnar nerves at the wrist produces nerve action potentials that propagate in opposite directions, proximally and distally. The distally propagated nerve impulses ultimately excite the target muscles, thereby producing an observable twitch and an electrically recorded muscle action potential. The propagation of the nerve impulse in the proximal direction (retrograde or antidromic direction) ultimately reaches the motor neuron in the spinal cord. Some of the impulses will be reflected back down the axon in an orthodromic direction to produce secondary action potentials recorded from target muscles in the hand. This "reflected" potential is called an F-wave. For an F-wave to be elicited, there must be successful antidromic and orthodromic impulse propagation occurring in an individual axon; this necessarily requires propagation of the impulse across the root and proximal portions of the brachial plexus. Consequently, this technique could be used to test the proximal sites of compression as required in the diagnosis of thoracic outlet syndrome.

The standard technique is based on taking the shortest latency response observed after approximately 20 repetitions; this latency is then compared to the response from the contralateral limb or compared to responses from a reference population. Unfortunately, if even some of the nerve fibers are functioning normally, then a normal minimal F-wave latency will be recorded. Nevertheless, in some cases of thoracic outlet syndrome, a delayed F-wave latency may be determined (Figure 10).[13,24,27] Greater sensitivity may be obtained if additional F-wave parameters are measured, such as variability of latencies (chronodispersion) or average

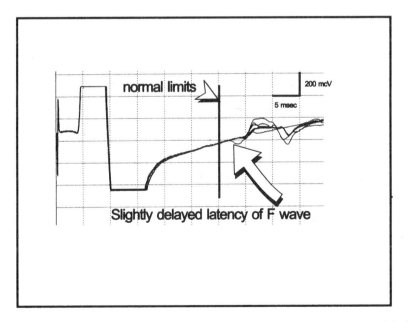

Figure 10. F waves vary with repeated trials. The shortest in 10 to 20 trials is taken as the reported value. In this patient with thoracic outlet syndrome, a slight slowing of latency is seen. Only 7 trials are shown in this partial sample, a total of 20 were taken to make sure that a spurious value was not obtained.

latency.[28] These latter parameters have not been thoroughly investigated in the setting of thoracic outlet syndrome.

Electrophysiologically Guided Anterior Scalene Blocks

Anterior scalene muscle injections are useful in confirming the diagnosis of thoracic outlet syndrome and in determining which patients may respond favorably to surgery. Routine techniques have relied on surface landmarks. Considering the wide variation in neck subcutaneous fat and muscle development, hypodermic needle placement is often uncertain so that inadvertent anesthesia of the brachial plexus or sympathetic ganglia may occur in up to 10% of attempts. With routine techniques, the interpretation of a negative test is uncertain because there is no confirmation of effective neuromuscular block of the anterior scalene muscle. Furthermore, in the interpretation of positive test results, the routine technique does not account for placebo effects, which may be high in patients with chronic pain syndromes. Recently developed methods of performing anterior scalene blocks utilize electromyographic recording and stimulation techniques that improve the accuracy of needle tip placement in performing anterior scalene blocks, thereby avoiding injury or inadvertent anesthesia of the brachial plexus or sympathetic ganglia. Furthermore, with the inclusion of control injections diagnostic accuracy is improved in what remains a test that relies on subjective responses. Similar electrophysiological techniques improved on the results of selective botulinum toxin injections into cervical muscles for the treatment of dystonia. In patients presenting with chronic neck and shoulder pain, overlapping problems may coexist, making it difficult to decide which treatment plan is most likely to result in a good outcome. Of all the electrophysiological tests and imaging tests discussed elsewhere in this book, a selective anterior scalene block may be in a unique position to serve as a dress rehearsal" for a more definitive surgical treatment. By temporarily relaxing the anterior scalene muscle, the block may partially simulate the results of surgical decompression and may afford the patient an opportunity to experience to what extent the overall pain syndrome may be relieved. In such a manner, anterior scalene blocks determine if temporary relief of symptoms after anterior scalene block predicts a good surgical outcome.

Before anterior scalene block, each patient should have a baseline examination, which includes an assessment of tenderness of the scalene muscles, and symptoms with elevated arm stress testing. Discomfort induced by stress maneuvers was rated according to a 101-point numerical scale. A Teflon-coated 25-gauge hypodermic needle, bared at the tip, is advanced in the sternocleidomastoid muscle, the patient would be asked if pain was produced and whether insertion at this depth reproduced pains that were similar in quality and location to the usual pains described historically (Figure 11). After a control injection of 2 cc of 2% lidocaine, the arm is placed into a stress position and exercised for 1 minute; the patient is again asked to rate the pain. The anterior scalene muscle was identified deep to the sternocleidomastoid muscle and could be activated with lateral neck bending against resistance and with deep inspiration. Final depth is adjusted with stimulation to make sure that the needle tip is not in the brachial plexus. Lidocaine in a total of 3 cc of volume is injected into the anterior scalene muscle. A positive test result is scored if the patient has greater than 50% improvement in the elevated arm stress test pain scores after anesthetic injection of the anterior scalene muscle as compared with the control injections.

In our experience with 122 patients with anterior scalene blocks, there were no complications and no instances of inadvertent somatic or sympathetic ganglionic blockade that could have interfered with the interpretation of the test results. Overall, 93 (72%) of these patients had a positive test. Twenty patients were ultimately diagnosed to have conditions other than thoracic outlet syndrome such as cervical myeloradiculopathy, peripheral compression neuropathy, and shoulder impingement. In the latter group, 1 patient (5%) had a positive block. Of patients with a clinical diagnosis of thoracic outlet syndrome, 92 out of 102 (90%) had a positive response to anterior scalene block.

In our experience, 32 of 38 patients (84%) had a positive response to anterior scalene block prior to thoracic outlet surgery. By comparison only 15 of 33 patients (45%) had an abnormal preoperative somatosensory evoked response consistent with a diagnosis of thoracic outlet syndrome; and 12 of 35 patients (38%) had an abnormal standard EMG and nerve conduction study of the upper limbs. Overall, 30 of the 38 patients had a good outcome (79%). Of patients with a positive anterior scalene block, surgery was successful in 30 of 32 cases (94%); in contrast, in patients with a negative block only 3 out of 6 (50%) had a good outcome.

In the performance of anterior scalene muscle blocks, electrophysiological guidance can improve the accuracy of needle tip placement, avoiding inadvertent brachial plexus blocks or sympathetic blocks, which could interfere with the interpretation of, test results. Test sensitivity compares favorably to other tests, which are often used to confirm a clinical diagnosis of thoracic outlet syndrome. In patients referred with a diagnosis of possible thoracic outlet syndrome, a negative anterior scalene block should make the examiner consider alternative diagnoses; most of the patients with a negative block in this study ultimately were diagnosed with a condition other then thoracic outlet syndrome such as cervical myeloradiculopathy. Furthermore, a positive anterior scalene block does predict a good outcome to surgical decompression.

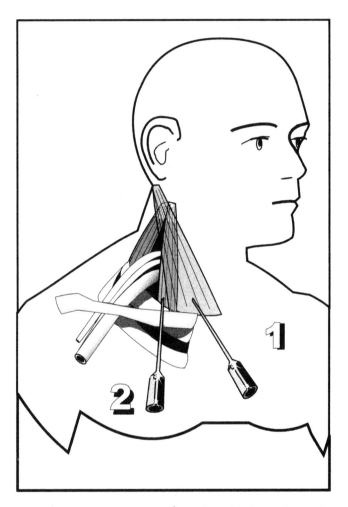

Figure 11. In performing electrophysiologically guided anterior scalene muscle blocks, a Teflon-coated hypodermic needle is placed first in the sterocleidomastoid (SCM) muscle as a control injection site 1. The anterior scalene muscle (ASM) at site 2 is found just behind the sternal portion of the SCM. EMG activation with lateral head tilt and deep inspiration helps identify the proper depth. Stimulation through the needle tip will often activate the phrenic nerve (hiccup motion), however, limb muscle twitch with 2 mA or less current would suggest a placement that is too close to the main portion of the brachial plexus.

Conclusions

A model basic electrophysiological protocol is listed in Table 1. The suggested battery of electrophysiological tests could be used to fulfill two roles: (1) to confirm the diagnosis of thoracic outlet syndrome and (2) to help discover other causes of limb pain and numbness, in particular, cervical radiculopathy and median or ulnar compression neuropathies. In both roles, test sensitivity and specificity can be problematic; however, if these limitations are kept in mind and the results are interpreted in light of clinical data, then these techniques can be helpful in diagnosing cases

---

Table 1
Electrophysiological Protocol for Thoracic Outlet Syndrome

  I. EMG
   A. Quantitative analysis of motor units in affected limbs with particular attention to abductor pollicis (median nerve, lower trunk) and abductor digiti minimi (ulnar nerve, lower trunk). Note amplitude, duration, polyphasics.[11]
   B. Include paraspinal muscle examination to evaluate possible radiculopathy.
 II. Sensory Nerve Conduction Studies
   A. Keep limb warm in order to avoid spurious latency prolongation.
   B. Median and ulnar nerves at wrist (orthodromic or antidromic technique).
     1. Median sensory conduction tests would help screen for carpal tunnel syndrome.[28]
     2. Watch for reduced amplitude of ulnar sensory potentials as a sign of thoracic outlet syndrome.[23]
   C. Add sensory conduction determination across wrist for median nerve if carpal tunnel syndrome is likely.
     1. Palmar sensory distal latency,[28] or
     2. "Inching" technique.[29,30]
III. Motor Nerve Conduction Studies
   A. Median motor conduction test
     1. Observe prolonged distal latency as a screening test for carpal tunnel syndrome.
     2. Add transcarpal motor conduction test if carpal tunnel syndrome is likely.[29,30]
   B. Ulnar motor conduction test must include segmental conduction velocity determination across elbow to evaluate possible ulnar entrapment neuropathy.
   A. Be cautious in the overinterpretation of minor abnormalities.
IV. F-Wave Tests
   A. Ulnar F-waves (median Fs may be added).
   B. At least 20 supramaximal stimulations.
   C. This test is uncomfortable for patients and should be done last and avoided if convincing results are obtained with previous tests.
 V. Somatosensory Evoked Potentials of Median and Ulnar Nerves With and Without Arm Hyperabduction

---

of thoracic outlet syndrome. Recently developed electrophysiologically guided anterior scalene blocks can be useful in confirming a diagnosis of thoracic outlet syndrome; this procedure compares favorably in terms of sensitivity and specificity with other tests. Furthermore, the anterior scalene muscle block potentially simulates the effects of thoracic outlet syndrome surgery that may be helpful in selecting patients for an operative approach.

References

1. Carroll RE, Hurst LC: The relationship of thoracic outlet syndrome and carpal tunnel syndrome. *Clin Orthop* 164:149–153, 1982.
2. Gergoudis R. Barnes RW: Thoracic outlet arterial compression: Prevalence in normal persons. *Angiology* 31:538–541, 1980.
3. Gilroy JS, Meyer JS: Compression of the subclavian artery as a cause of ischemic brachial neuropathy. *Brain* 86:733, 1963.
4. Wright IS: The neurovascular syndrome produced by hyperabduction of the arms. *Am Heart J* 29:1, 1945.
5. Schwartz MS, Gordon JA, Swash M: Slowed nerve conduction with wrist flexion in carpal tunnel syndrome. *Ann Neurol* 8:69, 1980.
6. Marin EL, Vernick S. Friedman LW: Carpal tunnel syndrome: Median nerve stress test. *Arch Phys Med Rehab* 64:206–208, 1983.
7. Fine EJ, Wongjirad C: The ulnar flexion maneuver. *Muscle Nerve* 8:612, 1985.
8. Redmond MD, Rivner MH: False positive electrodiagnostic tests in carpal tunnel syndrome. *Muscle Nerve* 11:511–517, 1988.
9. Stewart JD, Eisen A: Tinel's sign and the carpal tunnel syndrome. *Br Med J* 2: 1125, 1978.
10. Longstreth WT Jr Barnhart S. Rosenstock L: Reliability and validity of Tinel's and Phalen's signs in carpal tunnel syndrome. *Neurology* 37:291, 1987.
11. Smith T. Trojaborg W: The diagnosis of thoracic outlet syndrome: Value of sensory and motor conduction studies and quantitative electromvography. *Arch Neurol* 44:1161–1163, 1987.
12. Morales-Blanquez G. Delwaide PJ: The thoracic outlet syndrome: An electrophysiological study. *Electromyogr Clin Neurophysiol* 22:255–263, 1982.
13. Gilliatt RW: Thoracic outlet syndrome. In: Dyck PJ, Thomas PK, Lambert EH, Burge R, eds. *Peripheral Neuropathy*. Philadelphia, PA: WB Saunders Co; 1984, pp. 1409–1424.
14. Gilliatt RW: Acute compression block. In: Summer AJ, ed. *The Physiology of Peripheral Nerve Disease.*Philadelphia, PA: WB Saunders; 1980; pp. 287–339.
15. Gilliatt RW: Chronic nerve compression and entrapment. In: Summer AJ, ed. *The Physiology of Peripheral Nerve Disease*. Philadelphia, PA: WB Saunders; 1980; pp. 316–339.
16. Urshel HC, Razzuck MA: Management of the thoracic outlet syndrome. *N Engl J Med* 286:1140–1143, 1972.
17. Urshel HC, Razzuck MA: Objective diagnosis and current therapy of the thoracic outlet syndrome. *Ann Thorac Surg* 12:608–620, 1972.

18. Caldwell JW, Crane CR, Hrusen EM: Nerve conduction studies: An aid in the diagnosis of thoracic outlet syndrome. *South Med J* 64:210–212, 1971.
19. London GW: Normal uluar nerve conduction velocity across the thoracic outle\: Comparison of the measuring techniques. *J Neurol Neurosurg Psychiatry* 38: 756–760, 1975.
20. Cherington, M: Ulnar conduction velocity in thoracic outlet syndrome. *N Engl J Med* 294:1185, 1976.
21. Wilbourn AJ, Lederman RJ: Evidence for conduction delay in thoracic outlet syndrome is challenged. *N Engl J Med* 310:1052–1053, 1984.
22. Daube JR: Nerve conduction studies in the thoracic outlet syndrome. *Neurology* 25:347, 1975.
23. MacLean IC, Tavlor RS: Nerve root stimulation to evaluate brachial plexus conduction. Abstracts of Communications of the Fifth International Congress of Electromyography, Rochester, Minnesota, 1975, p. 47.
24. Gilliatt RW, Willison RG, Dietz V, et al: Peripheral nerve conduction in patients with a cervical rib and band. *Ann Neurol* 4:124–129, 1978.
25. Eisen A, Schomer D, Melmed C: The application of F-wave measurements in the differentiation of proximal and distal upper limb entrapment. *Neurology* 27:662–668, 1977.
26. Dorfmann LJ: F-wave latency in the cervical rib and band syndrome. *Muscle Nerve* ??:150, 1979.
27. Wulff CH, Gilliatt RW: F-waves in patients with hand wasting caused by a cervical rib and band. Muscle Nerve 2:452, 1979.
28. Fisher MA: F response latency determination. *Muscle Nerve* 5:730–734, 1982.
29. Stevens JC: The electrodiagnosis of carpal tunnel syndrome *Muscle Nerve* 10: 99–113, 1987.
30. Kimura J: The carpal tunnel syndrome: Localization of conduction abnormalities within the distal segment of the median nerve. *Brain* 102:619–635, 1979.
31. Kimura J: A method for determining median nerve conduction velocity across the carpal tunnel. *J Neurol Sci* 38:1–10, 1978.
32. Sanders RJ. *Thoracic Outlet Syndrome*. Philadelphia, PA: Lippincott, 1991.
33. Verdugo RJ, Ochoa JL. Use and Misuse of Conventional Electrodiagnosis, Quantitative Sensory Testing, Thermography, and Nerve Blocks in the Evaluation of Painful Neuropathic Syndromes. Muscle Nerve 16: 1056–1062, 1993
34. Comella CL, Buchman, AS, Tanner AS, et al. Botulinum toxin injection for spasmodic torticollis: increased magnitude of benefit with electromyographic assistance. Neurology 1992; 42: 878–882.

7

Somatosensory Evoked Potentials in the Assessment of Upper Extremity Neurovascular Compression

Marc R. Nuwer, MD, PhD

Evoked potentials (EPs) are electrical voltages, or potentials, that can be recorded after a brief stimulus. The stimuli may be auditory, visual, or sensory of a wide range of types. In fact, almost any very brief stimulus will cause a change in voltages over some portion of the nervous system. These EPs, ie, voltages evoked by some stimulus, can be used clinically to ascertain information about the function of the pathways involved. This information can help determine the anatomic site or category of pathology responsible for a patient's signs and symptoms.

EPs are very sensitive, objective, reproducible tools. They are sufficiently sensitive to show abnormalities even in the absence of signs and symptoms. Such a subclinical electrical abnormality is one of the key features of these tests, responsible for vaulting them into the mainstream of neurological testing. In general neurology, this ability to find subclinical abnormalities has been used especially in evaluation of patients who may have multiple sclerosis. In such an evaluation, EPs can sometimes find evidence of a second or third lesion, thereby helping to make the diagnosis of multiple sclerosis. EPs are objective because the results are independent

From Machleder HI, (ed): *Vascular Disorders of the Upper Extremity*. Third Revised Edition. Futura Publishing Company, Inc., Armonk, NY, © 1998.

of whether the subject is cooperating or not, or even whether the subject is awake or asleep. The potentials are reproducible and very similar results can be obtained in general even when retested after a 1-year interval.

The typical EP used for upper extremity evaluations begins with stimulation of the median nerve at the wrist. In some settings, additional information can be gained by stimulating the ulnar nerve at the wrists. The peaks occurring in the 30 ms after the stimulus are called median nerve and ulnar nerve short latency somatosensory EPS (SEPs).

Principal Peaks

Median and ulnar short-latency SEPs consist of several typical peaks generated at successively more rostral anatomic way stations along these pathways. Typical recordings are shown in Figure 1.

The brachial plexus gives cause a high-amplitude negative potential that is most easily recorded over the shoulder. The classic recording site is at Erb's point, which is found just above the clavicle and just lateral to the insertion of the sternocleidomastoid muscle. This peak is officially called N9, although it is often referred to as the Erb's point peak, the brachial plexus peak, or the peripheral peak. The exact location of this peak's generator is still somewhat unclear. It probably arises from within the brachial plexus. The axons responsible for this peak have a cell body at the dorsal horn nucleus, on the dorsal root of the spinal cord. As long as the pathway from the wrist to the cell body remains intact, this sensory pathway will continue to conduct in a relatively normal fashion. Thus, the Erb's point peak may persist even if the pathway is severed proximal to the dorsal horn nucleus. Motor axons can also contribute to the Erb's point peak. This occurs through antidromic conduction, in which an axon potential can travel backward up the arm along a motor pathway, all the way through the brachial plexus to the anterior horn cells. At that point, the antidromic motor conduction ceases because it cannot pass more rostrally in a wrong—way direction across a synapse. In the sensory pathways, the potentials can cross successive synapses in the normal physiological direction and can continue their conduction all the way to the cerebral cortex. The conduction occurs principally along the lemniscal system, the large-fiber sensory pathway usually most associated with vibration and joint-position sense. Notice that these pathways are distinct from the spinothalamic pathways that conduct pain and temperature sense. The latter pathways do not contribute in any substantial way to any of the ordinary EPS.

Several SEP peaks occur in the cervical region. These can be recorded from skin over the cervical spinal column. Several sets of nomenclature have been used, usually derived from the peak polarity and average la-

MEDIAN NERVE
SOMATOSENSORY EVOKED POTENTIAL

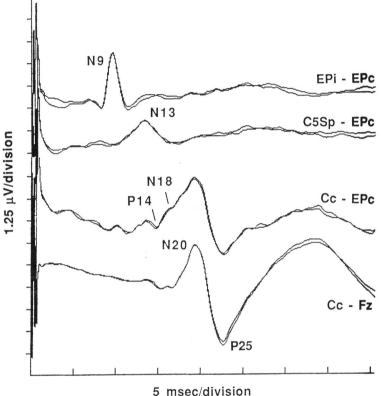

Figure 1. Example of an upper extremity somatosensory evoked potential (SEP). Stimulus was at the median nerve at the wrist. The channels, from top to bottom, record peripheral, cervical brain stem, and cortical activity. The N9 peak, in the top channel, represents conduction at the brachial plexus. EPi, EPc indicates Erb's point ipsilateral and contralateral, respectively; C5Sp, neck over the fifth cervical spine; Cc, scalp contralateral to the arm stimulated; Fz, frontal midline scalp. The several standard peaks are identified by name. (Reproduced with permission from Reference 1.)

tency. The most common type of nomenclature is used here. The three most prominent cervical peaks are referred to as N11, N13, and P14. The N11 peak is probably generated at the middle to lower cervical spinal cord, probably at the dorsal root entry zone. Traveling more rostrally, the N13 peak is generated around the foramen magnum level. It probably actually occurs in the rostral cervical spinal cord around the cuneate nucleus at the top of the posterior column. The third peak, P14, probably arises at a brain stem level, although the generator for this is still in dispute. A subsequent broad downgoing deflection in EP recordings probably represents conduction up the medial lemniscus in the brain stem.

At the scalp, several peaks can be seen around the contralateral primary somatosensory cortex. Sometimes the initial negative polarity peak at the scalp can be seen to break up into several subcomponents. This includes N18, a farfield component with broad representation over the scalp, and N20, a potential generated at the central fissure and identified by its reversal of electrical polarity at opposite sides of the central fissure region. Following this set of negative peaks, there is a broad positive polarity peak recorded from just behind the central scalp region.

By understanding the relations among the EPs, their physiological basis, and their anatomic generators, the clinician can learn to use the EPs to study the normal or pathological function along these sensory pathways. This can help localize a disruption along the peripheral, cervical cord, brain stem, internal capsule, or cortical levels of the pathway. The tests are complementary to electromyographic (EMG) tests, which evaluate motor pathways and distal sensory pathways. The tests are also complementary to the exquisite neuroimaging tests now available, such as magnetic resonance imaging (MRI), because the EPs tell about physiology rather than anatomy.

International standards for testing and peak identification are published in Nuwer et al.[1]

Techniques

Stimulation

The median nerve at the wrist is the site most frequently chosen for stimulation. That nerve serves a sensory function for the thumb and the two to three adjacent fingers. That sensory region is very generously represented on the cortical homunculus, corresponding to the importance of the thumb in human activities. Both the peripheral and central portions of this pathway reduce large, well-defined EPs. The ulnar nerve at the wrist serves sensory functions for the fourth and fifth fingers. Corresponding to the lesser importance of these fingers, the size of this nerve pathway and the EPs generated from this pathway are somewhat smaller than those from the median nerve. It should be noted that EPs can also be generated from other sites, such as the radial nerve at the wrist, the median or ulnar nerve at the elbow, or the sensory nerves along the fingers themselves.

Stimulus intensity is usually set to occur substantially above motor threshold for that individual patient. This is often in the range of 10 to 15 mA. This produces a very noticeable twitch of the muscles innervated by these nerves. For the median nerve, there is a movement of 1 to 2 cm when the stimulus is set appropriately. In that movement, the thumb is adducted. For the ulnar nerve stimulation, the fifth finger twitches in an abducted direction along with contraction of the hypothenar muscles.

Rate of stimulation is often limited by pain. Stimulation rates exceeding five per second often produce a moderately painful tightening or cramping of the muscles. It is important to reduce pain in this test because the patient must tolerate the test for substantial periods of time. Also, muscle artifact can substantially overwhelm the small EP signals themselves, therefore, a well-relaxed patient is very important to proper conduction of the test. Patients are often sedated because muscle tension is often decreased during sleep. A typical sedation is diazepam 10 mg orally.

Recording

Recording electrodes are usually placed at Erb's point on the shoulder, just above the clavicle and just lateral to the insertion of the sternocleidomastoid muscle. Cervical recording electrodes are placed on the skin overlying the cervical spinal column. Different investigators and clinical users have chosen different portions of the cervical spinal column to use for these recordings. This user chooses the skin over the seventh cervical spine for cervical recordings. The electrode for the contralateral scalp recording is placed on the scalp at a site overlying the hand region of the somatosensory cortex, determined by using the International 10- to 20-electrode system, at the site C3' which is 2 cm behind C3 (C4' is used on the right hemiscalp). A forehead reference electrode is used. Filters are set to 30 Hz and 3000 Hz, leaving the 60-Hz filter off.

General Clinical Uses

The peripheral Erb's point peak from the brachial plexus is a good indicator of peripheral nerve impairment. Peripheral neuropathies that disrupt myelin can slow conduction velocity and thereby delay the latency to the Erb's point peak. Neuropathies that impair axonal function without disrupting myelin are associated with decreased peripheral peak amplitude but relatively normal latency. Compression can result in a partial block of nerve function along a very brief stretch of the overall peripheral pathway. Such compression can cause a loss of amplitude from conduction block and loss of pathway fibers, but it does not usually result in a substantial increase in latency. The Erb's point peak is sensitive to disruptions occurring at any level of the pathway between the wrist and the dorsal horn nuclei of the spinal column. For the median nerve, common sites of impairment are the carpal tunnel and the spinal roots. For the ulnar nerve pathway, impairment can commonly occur at the cubital tunnel, thoracic outlet, or spinal roots. Usually radiculopathies at only one or two individual levels do not substantially alter the Erb's point SEP peaks. However, radiculopathies at multiple levels could result in alteration of that peak, and therefore should be included in the differential diagnosis of such changes.

Disorders of the cervical spinal cord can affect the conduction between the Erb's point peak and the N13 cervical peak. Patients with a cervical myelopathy or other damage to the cervical spinal cord will generally have a very normal Erb's point peak but an attenuated and delayed N13 cervical peak. This is most marked when the posterior columns are affected by the lesion. A small anterior cord lesion may fail to change somatosensory pathway function.

Lesions at the brain stem level can abolish the broad downgoing peak that follows the cervical peaks and can delay or abolish the recordings at the contralateral scalp. A brain stem lesion should spare the Erb's point and cervical N13 peak. A lesion at the internal capsule or somatosensory cortex itself, such as a stroke, will usually spare all the potentials up through the early farfield N18 recording from the contralateral scalp, but will abolish the subsequent EP activity in that channel.

As a result, the EPs can be used to anatomically determine the level of a lesion in the sensory pathway. The general level of impairment can be deduced to be at a peripheral, cervical, brain stem, or hemispheric level. Separate testing of median and ulnar nerve pathways can also help define impairments differentially affecting the peripheral course of those two nerve pathways. Changes in the latencies of peaks have a different meaning from changes in amplitude of the EPs, indicating a demyelinating rather than an axonal or compressive lesion.

Clinical settings for use of these potentials include a variety of disorders. One can use EPs to establish that there is an objective abnormality in a patient in whom no other test has provided such objective evidence. In multiple sclerosis, one could search for evidence of a second or third central nervous system lesion. In possible hereditary-degenerative neurological disorders, such as Friedreich's ataxia, diffuse bilateral slowing can occur. In coma, the sensory pathways can still be evaluated and evidence of serious cortical impairment can be discovered even in the presence of large doses of sedating drugs. There is an extensive literature on these various topics. In this chapter, only a superficial overview of these general applications can be provided, and the reader is referred to other works for a much more detailed review of outpatient and inpatient uses of SEPs. For example, there is an excellent review of this topic in *Evoked Potentials in Clinical Medicine* by Chiappa.[2] Uses of EPs in the operating room are reviewed in the book *Evoked Potential Monitoring in the Operating Room,* by Nuwer.[3]

Evoked Potentials in Thoracic Outlet Compression

The combined use of median and ulnar nerve SEPs is useful in the search for evidence of compression of the brachial plexus at the thoracic outlet. Such compression usually produces impairment primarily of the ulnar pathway with relative sparing of the median nerve pathway. This occurs because of the tendency for thoracic outlet compression to occur with a bony or fibrous band lifting the plexus from below, causing primarily a lower plexus impairment. The ulnar nerve pathway travels through this lower plexus, whereas the median nerve pathway does not. The effect of such compression is to cause a loss of amplitude of the Erb's point peak (N9) for the ulnar nerve.

Thoracic outlet compression of the brachial plexus can be worsened by placing the arm above the head and rotating the head. Such repositioning of the arm during SEP testing can be helpful because additional compression can cause worsening of the EPs. The loss of nerve function occurs within minutes of such repositioning in some patients. Repositioning can cause small changes in N9 latency and amplitude even among normal controls.[4,5] This needs to be taken into account when judging changes after repositioning.[6]

Other types of peripheral impairment should also be considered in the differential diagnosis of a thoracic outlet compression. Some of these do result in EP changes themselves. Compression of the ulnar nerve at the elbow can result in EP changes that mimic those described above. A principal way to differentiate ulnar pathway involvement at the two sites is through nerve conduction testing across the elbow. Demonstration of normal ulnar pathway conduction at the elbow in the setting of substantial impairment at the Erb's point peak would suggest a compression at the thoracic outlet. Another possibility is multiple radiculopathies at the lower cervical level. Radiographic or neuroimaging tests would be the principal way to evaluate for radiculopathies when the electrophysiological tests are already abnormal.

In patients with proven thoracic outlet compression, approximately 50% to 70% show SEP abnormalities.[6-16] The abnormalities are seen primarily for ulnar pathway testing (Figures 2 and 3). The most common changes are loss of amplitude of the Erb's point potential, accompanied also in some cases by diminished amplitude of the N13 cervical potential and occasionally also a delay in the latencies to the N13 peak.[17]

Abnormalities in these SEPs are more common in patients who also have abnormalities in the neurological physical examination and in EMG, nerve conduction, and F-wave testing.[11,18] Typical neurogenic thoracic outlet syndrome (TOS) signs include diminished pin and temperature sensation in a C8 distribution along with hand muscle atrophy and weakness. Patients may have an abnormal EMG showing neuropathic changes in intrinsic hand muscles. The fifth digit sensory nerve action potential (SNAP) may be diminished in amplitude.[19] Nerve conduction latencies are typically normal.[18,20-22] In such patients, ulnar SEPs are almost always abnormal because of a small or absent N9 peak.

In patients without signs of neurogenic TOS, SEP abnormalities are considerably less likely. Yiannikas[12] compared neurogenic TOS to TOS with only vascular signs (vasogenic) and to TOS patients who only had symptoms without signs. Those symptoms were of pain and hypoesthesia or dysesthesia. The latter group he termed symptomatic. He found that 15 of 15 (100%) of his neurogenic group has ulnar SEP N9 abnormalities. Of his symptomatic group, 7 of 33 (21%) had such SEP abnormalities. Of his vasogenic group, 6 of 17 (35%) had such SEP abnormalities. Among the neurogenic group, he also noted that 3 of 15 had normal EMG/nerve conduction velocity (NCV) testing. This demonstrated that SEP is sometimes abnormal, localizing, and confirmatory even when EMG/NCV is not helpful. This isan empirical answer to others who have asserted that SEP is always simply redundant with EMG/NCV testing.[18,23] It also answers the sometimes held belief that neurogenic TOS is rare.[24] These findings are consistent with reported normal SEPs in symptomatic or vasogenic types of TOS patients reported by others.[23,25] This breakdown also substantiates the various reports of abnormal ulnar SEPs in neurogenic TOS and recommendations for their clinical use.[7-9,13,14,16,22,26,27]

Occasionally other diagnoses are uncovered when using neurodiagnostic testing to evaluate a possible TOS patient. This ability of testing to find patients with other causes of their complaints is cited by some authors as reason to perform testing, either for EMG/NCV[28] or for SEPs.

Some patients with central nervous system problems have been diagnosed after SEP testing even when their presenting complaints favored a peripheral course of their problem.[29-31]

Some authors have tried to determine which type of testing becomes abnormal earliest in the average neurogenic patient. EMG/NCV testing has some advocates.[20,22] One set of investigations also proposed that the medial antebrachial cutaneous nerve was effected first in lower brachial plexopathies or TOS.[32]

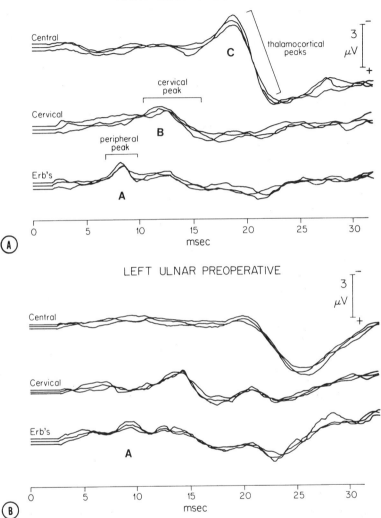

RIGHT ULNAR PREOPERATIVE

Central

thalamocortical
peaks

C

3
μV

cervical
peak

Cervical

B

peripheral
peak

Erb's

A

0 5 10 15 20 25 30
msec

(A)

LEFT ULNAR PREOPERATIVE

3
μV

Central

Cervical

Erb's

A

0 5 10 15 20 25 30
msec

(B)

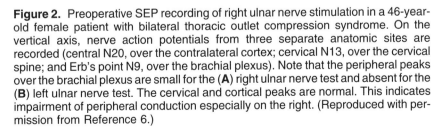

Figure 2. Preoperative SEP recording of right ulnar nerve stimulation in a 46-year-old female patient with bilateral thoracic outlet compression syndrome. On the vertical axis, nerve action potentials from three separate anatomic sites are recorded (central N20, over the contralateral cortex; cervical N13, over the cervical spine; and Erb's point N9, over the brachial plexus). Note that the peripheral peaks over the brachial plexus are small for the (**A**) right ulnar nerve test and absent for the (**B**) left ulnar nerve test. The cervical and cortical peaks are normal. This indicates impairment of peripheral conduction especially on the right. (Reproduced with permission from Reference 6.)

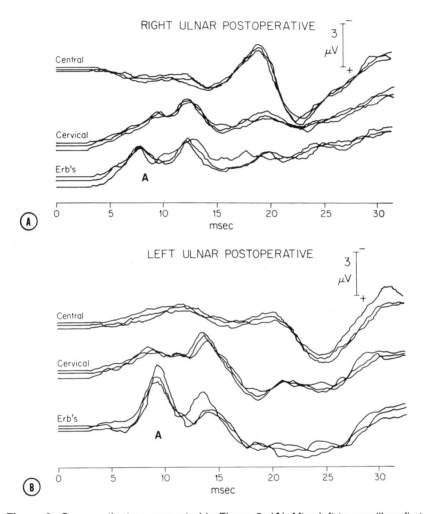

Figure 3. Same patient as presented in Figure 2. (**A**) After left transaxillary first rib resection, repeat SEP recordings show no significant change in amplitude on the unoperated (right) side. (**B**) Repeat recording of left ulnar SEP after left transaxillary first rib resection. Note improvement in the brachial plexus action potential peak at Erb's point "A". This amplitude is now normal and reflects improved nerve conduction through the brachial plexus, coincident with relief of radicular neuropathic symptoms. Compression of the inferior trunk of the brachial plexus was evident intraoperatively. (Reproduced with permission from Reference 6.)

Amplitudes are the criteria generally used in this setting. Latencies have failed to show clinical usefulness in TOS patients.[21] This is similar to the findings of decreased amplitude of distal SNAPs at the fifth digit, without conduction velocity change.[19]

A confounding factor is the variability in amplitude of all EPs between individuals. This makes it difficult to use absolute amplitude as a criterion for abnormality. The solution to this problem lies in using ratios of amplitudes within individual patients or subjects. Indeed, this approach has been taken by several of the investigative teams reporting on results in this field. In general, the ratios or comparisons used are between the left side and the right side or between the median nerve and the ulnar nerve. Another approach has been to compare peak amplitude with the arm in a neutral position along the patient's side, to the peak amplitude with the arm in a stressed position with the hand positioned above the head. The latter position tends to exacerbate the compression at the thoracic outlet and this exacerbation can be measured as a reduction in EPs in that position compared to the neutral position. Such changes in arm position may also cause some mild changes in peak latencies[4] and care must be taken not to allow the electrodes to move when the arm is repositioned. This can be a problem in patients who are obese or in patients whose skin is particularly loose, because of electrode movement or the interposition of further electrically insulating fatty tissue when the arm is placed in the stressed position. Care must also be taken to ensure that the stimulator continues to cause the same degree of thumb or fifth finger movement once the arm has been repositioned. The effect of such additional compression at the thoracic outlet may cause changes because of direct mechanical effects or because of compression of the vasa nervorum or because of ischemia to the limb from arterial compression. Limb ischemia itself can affect EPs.[33]

Several groups have evaluated the relative amplitude ratios of the SEP Erb's point peaks. The left-right asymmetry is the one most often used. For the median nerve, the limit of normal has been found to be 49%,[12] 54%,[11] 51%,[8] and 50%[6]; for the ulnar nerve it has been found to 48%,[12] 51%,[8] and 50%.[6] However, in patients with bilateral impairment, such left-right differences may not show a ratio beyond the 50% limit. In those cases, other criteria may be more useful.

The normal limit of the ratio between the peripheral peak amplitudes for the two nerves has been assessed as ulnar/median of 30%, with values lower than that implying an abnormally low ulnar amplitude. While other groups have not looked at this ratio per se, they have reported on other related amplitude data. Jerrett et al[9] considered their lower limits of absolute peripheral peak amplitude to be 2.1 μV for median and 1.4 μV for ulnar nerve. Yiannikas[12] described the average amplitude of the normal peripheral peaks to be 5.4 μV for median nerve and 2.9 μV for ulnar nerve.

It seems that the ulnar nerve peripheral peak is often only about two-thirds the height of the corresponding median nerve peak. The limit of normal of 30% ulnar/median would reflect a drop of one-half from the usual average. Reasons for the lower amplitude of ulnar peripheral peaks include a deeper location and a smaller size of that nerve compared to the median.

The effect of arm position on interpretation of clinical SEPs has only been assessed in one study. In that report, Machleder et al[6] found that commonly, the peripheral peak amplitude could change 20% to 30% with a change in position from neutral to an abducted, externally rotated (AER) stressed position. The limit of such normal variability appeared to be about 50%. A decrease of more than 50% was considered suggestive of compression. With thoracic outlet compression, such a change in position often completely abolished the peripheral peak despite no change in the stimulus or its associated abducting twitch of the fifth digit. This is not unexpected, especially when the fourth and fifth fingers became numb subjectively in that position.

Other criteria have also been applied. F-wave testing has been found useful by Jerrett et al[9] and this test is described by Jordan and Machleder in Chapter 6 of this book. An increase in the N9–N13 interpeak interval was also used by Jerrett et al.[9] Decreased amplitude of N13 has also been seen in some cases.[6,11]

Several studies have compared SEP results with surgical results from scalenectomy or rib resection. Most patients with abnormal preoperative EPs have symptomatic improvement postoperatively.[6–8,14] Postoperative improvement in symptoms was somewhat less common in patients who had normal EPs preoperatively. Interestingly, in one study, some patients who had normal preoperative EPs showed good improvement in symptoms postoperatively; in these cases, vascular compression may have been relatively more important than nervous system compression preoperatively.[6]

EP abnormalities tend to improve postoperatively. Indeed, Machleder and colleagues found a return to normal EPs in 95% of patients who had abnormal preoperative EPs and who had good or excellent postoperative relief of symptoms. Even in some patients who had normal preoperative EPs, a good or excellent postoperative improvement in symptoms sometimes corresponded with an increase in EP amplitudes over and above the previous normal amplitudes. Glover,[7] also found a postoperative return to normal in seven of their eight patients (88%) in whom both preoperative and postoperative EPs were recorded.

Case Discussion

A 28-year-old left-handed female nurse injured her left shoulder lifting a patient. She was seen by numerous physicians because of continuing

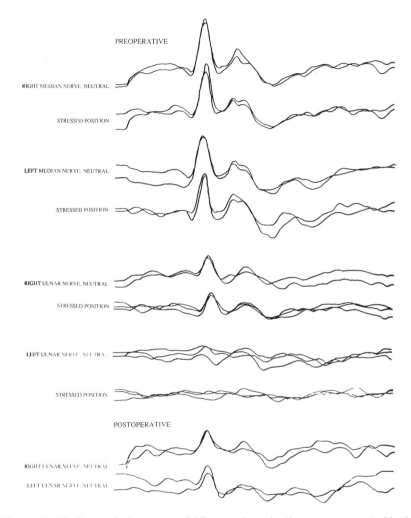

PREOPERATIVE

RIGHT MEDIAN NERVE, NEUTRAL

STRESSED POSITION

LEFT MEDIAN NERVE, NEUTRAL

STRESSED POSITION

RIGHT ULNAR NERVE, NEUTRAL

STRESSED POSITION

LEFT ULNAR NERVE, NEUTRAL

STRESSED POSITION

POSTOPERATIVE

RIGHT ULNAR NERVE, NEUTRAL

LEFT ULNAR NERVE, NEUTRAL

Figure 4. Median and ulnar nerve SEP recordings for the case presented in the text. Only the Erb's point (peripheral) channels are shown here. The recordings were made preoperatively except for the bottom two recordings, which were made postoperatively. The median nerve and the right ulnar nerve recordings were normal. The left ulnar peripheral peak was low amplitude preoperatively, and disappeared when the arm was placed into an overhead AER stressed position. Postoperatively, the left ulnar recordings had returned to normal, coincident with improvement in symptoms.

musculoskeletal discomfort, including a cramping myalgic discomfort radiating down the inner left arm with heaviness, weakness, and easy tiring, especially when the arms were outstretched or overhead. She also suffered from migraine headaches.

Routine physical examination was normal for power, reflex sensation, and range of motion while she sat in a neutral position. The Adson and similar maneuvers on the left reproduced her discomfort, heaviness, and tiredness, with a modest reduction of the palpated left radial pulse. Careful EMG examination and nerve conduction testing were entirely normal.

Cervical computed axial tomography (CAT) and x-rays were unremarkable, as well as the remainder of a general medical evaluation. Vascular testing did not confirm significant vascular compression. Conservative therapy included rest; nonsteroidal anti-inflammatory and muscle relaxant medications; cortisone injections and pulse high-dose oral steroids; physical therapy including traction, hot packs, ultrasound, and massage; transcutaneous electrical nerve stimulation (TENS); and a cervical collar and pillow.

Over a year, the patient's symptoms fluctuated in intensity without ever being resolved. She was unable to carry on with her normal nursing duties because they caused her symptoms to worsen.

SEPs were done, which showed an abnormally small peripheral potential for the left ulnar nerve testing, which was abolished with the arm in an overhead AER stressed position (Figure 4). This maneuver also resulted in a drop in amplitude of even the cervical and thalamocortical peaks. In contrast, the right-sided tests, the left median tests, and all the cervical spine, and the other thalamocortical peaks were normal in each position. The impression was of a myofascial pain syndrome and a left thoracic outlet level compression of the lower brachial plexus. The patient underwent a partial resection of the left first rib and a left anterior scalenectomy. Postoperatively, she continued to receive physical therapy, medications, and limitations on physical activity. Repeated SEPs demonstrated a return to normal of the left ulnar nerve test.

At 2-year follow-up, the patient had successfully returned to full-time employment and had been free of the ulnar pathway discomfort, weakness, and tiredness. Some should tenderness persisted, as did her migraine headaches.

References

1. Nuwer MR, Aminoff M, Desmedt J, et al: IFCN recommended standards for short latency somatosensory evoked potentials. *Electroencephalogr Clin Neurophysiol* 91:6–11, 1994.
2. Chiappa KH: *Evoked Potentials in Clinical Medicine.* Second Edition. New York: Raven Press; 1983.

3. Nuwer MR: *Evoked Potential Monitoring in the Operating Room*. New York: Raven Press; 1986.

4. Desmedt JE, Huy NT, Carmeliet J: Unexpected latency shifts of the stationary P9 somatosensory evoked potential far field with changes in shoulder position. *Electroenceph Clin Neurophysiol* 56:628–634, 1983.

5. Kameyama S, Yamada T, Matsuoka H, et al: Stationary potentials after median nerve stimulation: Changes with arm position. *Electroencephalogr Clin Neurophysiol* 71:348–356., 1988

6. Machleder HI, Moll F, Nuwer MR, et al: Somatosensory evoked potentials in the assessment of thoracic outlet compression syndrome. *J Vasc Surg* 6: 177–184, 1987.

7. Glover JL, Worth RM, Bendick PJ, et al: Evoked responses in the diagnosis of thoracic outlet syndrome. *Surgery* 89:86–93, 1981.

8. Siivola J, Sulg I, Pokela R: Somatosensory evoked responses as a diagnostic aid in thoracic outlet syndrome. *Acta Chir Scand* 148:647–652, 1982.

9. Jerrett SA, Cuzzone LJ, Pasternak BM: Thoracic outlet syndrome. *Arch Neurol* 41:960–963, 1984.

10. Hussein EA, El-Tayeb M: Transaxillary first rib resection for thoracic outlet syndrome: Follow-up of 9 cases. *Int Angiol* 14:404–409, 1995.

11. Yiannikas C, Walsh JC: Somatosensory evoked responses in the diagnosis of thoracic outlet syndrome. *J Neurol Neurosurg Psychiatry* 46:234–240, 1983.

12. Yiannikas C: Short-latency somatosensory evoked potentials in peripheral nerve lesions, plexopathies, radiculopathies and spinal cord trauma. In: Chiappa (ed): *Evoked Potentials in Clinical Medicine*. Second Edition. New York: Raven Press; 1990, pp. 439–468.

13. Synek VM: Diagnostic importance of somatosensory evoked potentials in the diagnosis of thoracic outlet syndrome. *Clin Electroencephalogr* 17:112–116, 1986.

14. Lai DT, Walsh J, Harris JP, et al: Predicting outcomes in thoracic outlet syndrome. *Med J Aust* 162:345–347, 1995.

15. Kunkel JM, Machleder HI: Treatment of Paget-Schroetter syndrome: A staged, multidisciplinary approach. *Arch Surg* 124:1153–1158, 1989.

16. Baran EM, Hunter J, Whitenack S, et al: Somatosensory evoked potential abnormalities in thoracic outlet syndrome. *Muscle Nerve* 13:859–860, 1990.

17. Chodoroff G, Lee DW, Honet JC: Dynamic approach in the diagnosis of thoracic outlet syndrome using somatosensory evoked responses. *Arch Phys Med Rehabil* 66:3–5, 1985.

18. Aminoff MJ, Olney RK, Parry GJ, et al: Somatosensory evoked potentials in suspected brachial plexopathy. *J Clin Neurophysiol* 4:216, 1987.

19. Smith T, Trojaborg W: Diagnosis of thoracic outlet syndrome: Value of sensory and motor conduction studies and quantitative electromyography. *Arch Neurol* 44:1161–1163, 1987

20. Simpson DM, Tagliati M: Pseudoneurogenic thoracic outlet syndrome (a reply). *Muscle Nerve* 17:1232, 1994.

21. Komanetsky RM, Novak CB, Mackinnon SE, et al: Somatosensory evoked potentials fail to diagnose thoracic outlet syndrome. J Hand Surg 21:662–666, 1996.

22. Passero S, Paradiso C, Giannini F, et al: Diagnosis of thoracic outlet syndrome:

Relative value of electrophysiological studies. *Acta Neurol Scand* 90:179–185, 1994.

23. Veilleux M, Stevens JC, Campbell JK: Somatosensory evoked potentials: Lack of value for diagnosis of thoracic outlet syndrome. *Muscle Nerve* 11:571–575, 1988.
24. Cherington M: A conservative point of view of the thoracic outlet syndrome. *Am J Surg* 158:394–395, 1989.
25. Newmark J, Levy SR, Hochberg FH: Somatosensory evoked potentials in thoracic outlet syndrome. *Arch Neurol* 42:1036, 1985.
26. Ozaki I, Baba M, Ogawa M, et al: Pseudoneurogenic thoracic outlet syndrome. *Muscle Nerve* 17:1231, 1994.
27. Huffman JD: Electrodiagnostic techniques for and conservative treatment of thoracic outlet syndrome. *Clin Orthop* 207:21–23, 1986.
28. Cherington M: Thoracic outlet syndrome: Reply from the author. *Neurology* 43:1270–1271, 1993.
29. Youl BD, Adams RW, Lance JW: Parietal sensory loss simulating a peripheral lesion, documented by somatosensory evoked potentials. *Neurology* 41: 152–154, 1991.
30. Simpson DM: Pseudoneurogenic thoracic outlet syndrome. *Muscle Nerve* 17: 242–244, 1994.
31. Wilbourn AJ, Porter JM: Thoracic outlet syndrome. In: Weiner MA, ed. *Spine: State of the Art Reviews*. Philadelphia, PA: Hanley and Belfus; 1988, pp. 597–626.
32. Nishida T, Price SJ, Minieka MM: Medical antebrachial cutaneous nerve conduction in true neurogenic thoracic outlet syndrome. *Electromyogr Clin Neurophysiol* 33:285–288, 1993.
33. Yamada T, Muroga T, Kimura J: Tourniquet-induced ischemia and somatosensory evoked potentials. *Electroencephalogr Clin Neurophysiol* 31:1524–1529, 1981.

8

Evaluation and Treatment of Repetitive Motion Disorders of the Upper Extremity in Office Workers and Musicians

Emil F. Pascarelli, MD

Repetitive motion disorders of the upper extremity is one of many terms used describe work-related soft tissue injuries.[1] Other names commonly used include repetitive strain injury (RSI),[2] cervicobrachial disorders, upper extremity musculoskeletal disorders (UEMSD), and occupational overuse syndrome (OOS). Cumulative trauma disorder (CTD) is often used by the scientific community.[3] Carpal tunnel syndrome is an inappropriate synonym, because it is actually one of many injuries that may be part of the total clinical picture.

Cumulative trauma is now the most common work-related illness in the United States, at least 5% of which occur in data entry jobs where there has been rapid computerization of the work force.[4] Controversy continues regarding the causal relation to work and other activities, as well as the pathophysiology of this disorder.[5] Evaluation and treatment of CTD does not come easily because it requires the fusing of knowledge from a number of disciplines including internal medicine, psychiatry, neu-

From Machleder HI, (ed): *Vascular Disorders of the Upper Extremity*. Third Revised Edition. Futura Publishing Company, Inc., Armonk, NY, © 1998.

rology, rheumatology, physical medicine, pain management, occupational medicine, public health, orthopedics, hand surgery, sports medicine, ergonomics, biomechanics, and physical and occupational therapy as well as a number of alternative disciplines. A detailed clinical examination combining these elements is necessary to evaluate the protean manifestations of this illness. Observers have noted that a basic present day problem is the reduction of direct physical involvement by the physician with the patient. This has led to an over-reliance on tests and a departure from what anthropologists call "local knowledge," which is wisdom accumulated over years of experience.[6] The intense and narrow focus on technical solutions to specific problems, does not serve the CTD patient well.

Therefore, evaluation should be based on the traditional medical approach: a complete history; a focused physical examination; appropriate laboratory and other tests; and an ergonomic assessment. The role of psychosocial factors and work environment should also be carefully weighed as contributing to symptoms and considered in the treatment plan.

This chapter focuses primarily on the work-related illness of office workers, about 50% of whom use computers and other input devices and many of whom work long hours for months or years, under adverse conditions as a prelude to their injury.[4] Another group to which this discussion applies is musicians, who injure themselves from a combination of incessant practicing, poor technique, poor physical condition, ill-fitting instruments, and demanding work schedules.[7] If left untreated or poorly treated, CTD can evolve into complex and painful neuromuscular illnesses of the upper body involving muscles, tendons, ligaments, connective tissue, nerves, and blood vessels resulting in partial or total disability.

History

Evaluation begins with a well-documented history. It is helpful to have patients fill out questionnaires and pain pictograms before their examination to serve as an adjunct to the oral history (Figure 1). The examiner will need to know the alleged origins of the problem, working conditions, hours of work, type of work, psychosocial factors, and past medical history including the presence of eyesight deficiencies, sleep, eating, exercise habits, and the use of medications. With computer users, information is needed about keyboard use, input devices, seating, monitor placement, and environmental factors such as lighting, ventilation, and crowding. Attention should also focus on activities of daily living that might contribute to the injury, especially those involving repetitive movement.[2] Photographs or a videotape of the actual work station can be very useful.[8]

Musicians need to discuss their practice habits, the instruments they use, lifestyle, exercise, past medical history, and other activities. Music students might also be avid computer users.

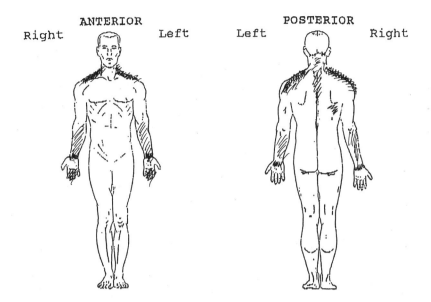

Figure 1. Pain pictograms filled out by the patient are a useful adjunct to the clinical diagnosis.

Physical Examination

The physical examination protocol we use is derived from a variety of specialties. The objective of the examination is to provide as accurate a set of clinical diagnoses as possible, supplemented by information gathered from specific tests, where indicated. Physical evaluation begins with vital signs followed by examination of the hands for finger length (Figure 2), swelling, tenderness, tremor, skin color and condition, temperature changes, and contraction of intrinsic muscles (Figure 3), Dupuytren's contracture,[9] ganglion cysts, functional anomalies such as Linburg's tendon[10] and trigger finger,[11] joint range of motion including hyperlaxity,[8] arthritic changes, and evidence of tendonitis including de Quervain's disease.[12] Loss of hand or arm function associated with pain, hyperesthesia, swelling, sweating and color or temperature changes should alert the clinician to the presence of reflex sympathetic dystrophy that may be caused by banal trauma, tight splints or casts, or brachial plexopathy associated with CTD.[13,14] This condition should be recognized early and treated without delay.

Wrist evaluation should focus on passive range of motion in flexion, dorsiflexion, radial, and ulnar deviation. Loss of range of motion and the physical characteristics of this loss during range of motion testing, sug-

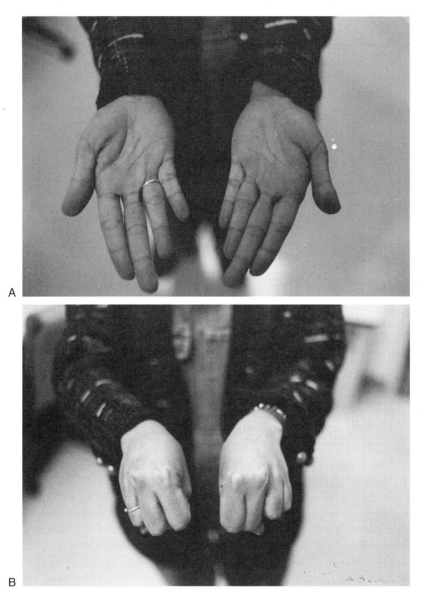

Figure 2A and 2B. Flutist with diminshed finger length due to shortened metacar-pals causing difficulty with finger movement while playing the flute.

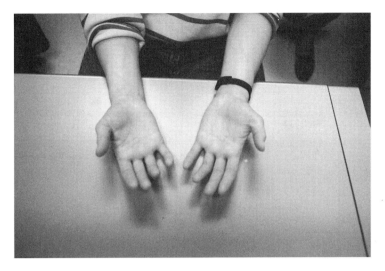

Figure 3. Patient with cumulative trauma showing evidence of contracted intrinsic musculature more marked on the right hand.

gests contraction of forearm muscles.[8] This can cause secondary loss of tendon slack and increased friction at peripheral sheaths and pulleys. Ulnar variance should be checked because it might be associated with a triangular fibrocartilaginous complex (TFCC) tear.[15] Elbow range of motion is measured in extension, flexion, supination, and pronation. At the elbow, carrying angle should also be measured,[16] because if extreme, it may cause computer users or musicians to assume awkward compensatory postures, particularly in pronation (Figure 4), and may even predispose the subject to cubital tunnel syndrome.[17] Shoulder examination should include testing for range of motion, bicipital tendinitis, bursitis, instability, impingement, and rotator cuff problems.[18] Postural deficiencies should be noted, including shoulder protraction, cervical and thoracic spine dysfunction as well as scoliosis and scapular winging and dynamic control, because proximal deficiencies will affect distal function of the extremities.[19–21]

Neck range of motion is evaluated noting the association of spasm and painful trigger points in neck and shoulder muscles. Palpation of muscles, particularly in the neck, shoulders, arms, and forearms is useful for assessing tenderness, muscle tone, and the presence of "jump signs" in the forearm from tendons that lack sufficient slack. The various entheses should be checked with particular attention paid to the lateral and medial epicondyles at the elbow.[22,23] Prolonged symptoms of "tennis elbow" might signify the presence of radial tunnel syndrome.[24]

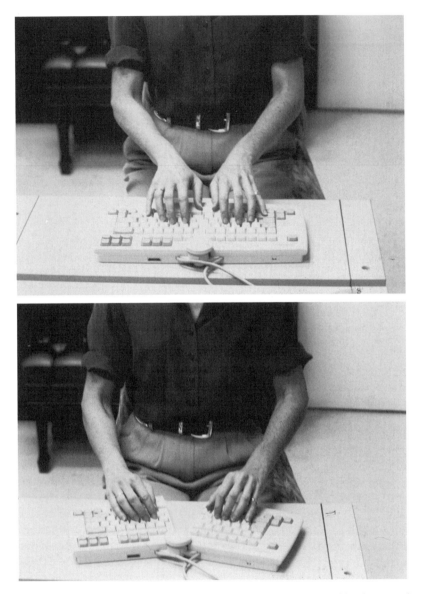

Figure 4. Patient with increased carrying angle (14°) showing position in pronation with ulnar deviation (**A**) and correction with a split keyboard (**B**).

Neurological evaluation should include observation for tremor, fasciculations, or movement disorders. Deep tendon reflexes are part of general neurological testing performed with specific tests deemed appropriate by the clinician. For example, a slow return phase of deep tendon reflexes might suggest hypothyroidism alerting the clinician to perform further tests.[25] The test for Tinel's sign, which consists of gentle tapping with the middle or index finger over various "mousetrap" areas of the median ulnar and radial nerves as well as the cervical and brachial plexus is extremely useful to test for traction or compression impairment of nerves.[26] Further testing to confirm suspicious findings might include Froment's sign for ulnar impairment, Phelan's 60-second test for carpal tunnel syndrome, or the middle finger test for radial tunnel syndrome. Other specific tests are performed by the attentive clinician where indicated.

Evaluation for the thoracic outlet syndromes, is important and consists primarily of clinical testing.[27] This should be carried out with care and precision because we have found the neurogenic variety present in approximately 80% of our patients with CTD.[28]

Diminished neck range of motion and poor posture often associated with tightened scalene muscles are capable of producing traction injuries to the nerves of the cervical and brachial plexus.[27] Gentle thumb pressure applied to the supraclavicular fossa medially and the infraclavicular fossa laterally can cause compromised nerves and muscles to release nociceptive substances causing pain that sometimes radiates to the neck, upper back, arms, and hands.[27] We have found this simple clinical test for "mechanoallodynia" to be very useful in evaluating for the thoracic outlet syndromes. The 3-minute Roos or elevated arm stress test (EAST) in the "surrender" position is another important basic clinical evaluation. During this test symptoms often mimic the patient's complaints.[27] Observing skin color or temperature changes, paresthesias, or pain is important for further defining the lesions in thoracic outlet syndromes. Wrights' maneuver, which consists of raising the extended arms overhead, essentially compresses the upper trunk and puts traction in the lower trunk of the brachial plexus and is a helpful confirmatory test.[27] Adson's maneuver is somewhat useful for determining whether a vascular component is present. Allen's test can determine if circulation is impaired in the ulnar artery, keeping in mind that vascular forms of thoracic outlet syndrome are found in less than 5% of persons with thoracic outlet syndrome, the majority being neurogenic in origin.[29] Vascular involvement, although less frequent can have serious complications and may necessitate further testing. The reader is referred to Chapters 4 and 11 of this book for further information on thoracic outlet syndromes and other vascular disorders.

The physical examination should also include testing of isometric muscle strength using the traditional five-point scale.[30,31] This adds another dimension to the diagnostic process. Testing should include muscles of the hands, thumbs, wrist, arms, shoulders, and trunk: grip strength is useful as a baseline on which to compare future values. Ideally all 5 positions of the Jamar dynamometer can be used, but we usually limit our testing to positions 2 and 3, especially if the patient complains of pain.[32] Pinch strength is also tested in the lateral, chuck, and tip positions using a pinch dynamometer.[33]

Spurling's maneuver to elicit neck pain coupled with other findings might suggest the need for cervical spine films or magnetic resonance imaging (MRI) to rule out compression, radiculopathy, spondylolysis, or spondylolisthesis. Cervical spine x-rays are also helpful in characterizing thoracic outlet syndromes by showing loss of the normal lordotic cervical curve associated with muscle spasm or pointing to other anomalies such as a cervical rib or elongated C7 transverse process that may predispose to brachial plexopathy. Trigger points can be checked in various locations for a painful reaction, suggesting the diagnosis of fibromyalgia.[34] Two-point discrimination and Semmes-Weinstein monofilament testing can help determine the status of peripheral nerve function.[35] After the physical examination, decisions are made to determine the need for other tests. These might include specific radiographs, computed tomography (CT) scans, MRIs, electromyograms (EMGs), nerve conduction velocities,[36] evoked potentials,[37] vibrometry,[38] thermography,[39] bone scans,[40] Doppler studies,[41] and blood tests to rule out thyroid disease, diabetes, collagen diseases, Lyme disease, and other suspected medical conditions that may be contributing to the cumulative trauma problem.

Performance Assessment

Once the history and physical examination are completed, subjects are assessed while performing various tasks that might contribute to their injury. An area of our examination room is set aside for this purpose. Videotaping the patient or viewing a workstation video are extremely useful because it permits a retrospective assessment and also enables the injured person to see the awkward postures or mannerisms that need correction as part of the treatment plan.[8] Because cumulative trauma is a work-related problem with causes that go beyond the specific major work function such as typing, it is difficult to impugn any one activity as the sole cause of the problem. Thus, a computer keyboard user should also be evaluated for typing skills, handwriting, input device, and telephone use and possibly injurious activities of daily living. Common sense dictates that if a person had no problems before using a keyboard or a mouse, then the major contributing cause will be the use of such devices. Computer keyboard users should also be assessed for technique. The principal technique deficiencies at the keyboard include typing in dorsiflexion, ulnar deviation, with hyperextended thumbs or fifth fingers or alienating the proximal musculature by placing the wrists on the table or on a wrist rest. Various intrinsic physical anomalies may facilitate injury. These include finger hyperlaxity, Linburg's tendon, short fingers, increased carrying angle at the elbow, slightness of build, and postural abnormalities. Even long nails can encourage hyperextension of the fingers, resulting in cocontraction of forearm flexors and extensors combined with loss of hand intrinsic muscle flexor activity.[42] Common anomalies in the neck such as scalene bands and less common ones such as cervical ribs or elongated transverse spinal processes can indirectly contribute to injury by compromising neurological function in the cervical or brachial plexus.[43]

Office workers should also be assessed for posture because poor posture may set the stage for the future development of CTD. An appropriate chair can help the user maintain good posture. Workers should be informed about what to look for in a good chair and instructed in its proper adjustment. The seat pan should tilt forward and extend no more than two-thirds of the thigh. The feet should be able to rest firmly on the ground, and chair arms should be avoided to allow freedom of arm movement. Most importantly, these adjustments should be easy to perform. Because standard desk height is adequate for writing but not for keyboard placement, we recommend an adjustable pullout keyboard tray (eg, Flex Rest, Inc., Worcester, MA). An important feature of a proper pullout tray is its potential for tilting the far end of the keyboard downward (negative tilt) to allow free shoulder movement, position the wrist in a more neutral position, and open the angle at the elbow beyond 90° (Figure 5). By having the elbow in this position, less traction is produced in the ulnar nerve at the sulcus. Because we have found a high incidence of cubital tunnel syndrome associated with CTD injuries, this is potentially a beneficial adaptation. During the evaluation and the ensuing retraining, patients are given a set of workstation measurements. Various keyboards and other devices are discussed and practical recommendations are made for their use. Contact is also made with worksite ergonomists and the physical and occupational therapists who will be caring for the injured person. We have also found it useful to give the patient a copy of our treatment protocol to give to their therapist along with their prescription. We always discuss the treatment plan with the therapists and re-evaluate patients periodically to assess their progress.

Musicians are examined and evaluated in much the same way because they have similar manifestations of cumulative trauma. It is beyond the scope of this chapter to discuss this subject in detail. It may be useful to know, however, that certain instruments, are potentially more likely to cause injuries. These include the piano and the string instruments such as the violin, viola, cello, double bass, and various guitars followed by

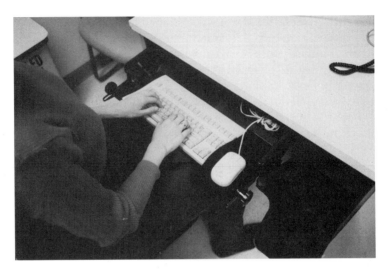

Figure 5. Positioning at the keyboard. Note the absence of chair arms, forward tilt of the seat pan, feet firmly on the ground, pullout tray with downward tilt, and location of the mouse. Elbow angle is greater than 90°, which diminishes ulnar nerve traction.

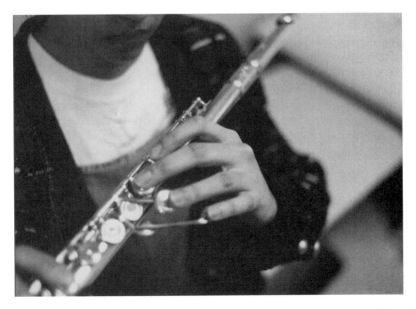

Figure 6. Flutist with short fourth and fifth fingers showing a more comfortable adaptation by moving and lenthening certain keys.

the wind instruments, which not only induce awkward positioning and difficulty of finger placement but can also create problems relating to the embouchure, which is the relation of the instrument to the lips, facial muscles, teeth, and oropharynx. Musicians must be observed playing their instrument to ferret out technique deficiencies. Certain of these instruments such as the flute, clarinet, bassoon and French horn are amenable to key and placement modifications that can make playing more comfortable and controlled (Figure 6). With instruments such as the piano, posture, positioning, technique, and conditioning are as important a remedial approach as they are with the computer keyboard. The basic treatment approach is the same. Establishing a dialogue with the musician's teacher is also desirable. Postural misalignment is common among musicians.

Pathophysiology

Given the complexity and confusion surrounding certain aspects of cumulative trauma, it is useful to speculate on the pathophysiology of these disorders because a better understanding can be the basis for an effective and successful treatment program. Cumulative trauma disorder is a serious and complex neuromuscular illness with principal manifestations in the upper body and proximal and distal manifestations that are linked.[28] The goal of an appropriate examination is to clarify the relation between the various injured soft tissues. These include muscles, tendons, ligaments, connective tissue, the circulatory system, and the nervous system with their various divisions. It is useful to hypothesize that the final common pathway in CTD is the lack of sufficient functional muscle to maintain adequate capacity to carry out necessary activities. This also implies that muscle regeneration capacity has been impaired. Therefore, the pivotal aspect of treatment will be to restore muscle regeneration to provide strength and endurance and a proper mix of fiber type necessary to carry out normal activities without fatigue or pain.

Muscle Injury and the Degeneration-Regeneration Cycle

The way in which muscles are used can accelerate injury. There is evidence to suggest that activating a lengthened muscle, a condition known as eccentric contraction,[44] increases the likelihood of injury.[45] This might occur in the lower extremities during intensive downhill running or in the smaller muscles of the forearms during computer use while striking the keys vigorously with bent wrists. The greater degree of length change occurring during eccentric muscle use, the greater degree of injury.[44,45] Therefore, the more malpositioning, the more potential for injury. Another contributing factor postulated as being responsible for muscle injury during eccentric exercise is high-force change, especially during the first contraction. These high-force changes can occur with keying and is also a characteristic of playing certain musical instruments. Fiber type specificity of injury may also account for the loss of endurance in patients with cumulative trauma disorders.[46] There is evidence that the largest muscle fibers are most vulnerable to injury. In humans, these are the type II fibers that are the fast-twitch, nontonic fibers that are essential to repetitive activity.

Loss of calcium homeostasis has been implicated in muscle fiber injury. Injured muscle also shows loss of desmin cytoskeletal protein which is the component of the inter-Z bands.[48] The myofibrillar changes that occur after repetitive eccentric contractions include disorganization of the myofilbrillar Z band, focal disruption of the A band and clotted fibers.[44,47] These observations suggest that substantial structural changes follow eccentric exercise.

Muscle injury can also occur without a major eccentric component if the milieu for regeneration is poor and muscle use is excessive.[49] In the computer work environment as well as among musicians, the upper extremity muscles are often subjected to sustained activity in awkward positions. A typical pain pattern indicated by the patient with CTD is shown in the pictogram (Figure 1). Clinically, in injured patients, palpation of these muscles in the hands, forearm, neck, and upper back often reveals soreness and contraction or spasm. In the forearm muscle groups, this results in limited range of motion in flexion and dorsiflexion and often in supination and pronation. Contraction of hand intrinsics may also be present (Figure 3). A study by Machleder and associates[50] in patients with thoracic outlet syndrome and chronic scalene muscle spasm revealed hypertrophy and recruitment of type I slow-twitch fibers. The clinically observed muscle contraction and spasm causing diminished circulation contributes to muscle soreness by trapping nociceptive metabolites such as prostaglandins, calcium and hydrogen ions, histamine, and lactic acid. This also creates an unfavorable environment for muscle regeneration because of impairment of metabolic processes.

Evaluation of muscle injury also requires a closer look at the degeneration-regeneration process and its relation to the nervous system. This important linkage resides in the satellite cell.[51,52] The muscle fiber complex consists of three basic components: the multinucleated skeletal muscle fiber; its surrounding basal lamina; and a population of mononuclear stem cells, the satellite cells. The latter are interspersed between the muscle fiber and the basal lamina. A fiber complex interacts with other tissue components such as motor nerve terminations, connective tissue cells, and fibers at the myotendinous junctions as well as capillaries that run parallel to the muscle fiber and the mechano-sensory apparatus. This relation between the muscle fibers, capillaries, and the nervous system is crucial to understanding CTD.

Because the muscle fiber cell is postmitotic, it has lost the capacity to divide. Satellite cells, however, retain this capacity and are the source of new muscle fiber during regeneration and growth.[53] At birth, immature muscle fibers are associated with a large population of satellite cells. These diminish in number with aging,[54] although even older muscle has a sufficient number of satellite cells to permit regeneration. Damage to muscle fiber units results in a series of degenerative changes followed by phagocytosis of the degenerating fibers by macrophages. This is a normal physiological process that occurs not only to allow replacement of muscle but also to facilitate the adaptive changes of the kind seen in training. Macrophages also activate satellite cells that proliferate, forming myotubes that ultimately differentiate into muscle fibers provided the circumstances are favorable.[53] Adequate circulation, a supply of humoral substances and unimpeded innervation are necessary for regeneration. Disturbances of innervation can impair regeneration.[54] Clinically, the two areas of nerve damage that need to be considered are the proximal and distal components. Seddon[55] proposed three categories of nerve injuries while Sunderland[56] expanded this to five. These range from neuropraxia where the nerve is temporarily not conducting at the site of a lesion, but axon continuity is maintained to total disruption of function. Proximally, cervical radiculopathy or the thoracic outlet syndromes can disturb nerve functions to varying degrees. Very little research has focused on the role of repetitive motion in the pathophysiology of nerve damage peripherally. It has been postulated that peripheral nerve damage is a multifactorial process that includes: varying longitudinal force on the nerve; mechanical damage caused by repetitive gliding through narrow canals or tendinous arches; external compression from hypertrophied muscle, edema, synovial thickening, tendinitis; biomechanical factors such as histamine release causing angioedema[57]; systemic humoral factors such as pregnancy increasing the likelihood of carpal tunnel syndrome; and medical conditions such as diabetes,[58] hypothyroidism, rheumatoid arthritis, alcoholism, and malnutrition.[59]

Nerve Injuries

Because of their relation to muscular and vascular function, nerves play an important role in the pathophysiology of cumulative trauma disorders. One of many important nerve functions is to carry pain messages from the site of peripheral tissue damage to the central nervous system. Injury to the nerve itself can also manifest itself as pain, which can persist even after muscle injury has subsided. In addition, the nerve's role in muscle regeneration is critical. While we have some knowledge of the mechanisms causing "mousetrap" injury to median, ulnar, and radial nerves in the arm and hand, little work has been done to define changes in nerves that are subject to repetitive movement. Proximally, traction and compression can cause neurogenic thoracic syndromes. Normally there is approximately 15 mm of longitudinal excursion in the brachial plexus, which may be impaired in the thoracic outlet syndrome. Eighty percent of 150 patients we examined were found to have evidence of thoracic outlet syndrome using Roos' diagnostic criteria[27] (Table 1). Their average age was 39 years, with a slight predominance of women (Table 2). All of these patients also had evidence of postural misalignment. Obviously, not all persons with postural syndromes develop thoracic outlet syndrome. One answer may lie in the presence or absence anatomic anomalies. Congenital fibromuscular bands between scalene muscles are found in approximately 30% of the population while cervical ribs or enlargement of the C7 transverse process are less common.[60]

Vascular types of thoracic outlet syndrome constitute less than 5% of the total although induced vascular manifestations by the sympathetic nervous system such as cooling of the hands and fingers are not uncommon in the CTD patient. Occasionally the more draconian complication of reflex sympathetic dystrophy can occur in the more severely injured person. The reader is referred to Chapter 11 by Dr. Roos for a further discussion of thoracic outlet syndromes.

Postural misalignment that is associated with thoracic outlet syndrome in our cumulative trauma patients consists primarily of rounded protracted shoulders with head-forward position often associated with tight painful scalenes, sternocleidomastoid, and trapezius muscles, resulting in loss of neck range of motion. Cervical spine radiographs will often show straightening of the cervical spine with loss of the normal lordotic curve. Straightening of the thoracic spine is often noted clinically. Scapular control and weakness and occasional rotator cuff deficiencies resulting in impingement are also found. With these postural changes one can postulate continuing compromise of nerve and musculoskeletal function resulting in a cyclical deterioration and the peripheral manifestations of muscle injury and compromised muscle regeneration. Accurate diagnosis is based on a carefully obtained history and physical examination that rules out other lesions such as tumors or cervical radiculopathy. Peripheral nerve lesions can be evaluated by various tests including the Tinel's percussion test; the Phelan 60-second test; and strength testing, EMGs, and nerve conduction velocities can be obtained if considered necessary but will be of limited use in the diagnosis of the thoracic outlet syndromes.[24]

Peripheral nerve impairment is not infrequently associated with thoracic outlet syndromes. The theory of a "double-crush" injury has been

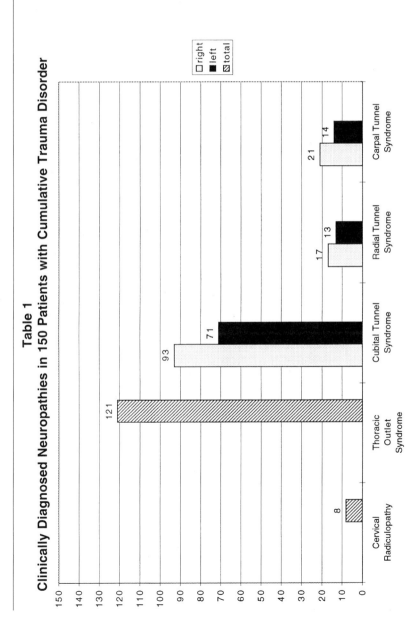

Table 1
Clinically Diagnosed Neuropathies in 150 Patients with Cumulative Trauma Disorder

n=150

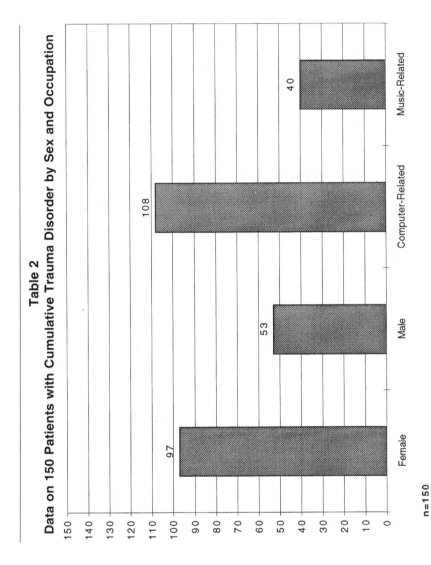

Table 2

Data on 150 Patients with Cumulative Trauma Disorder by Sex and Occupation

n=150

proposed to explain this phenomenon.[61] Carpal tunnel syndrome was found in 11% of 150 patients we studied (Table 1), and the most common peripheral nerve symptom based on our clinical evaluation was cubital tunnel syndrome, which we detected in up to 62% of 150 subjects (Table 1). The relation between cubital tunnel syndrome and thoracic outlet syndromes needs further study, suggesting a possible traction injury at both sites. In addition there is some speculation about the existence of a reversed double crush syndrome where the distal entrapment may contribute to the genesis of an entrapment neuropathy of the same nerve proximally.[62]

Tendons and Ligaments

Tendons and ligaments should be viewed as dynamic rather than static structures that are critical for joint movement and joint stabilization. Both tendons and ligaments have a rich afferent nerve supply to mediate proprioception as well as a substantial blood supply. Some regions of tendon have less vascularity than others and are more vulnerable to injury.[63] As such they can be injured when subjected to sustained repetitive forces. Because of their size, tendons of the upper extremity are particularly at risk for tendinitis (inflammatory reaction) or tendinosis (degeneration). Microscopically, tendons and ligament cells are fibroblasts lying longitudinally between bundles of collagen fibers. With injury, these tissues sustain changes that are often irreversible resulting in scarring and shortening.[64] Tendons are attached to muscle at the muscle tendon junction and convey the mechanical movement of the muscle through its attachment to bone (the entheses), both distally and proximally. Ligaments and tendons are viscoelastic tissues that have nonlinear biomechanical properties.[65] The biomechanics of tendon injuries is poorly understood. As with other soft tissues there is evidence to suggest that passive motion results in superior healing properties Benjamin and Ralphs[66] describe the essential role of tendons and ligaments.

Tendons

- To allow the muscle to be some distance from its site of action and permit pull through a narrow space (eg, carpal tunnel).
- Enable the muscle pull to be focused onto single or multiple sites or for several muscles to act on one site.
- Eliminate the need for unnecessary length of muscle between origin and insertion.

- Change the direction of pull of a muscle by wrapping around a bony pulley.
- Reinforce or replace part of a joint capsule.
- Act as spring that stores energy in locomotion.
- Holds other tendons in position.

Ligaments

- Guide and limit movements of synovial joints, limiting allowable movements, and prohibiting unwanted ones.
- Provide attachment for muscles (interosseous membrane).
- Send signals to the brain important for proprioception and play an active role in maintaining joint stability.
- May act as guy wires to tie down other soft tissues to bone.
- Are modified to form articular disc and synovial surfaces.
- Loose ligaments tend to destabilize joints which may explain why hyperlax individuals are more at risk for injury because they cocontract extensor and flexor muscles and therefore have to work harder to maintain a stable hand (Table 3).

Anatomic variations can occur in ligaments and tendons that can contribute to problems of cumulative trauma. We have noted that Linburg's anomaly where fibrous or tendinous bands connect the flexor pollicis longus and flexor digitorum profundus of the index finger can cause problems of finger action in computer users and musicians. Various forms of tendinitis accompany cumulative trauma disorders. In our analysis of 150 patients, medial epicondylitis occurred in 88 persons on the right and 78 on the left. Lateral epicondylitis occurred in 44 on the right and 31 on the left. de Quervain's tenosynovitis occurred in 33 persons on the right and 14 on the left (Table 4). Hyperlaxity of the fingers in extension was extremely common (Table 3).

Treatment

Treatment of CTD is based on the findings of the history, physical examination, and biomechanical and ergonomic evaluation, combined with an understanding of the pathophysiology. Basically an attempt should be made to treat these soft tissue injuries conservatively yet aggressively with the physical and occupational therapists playing a pivotal role in guiding therapy in cooperation with the physician.[60] Success in treatment can only be achieved if the patient cooperates by performing stretching and strengthening exercises daily at home and follows other instructions such as limiting or changing work activity.

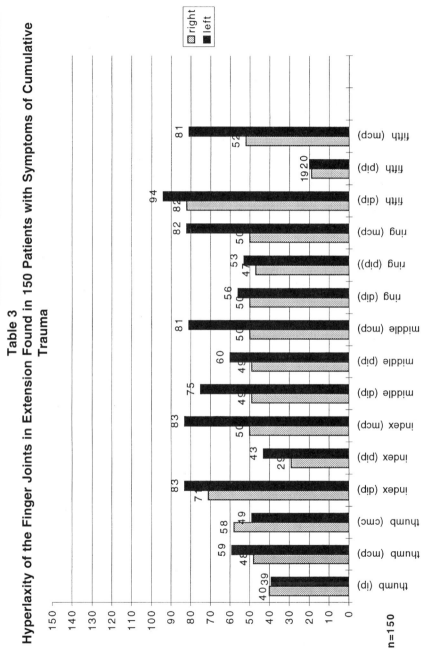

Table 3

Hyperlaxity of the Finger Joints in Extension Found in 150 Patients with Symptoms of Cumulative Trauma

n=150

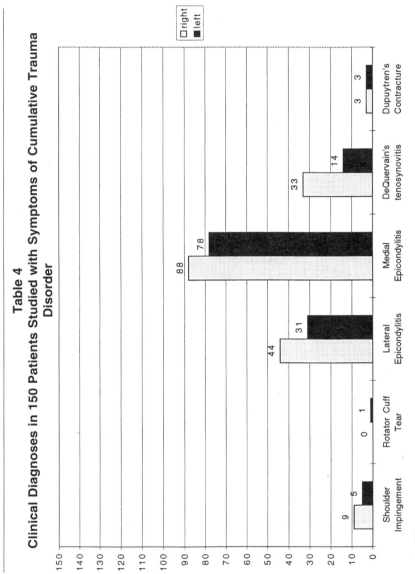

Table 4
Clinical Diagnoses in 150 Patients Studied with Symptoms of Cumulative Trauma Disorder

n=150

The question of splint use often arises. We feel strongly that they should be used sparingly, if at all, for patients with CTD because the soft tissues need to remain mobile and functional despite injury.[2] Wrist splints should be limited to night use for persons with carpal tunnel syndrome and never used during work activity. If a patient needs splints in order to work, then he or she probably shouldn't be working. Thumb spica splints for de Quervain's tenosynovitis should only be used during the acute phase and removed as soon as feasible. Elbow splinting for cubital tunnel syndrome is usually poorly tolerated. Stretching tightened muscles is an important part of the therapeutic program and is inhibited by splinting.

In some cases ancillary treatment may be necessary for pain management or for specific therapies such as nerve blocks, while other modalities such as massage, rolfing, myofascial release, craniosacral therapy, Alexander technique, Feldenkreis technique, acupuncture, and chiropractic may be helpful in specific cases as adjuvant therapy. Psychiatric consultation or psychological counseling are often necessary to treat the common complications of anxiety and depression. There is frequently a need for ergonomic intervention or biomechanical retraining which is then made an integral part of the treatment plan.

Physical and Occupational Therapies

The initial approach for the physical or occupational therapist should be to involve the patient immediately in active participation. The patient is instructed in an intensive graduated home exercise program stressing the concept of constant training and the fact that they are upper body athletes. Therapy should begin with stretching of forearm, shoulder, cervical, and pectoral musculature. The specific focus, initially should be on pectoralis minor and major, scalenes, upper trapezius, and rhomboid muscles. Postural and biomechanical retraining is integrated early in the treatment program. Cervical and upper extremity range of motion are a prelude to an aggressive upper extremity and abdominal strengthening program with special emphasis on the posterior shoulder girdle and upper back musculature. Proximal stabilization and muscle balance are begun assisted by use of the UBE (upper body ergometer; Cybex Medical Systems, Ronkonkoma, NY) and the Body Blade (Hymanson, Inc., Los Angeles, CA) as well as other appropriate equipment. Breathing exercises include diaphragmatic breathing, lateral costal expansion, and relaxation of accessory inspiration muscles such as the scalenes and pectoralis minor muscles. Soft tissue and joint mobilization are carried out on the pectoralis minor muscles with mobilization of clavicles and upper ribs. An important caveat; minimize passive exercises and dependency on the therapist and stress home-based exercise. Based on the high number of persons with thoracic outlet syndrome in our experience, this course of therapy is usually prescribed for 8 weeks after which the patient is re-evaluated to refocus the treatment and to determine the degree of treatment success. The most frequent cause of slow response or failure is lack of compliance to home therapy followed by lack of appropriate supervision by the therapist. Other causes that might make therapeutic outcome less favorable are longstanding symptoms, associated medical problems, multiple operations, psychosocial problems and involvement in litigation.

Pain Management

Pain is a cardinal symptom of CTDs. Pain management is an essential part of the treatment program. If pain is adequately controlled, physical therapy and exercises can be carried out more easily, sleep patterns will improve and coping with work and activities of daily living becomes more tolerable. With a focused physical therapy program that includes stretching and strengthening, pain levels should gradually diminish.

Constant pain in the hands, forearms, arms, neck, and upper back sometimes described as aching and burning is the most common complaint of persons we see with CTD. This type of pain is probably due to irritation of nociceptive pain fibers from a variety of metabolic products trapped in the soft tissues as well as local nerve damage. Nonsteroidal anti-inflammatory medications can be tried for relief, but are often ineffective because they work primarily by inhibiting prostaglandin synthesis, one of many nociceptive substances contributing to this disorder. For more acute pain symptoms we have found acetaminophen with codeine useful for short periods although many clinicians have found a variety of medications useful.

Ice massage can be used to desensitize the nociceptive nerve fibers several times daily for temporary relief. Using ice frozen in a paper cup directly applied to the skin for 30 to 45 seconds is often effective. Alternating heat and cold applications also works well in some circumstances. Tricyclics or serotonin re-uptake inhibitors that are antidepressant medications, tend to raise the pain threshold and improve sleep patterns in low doses. Where there is severe muscle spasm associated with cumulative trauma, massage, rolfing, trigger-point injection or a transcutaneous electrical nerve stimulation (TENS) unit might be helpful. When splints are applied to immobilize injured tissues, transitory relief of pain may occur, but the soft tissues contract further causing fibrosis and stiffness of muscles and joints with more pain ensuing when the splints are removed and mobilization is attempted.

Ice should not be applied to extremities when reflex sympathetic dystrophy is present. In these cases pain levels and sensitivity are likely to be extremely high because of sympathetic enhancement of pain perception. With RSD, pain patterns can become complex and may necessitate intervention by pain management specialists. Intervention may include a variety of medications, biofeedback, sympathetic nerve blocks, or even sympathectomy. With properly focused physical and occupational therapy coupled with home exercises, biomechanical retraining, and ergonomic changes in workstations, pain levels should diminish and ultimately allow the patient to improve function, provided the proper diagnoses are made and the patient is viewed in terms of total body function rather than a specific lesion.

In summary, the focus of cumulative trauma treatment should combine an active exercise-oriented program including intensive home exercise with a change in work habits and techniques and psychological counseling if needed. The ultimate goal is to strengthen the upper body musculature by facilitating muscle regeneration, correcting nerve impairment and retraining the patient for a pain free functional existence, which may mean a substantial modification of work habits.

References

1. Gordon SL, Blair SJ, Fine LJ (ed): *Repetitive Motion Disorders of the Upper Extremity.* Rosemont, IL: American Academy of Orthopedic Surgeons; 1995.
2. Pascarelli EF, Quilter D. *Repetitive Strain Injury: A Computer User's Guide.* New York: John Wiley & Sons; 1994.
3. Stone WE. Occupational overuse syndrome in other countries. *J Occup Health Safety Aust NZ* 3(4):400, 1986.
4. *Occupational Injuries and Illnesses in the United States, 1992.* Washington DC: US Department of Labor, Bureau of Labor Statistics, doc no. L 2.2: OCI/153, 1994.
5. Hadler NM: Cumulative traurna disorders: An iatrogenic concept. *J Occup Med* 32:38–41, 1990.
6. Tenner E: *Why Things Bite Back: Technology and the Revenge of Unintended Consequences.* A. Knopf; 1996.
7. Fishbein M, Middlestadt SE, with Oltati V et al. Medical problems among ICSOM musicians: Overview of a national survey. *Med Probl Perform Art* 3: 1–8, 1988.
8. Pascarelli E, Kella J: Soft-tissue injuries related to use of the computer keyboard: A clinical study of 53 severely injured persons. *J Occup Med* 35:5, 1993.
9. McFarlane RM: Dupuytren's disease: Relation to work and injury. *J Hand Surg* 16A:775–779, 1991.
10. Linburg RM, Comstock BE: Anomalous tendon slips from the flexor pollicis longus to the flexor digitorum profundus. *J Hand Surg* 4A:79–83, 1979.
11. Fahey JJ, Bollinger JA: Trigger finger in adults and children. *J Bone Joint Surg* 36A:1200–1218, 1954.

12. Lapidus PW, Fenton R: Stenosing tenovaginnitis at the wrist and fingers: Report of 423 cases in 369 patients with 354 operations. *Arch Surg* 64:475–487, 1952.
13. Wilson PR: Sympathetically maintained pain: Diagnosis, measurement and efficacy of treatment. In: Stanton-Hicks M, ed. *Pain and the Sympathetic Nervous System.* Boston, MA: Kluver Academic Publishers; 1990; pp. 191–123.
14. Hooshmand H: *Chronic Pain, Reflex Sympathetic Dystrophy Prevention and Management.* Boca Raton, FL: CRC Press; 1991.
15. Palmer AK, Werner FW: The triangular fibrocartilage complex of the wrist: Anatomy and function. *J Hand Surg* 6:152, 1981.
16. Beals RK: The normal carrying angle of the elbow. *Clin Orthop* 119:194, 1976.
17. Conwell HE: Injuries to the elbow. *Clin Symp* 22:35, 1970.
18. Yocum LA: Assessing the shoulder: History, physical examination, differential diagnosis and special tests used. *Clin Sports Med* 2:281, 1983.
19. Rose MJ. Keyboard operating posture and activation force: Implications for overuse. *Appl Ergonomics* 22:198–203, 1991.
20. Keur P, Wills R: The effect of typing posture on wrist extensor loading: Proceedings of the Biannual Conference of the Canadian Society for Biomechanics. Kingston, Ontario: Queens University, 1994.
21. Serina E, Tal R, Rempel D: Wrist and arm angles during typing. Proceedings of the Marconi Keyboard Research Conference. Ann Arbor, MI: University of Michigan, 1994.
22. Leach RE, Miller JK: Lateral and medical epicondylitis of the elbow. *Clin Sports Med* 6:259–272, 1981.
23. Morrey BF, Regan WD: Tendinopathies about the elbow. In: DeLee JC, Drez D Jr, eds. *Orthopedic Sports Medicine: Principles and Practice.* Philadelphia PA: WB Saunders; 1994, pp. 860–881.
24. Roles NC, Maudsley RH: Radial tunnel syndrome: Resistant tennis elbow as a nerve entrapment. *J Bone Joint Surg* 54B:499, 1972.
25. DiMauro S: Metabolic myopathies. In: Vinken PJ, Bruyn GW, eds. *Handbook of Clinical Neurology.* Volume 41. Amsterdam: North Holland; 1980, pp. 175–234.
26. Moldover V: Tinel's sign—Its characteristics and significance. *J Bone Joint Surg* 60A:412, 1978.
27. Roos DB: Overview of thoracic outlet syndromes in vascular disorders of the upper extremity. In: Machleder HI, ed. *Vascular Disorders of the Upper Extremity.* Second edition. Mt. Kisco, NY: Futura Publishing Company; 1989, pp. 155–177.
28. Pascarelli EF: Proceedings of the Second International Conference on the Neurovascular Comprehensive and Cumulative Trauma Disorders. Boston, MA: 1996.
29. American Society for Surgery of the Hand: *The Hand: Examination and Diagnosis.* Aurora: 1978.
30. Lister G: *Muscle Testing in the Hand, Diagnosis and Indications.* New York: Churchill Livingstone; 1984, pp. 351–386.
31. Kendall EP, McCreary BK: *Muscles: Testing and Function.* Baltimore: Williams & Wilkins; 1983.
32. Hazelton FT, Smidt GL, Flatt AE, et al: The influence of wrist position on the force produced by the flexors. *J Biomech* 8:301, 1975.

33. Tubiana R: Paralysis of the thumb. In: Tubiana R, ed. *The Hand*. Philadelphia, PA: W.B. Saunders; pp. 182–187, 1993.

34. Goldenberg DL: Controversies in fibromyalgia and myofascial pain syndrome. In: Arnoff GM, ed. *Evaluation and Treatment of Chronic Pain*. Second edition. Baltimore: Williams & Wilkins; 1992, pp. 165–175.

35. Guerra JJ, Shapiro DB: Diagnosis and treatment of carpal tunnel syndrome. *Hosp Physician* 28(4):29–41, 1992.

36. Daube JR: *Quantative EMG in Nerve Muscle Disorders in Clinical Neurophysiology*. London: Butterworths; 1981.

37. Halliday AM: *Evoked Potentials in Clinical Testing*. Bath: Churchill Livingstone; 1982.

38. Lundborg G, Liestenstrom AK, Sollerman C, et al: Digital vibrogram: A new diagnostic tool for sensory testing of compression neuropathy. *J Hand Surg Am* 11A(s):693–699, 1986.

39. Hooshmand H: *Chronic Pain, Reflex Sympathetic Dystrophy, Prevention and Management*. Boca Raton, FL: CRC Press; 1993, pp. 14–17.

40. Demanglat J, Constantinesco A, et al: Three phase bone scanning in reflex sympathetic dystrophy of the hand. *J Nucl Med* 29:26–32, 1988.

41. Sumner DS, Lambeth A, Russell JB: Diagnosis of upper extremity obstructive and vasospastic syndromes by Doppler ultrasound, plethysmography and temperature profiles. In: Puel P, Boccalon H, Enjalbert A, eds. *Hemodynamics of the Limbs*. Toulouse, France: GEPESC; 19??, pp. 365–373.

42. Pascarelli EF, Quilter D: *Repetitive Strain Injury. A Computer User's Guide*. New York: John Wiley & Sons; 1994, pp. 00–00.

43. Roos DB: Congenital anomalies associated with thoracic outlet syndrome: Anatomy, symptoms, diagnosis and treatment. *Am J Surg* 132:771–778, 1976.

44. Armstrong RB, Warren GL III, Lowe A: Mechanisms in the initiation of contraction-induced skeletal muscle injury. In: Gordon S, Blair S, Fine L, eds. *Repetitive Motion Disorders of the Upper Extremity*. Rosemont, IL: American Academy of Orthopedic Surgeons Symposium; 1995, pp. 339–348.

45. Fridén J, Sjöström M, Erblom B: Myofibrillar damage following intense eccentric exercise in man. *Int J Sports Med* 4:45–51, 1983.

46. Lieber RL, Fridén J: Selective damage of fast glycolytic muscle fibers with eccentric contraction of the rabbit tibialis anterior. *Acta Physiol Scand* 133: 587–588, 1988.

47. Armstrong RB, Warren GL, Warren JA: Mechanisms of exercise induced muscle fiber injury. *Sports Med* 12:184–207, 1991.

48. Fridén J, Thornell LE, Lieber R: Muscle cytoskeletal disruption occurs within the first 15 minutes of cyclic eccentric contraction. *Med Sci Sports Exerc* 26:526, 1994.

49. Lieber RL, Fridén J: Skeletal muscle metabolism, fatigue and injury. In: Gordon SL, Blair SJ, Fine LJ, eds. *Repetitive Motion Disorders of the Upper Extremity*. Rosemont, IL: American Academy of Orthopedic Surgeons Symposium; 1995, pp. 287–300.

50. Machleder HI, Moll F, Verity MA, The anterior scalene muscles in thoracic outlet compression syndrome. *Arch Surg* 121:1141–1144, 1986.

51. Mauro A: Satellite cell of skeletal muscle fibers. *J Biophys Biochem Cytol* 9: 493–495, 1961.

52. Campion DR: The muscle satellite cell: A review. *Int Rev Cytol* 87:225–251, 1984.
53. Snow MH: Myogenic cell formation in regenerating rat skeletal muscle injured by mincing: II. An autoradiographic study. *Anat Rec* 188:201–217, 1977.
54. Carlson BM: The satellite cell and skeletal muscie regeneration: The degeneration and regeneration cycle in repetitive motion disorders of the upper extremity. American Academy of Orthopedic Surgeons Symposium, Rosemont, IL: 1995, pp. 313–322.
55. Seddon HJ: Three types of nerve injury. *Brain* 66:237–288, 1943.
56. Sunderland S, ed. *Nerves and Nerve Injuries.* First edition. Baltimore: Williams & Wilkins; 1968.
57. Wener MH, Metzger WJ, Simon RA: Occupationally acquired vibratory angioedema with secondary carpal tunnel syndrome. *Ann Intern Med* 48:44–46, 1983.
58. Mulder DW, Lambert EH, Bastion JA, et al: The neuropathies associated with diabetes mellitus: A clinical and electrographic study of 103 unselected diabetic patients. *Neurology* 11:275–384, 1961.
59. Marshall SC, Murray WR: Deep radial nerve palsy associated with rheumatoid arthritis. *Clin Orthop* 103:157–162, 1974.
60. Smith KF: The thoracic outlet syndrome: A protocol of treatment. *J Orthop Sports Med* 1:89–98, 1979.
61. Upton AR, McComas AJ: The double crush in nerve entrapment syndromes. *Lancet* 2:359–362, 1973.
62. Dahlin LB, Lundborg G: The neuron and its response to peripheral nerve compression. *J Hand Surg* 15B:5–10, 1990.
63. Hirasway L, Katsumi Y, Akiyoshi T, et al: Clinical and microangiographic studies on rupture of the EPL tendon after distal radial fractures. *J Hand Surg* 15B:51–57, 1990.
64. Woo SL, Inove M, McGurk-Burleson et al: Treatment of the medial collateral ligament injury. II. Structure and function of canine knees in response to differing treatment regimens. *Am J Sports Med* 15:22–29, 1987.
65. Fronek J, Frank C, Amiel D, et al: The effect of intermittent passive motion (IPM) on the healing of the medial collateral ligament. *Trans Orthop Res Soc* 8:13, 1983.
66. Benjamin M, Ralphs J: Functional and developmental anatomy of tendons and ligaments. In: Gordon SL, Blair SJ, Fine LJ, eds. *Repetitive Motion Disorders of the Upper Extremity.* Rosemont, IL: American Academy of Orthopedic Surgeons; 1995; pp. 185–203.

9

Arterial Compression at the Thoracic Outlet

Herbert I. Machleder, MD

From the extensive literature discussing symptomatic cervical ribs, came the recognition that ischemic symptoms of the hand could follow as a consequence of thoracic outlet compression. Initial explanations focused on sympathetic innervation of the arm via the C8-T1 nerve roots, postulating that compression of these roots as they rest on the first rib leads to sympathetic induction of vasospasm and Raynaud's symptoms.[1] It was subsequently recognized that the subclavian artery can be compressed, either against a cervical rib by the anterior scalene muscle or between the normal first thoracic rib and overlying clavicle. At the site of compression, a spectrum of changes can be observed ranging from mild intimal injury and irregularity, which can give rise to mural thrombus and subsequent embolization, to post-stenotic dilatation and small aneurysm formation.[2] Repetitive episodes of embolization with progressive obliteration of the distal vessels accounts for the attacks of Raynaud's symptoms that in some cases are followed by ischemia and digital gangrene (Figures 1A and 1B and 2A through 2C).

The angiographic appearance may underestimate the pathological changes by disclosing only very subtle luminal abnormalities, particularly when the patient is supine. This disparity between the angiographic appearance and operative findings reflects the similar underestimation of the magnitude of mural thrombus, propagating clot, and post-stenotic dilatation. On occasion, minor areas of irregularity with associated thrombus may be more demonstrable on computed tomographic (CT) or magnetic resonance imaging (MRI) scan. The CT scan is often difficult to interpret because the subclavian artery course is such that in the sagittal sections, it moves in and out of the field. The coronal sections of the MRI

From Machleder HI, (ed): *Vascular Disorders of the Upper Extremity*. Third Revised Edition. Futura Publishing Company, Inc., Armonk, NY, © 1998.

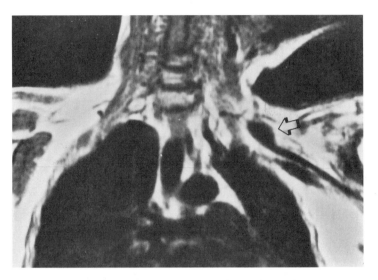

Figure 1A. Magnetic resonance imaging (MRI) of left subclavian aneurysm, or post-stenotic dilatation, in a patient with left cervical rib and ischemia of the left hand.

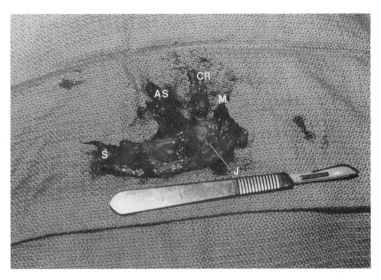

Figure 1B. Operative specimen of first thoracic rib and accompanying cervical rib. (S indicates sternal articulation of rib; AS, anterior scalene muscle inserting on rib; CR, cervical rib. J and arrow, the little joint (with cartilaginous surface, and capsule) where cervical rib articulates with first thoracic rib; M, stump of middle scalene muscle at its insertion. Refer to transaxillary illustrations to orient anatomy. The brachial plexus and subclavian artery are compressed and displaced antero-superiorly by the cervical rib.

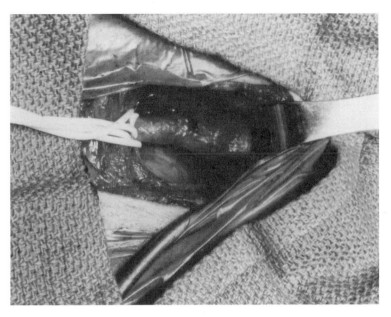

Figure 2A. Small subclavian aneurysm associated with a cervical rib, seen from a small supraclavicular incision. The aneurysm is exposed after the first and cervical rib have been resected via the transaxillary route. This sequential exposure limits the dissection in the neck and protects the brachial plexus both from operative injury, and from postoperative scar or fibrosis.

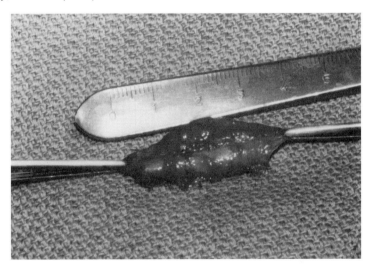

Figure 2B. Operative specimen of the subclavian aneurysm. Prior resection of the first and cervical rib facilitates primary end-to-end anastomosis of the subclavian artery. If the remaining vessel is inadequate for primary anastomosis, a small interposition graft can be used.

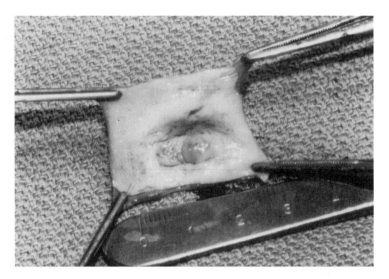

Figure 2C. The opened specimen shows the rough granular surface. Mural thrombus forms in this area and embolizes distally. The consequences of the distal embolization are usually the only manifestation of this disorder. In a thin patient, the post-stenotic dilatation and cervical rib can often be palpated in the supraclavicular area.

provide a better picture for interpretation. Often, no bony abnormality is encountered, and post-traumatic changes in the anterior scalene muscle may account for the compression.

Earliest Descriptions

Injury to the subclavian artery as a consequence of anatomic variation was first reliably described in 1860 by Holmes Coote in *The Lancet*.[3] In 1958, Robb and Standeven[4] reported 10 cases of arterial occlusion as a complication of what they termed, thoracic outlet compression syndrome. They remarked at the often delayed diagnosis of thoracic outlet problems, suspecting that the subtle early manifestations of arterial compression were often masked by collateral formation. They further observed that, "Three cases have been recorded in the literature in which proximal spread of arterial thrombosis had reached the bifurcation of the innominate artery and caused hemiplegia."

Almost three decades later, major league pitcher J.R. Richards suffered this identical consequence during a playoff game for the World

Series. He developed a sudden left-sided hemiparesis. W.S. Fields, the neurologist, recognized that the preceding cramping pain in the arm had been diagnosed as tendonitis when in reality the pitcher had subclavian artery occlusion from thoracic outlet compression syndrome. As the clot propagated in a retrograde fashion, the tail reached the innominate artery and subsequently embolized up the right carotid system. Both Robb[4] in 1958 and Fields[12] in 1986 decried the lack of diagnostic awareness when physicians encountered these neurovascular compression disorders.

More recently, after the work of Cormier et al[5] and Durham et al[6] it has come to be recognized that arterial injury at the thoracic outlet area is a consequence of repetitive stress, or cumulative trauma. Each of the three portions of the subclavian and axillary arteries develop characteristic abnormalities, associated with unique anatomic variations as well as distinctive predisposing activities. These disorders affect industrial workers and competitive athletes with markedly increased frequency, when compared with the general population. Anatomic variations such as cervical ribs, supernumerary scalene muscles, and residual fibrocartilaginous bands have been identified as predisposing anomalies in work and recreational settings of increased upper extremity stress (Figures 3A through 3D).[7-9]

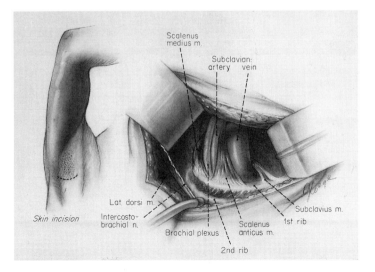

Figure 3A. Appearance of the anatomy as seen from the transaxillary approach.

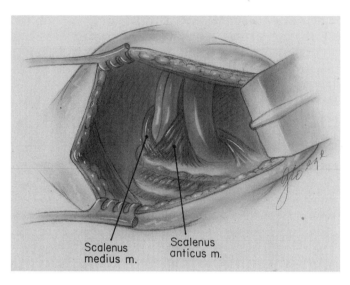

Figure 3B. Compression of the subclavian artery and brachial plexus by abnormal insertion of the anterior and middle scalene muscles. This anomaly is referred to as intercostalization, from the arrest in the embryological differentiation of the scalene muscle mass.

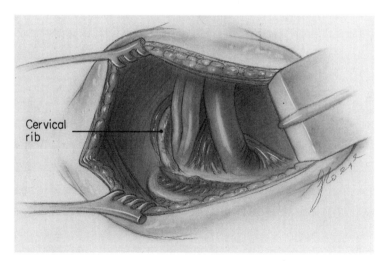

Figure 3C. Compression and displacement of the brachial plexus and subclavian artery by a right-sided cervical rib. This cervical rib articulates in the center of the first thoracic rib, much like the specimen seen in Figure 1B, which is from the left side.

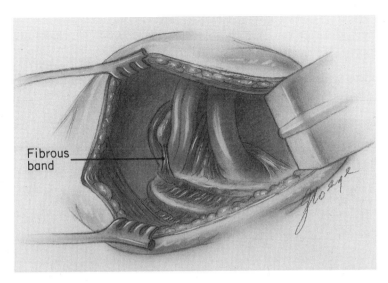

Figure 3D. A fibrocartilaginous band from the tip of the seventh cervical transverse process. This abnormality can compress the brachial plexus and subclavian artery, causing symptoms identical to those resulting from a cervical rib. The fibrocartilaginous band commonly occurs with an elongated C7 transverse process, and represents partial formation of a cervical rib.

Anatomy

The surgical anatomy of the subclavian artery is described in three distinct sections. The first part of the subclavian artery extends to the medial border of the anterior scalene muscle, and gives rise to the vertebral and internal mammary arteries as well as the thyrocervical trunk. This arterial segment is not primarily involved in cumulative trauma (thoracic outlet) injuries. Secondary thrombosis, propagating retrograde from the second and third portions can reach the innominate junction, then embolize up the right carotid causing left hemiplegia. As indicated above, this phenomenon has been recognized and reported, most strikingly in the case of baseball pitcher J.R. Richards.[5,8]

The second portion of the subclavian artery is the retroscalene portion, which is often the site of stricture, positional compression, or the most proximal area of post-stenotic dilatation and aneurysm formation. These later abnormalities most commonly also involve the third portion of the subclavian artery, which extends from the lateral border of the anterior scalene muscle to the lateral border of the first thoracic rib (Figure 4).

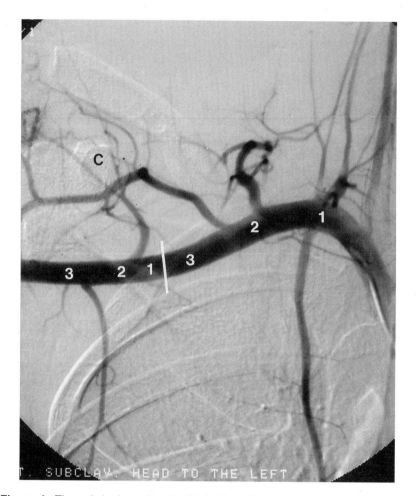

Figure 4. The subclavian artery is divided into three segments. Lesions in each segment usually arise from discrete and stereotypical causes, and require a specific therapeutic approach. Likewise, the axillary artery is divided into three sections with characteristic abnormalities confined to each region. C indicates the coracoid process, into which the pectoralis minor tendon inserts. Segment 2 of the subclavian artery represents the retroscalene segment. Segment 2 of the axillary artery identifies the retropectoral region. Characteristic compressive abnormalities specific to the anatomic regions are described later in this chapter.

The axillary artery is likewise divided into three sections. The first section, from subclavian artery to medial border of pectoralis minor muscle, gives rise to the superior thoracic artery. The second portion lies beneath the pectoralis minor tendon, and the third portion extends to the lateral border of the teres major muscle. Major branches are the thoracoacromial, lateral thoracic, humeral circumflex, and the subscapular arteries.

It must be recognized that the arterial symptoms in these anatomic regions are a manifestation of the thoracic outlet compression syndrome, and consequently, frequently have concomitant signs and symptoms derived from simultaneous compression of the brachial plexus. The artery and brachial plexus travel together, through the interscalene triangle (between anterior and middle scalene), as they traverse the thoracic outlet and costoclavicular space. They are even more intimately associated at the level of the axillary artery. In contradistinction, the axillosubclavian vein travels in a separate course, medial to the anterior scalene muscle (Figures 1A, 1B, 2A through 2C, and 3A through 3D).

Presenting History and Physical Signs

Patients with arterial compression may in the early stages have symptoms suggestive of autonomic dysfunction such as unilateral cold hypersensitivity, Raynaud's phenomenon, episodes of rubor, and recurrent mild edema. The disorder may often be attributed erroneously to a collagen vascular disease. The unilaterality of the symptoms must be the warning that this is more likely an embolic or neurovascular compressive process (Figures 5A and 5B).

As the disorder progresses, there will be episodes of cold-induced ischemia, fingertip pain, and frank punctate ischemic ulcers at the paronychial area. Examination will occasionally show splinter hemorrhages in the nail beds. Digital plethysmography will often show dampened waveform shapes in the affected fingers with evidence of digital artery occlusion. Once again the unilaterality must suggest to the examiner the possibility of an axillosubclavian artery lesion or central embolizing source (Figure 6A and 6B).[9]

Alternatively, in the face of complete occlusion, patients will complain of aching in the hand and arm with exercise. This is usually associated with cold hypersensitivity or cold intolerance in the hand and fingers. Although a misnomer, this symptom is often referred to as "arm claudication" because of its similarity to the exercise-induced lower extremity symptoms of arterial insufficiency. At this stage, Doppler derived segmental arterial pressures of the upper extremities will be clearly abnormal.

Arteriography is almost invariably required, recognizing the problems of interpretation discussed previously. The studies should be done

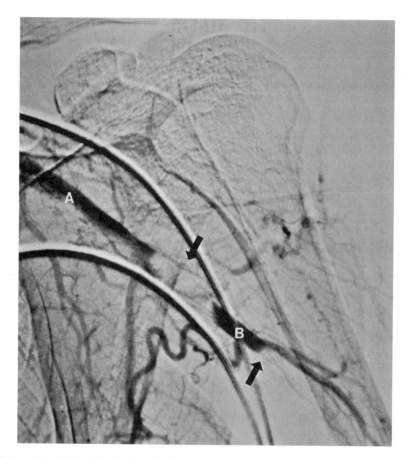

Figure 5A. Emboli occluding distal axillary artery (**A**) and proximal brachial artery (**B**).

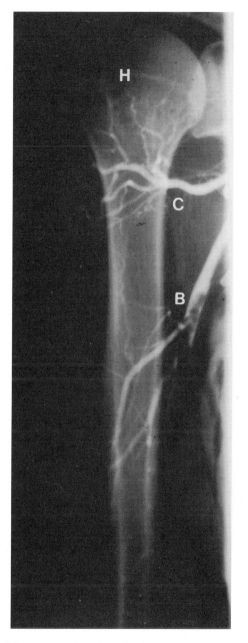

Figure 5B. Emboli from second portion of subclavian artery occluding the brachial artery (B). H indicates humeral head; C, circumflex humeral artery.

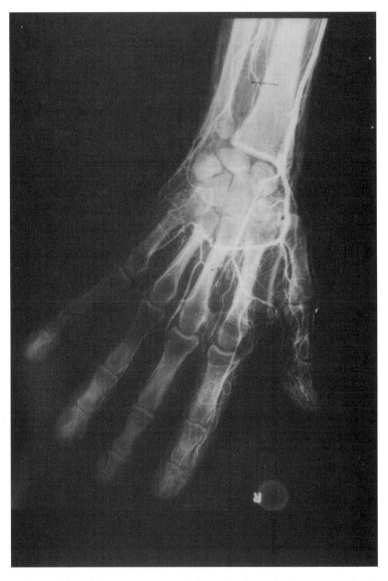

Figure 6A. Emboli from a proximal subclavian lesion, obstructing the distal ulnar artery and digital arteries on the ulnar side of the hand.

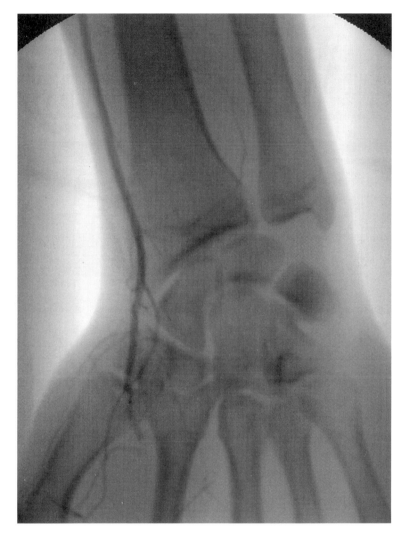

Figure 6B. Emboli from a circumflex humeral aneurysm in a young volleyball player, obstructing the ulnar artery and the distal portion of the radial artery. The sole presenting symptoms, from the lesion of the second portion of the axillary artery, were severe cold hypersensitivity of the hand and progressive Raynaud's phenomenon.

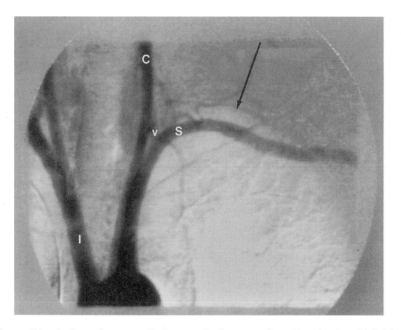

Figure 7A. Arch angiogram with the arm in the neutral position (at the side). Note the normal appearance of the subclavian artery. C indicates carotid; S, subclavian; I, innominate; V, vertebral.

with the arm in the neutral position and then with the arm place in abduction, at a right angle to the thorax. Failure to utilize stress positions will result in many false-negative or incomplete studies (Figures 7A and 7B).

Treatment

Treatment of these patients should be prompt surgical repair, to avoid progressive loss of the outflow vessels from repetitive embolization. Our standard approach has been removal of the first thoracic rib, to decompress the thoracic outlet and facilitate a normal anatomic reconstruction. When there is post-stenotic dilatation of the axillosubclavian artery, aneurysmal formation, or complete obstruction, resection, and direct repair or interposition graft will provide durable correction of the abnormality. In patients who have developed severe autonomic changes or reflex sympathetic dystrophy, cervicothoracic sympathectomy will provide additional relief of symptoms when coupled with vascular reconstruction.

Typical demographic and clinical characteristics of arterial compression at the thoracic outlet are illustrated by the following group of patients.

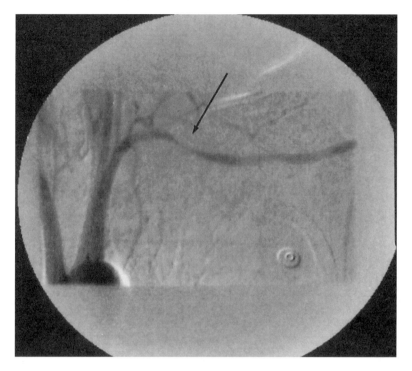

Figure 7B. Arch angiogram of the same patient in Figure 7A, with the left arm in abduction (arm extended). Note the area of compression at the second (retro-scalene) segment of the subclavian artery. In a tradesman who works with the arms in the overhead position, this abnormality can be restricting or disabling, and can lead to intimal arterial damage with embolization. When studying the upper extremity arterial system positional views can be critical to establishing the correct diagnosis.

Between 1984 and 1995, 23 patients were seen at the UCLA Medical Center, with acute symptoms of arterial occlusion or embolization, found to be originating from the axillosubclavian arterial segment.[10] The group comprised 14 females and 9 males, ranging from 15 to 74 years, with an average age of 37 years. There were 7 competitive athletes, 3 industrial workers, and 13 home, office, or service workers. The most severe present-ing symptoms, occurring alone or in combination, and ranked in order of frequency observed, were: arm claudication (74%); hand ischemia (48%); and digital gangrene (44%). Transaxillary thoracic outlet de-compression was undertaken in 22 cases. This was combined with arterial reconstruction in 8 cases and sympathectomy for ischemic causalgia in 7 cases. Transaxillary resection of a cervical rib was accomplished in 11 cases. There was 1 postoperative graft occlusion (PTFE), corrected by thrombectomy, with cumulative secondary patency (to 64 months), and 1 secondary embolic occlusion. Except for the 2 secondary procedures, no patient had recurrent symptoms at a mean follow-up of 61 months.

All of these patients were right-hand dominant. However, 13 presented with left-sided symptoms and 9 with right-sided symptoms. One patient had bilateral upper extremity ischemic symptoms presenting nonconcurrently. Arterial symptoms were associated with an abnormality of brachial pressure in 13 patients (57%), and an axillosubclavian artery bruit in thoracic outlet stress positions in 15 patients (65%). Eighteen patients had an absent radial or ulnar pulse in either the neutral or the abducted externally rotated (thoracic outlet stress) position. Digital plethysmography was abnormal in 13 patients (57%). Seven patients had typical symptoms of Raynaud's phenomenon.

Nine patients had symptoms of adjacent brachial plexus compression, identified by typical symptoms and/or confirmatory electrophysiological tests. These conduction abnormalities were identified among 11 cases with complete somatosensory evoked responses of median and ulnar nerves. In 9 cases, the somatosensory evoked responses were abnormal, indicting a level of compression consistent with brachial plexus injury. Three patients had evidence of muscle wasting in the intrinsic muscles of the hand.

Raynaud's symptoms are not uncommon in patients suffering from neurogenic thoracic outlet syndrome. These "vascular" symptoms result from intermittent compression of the inferior trunk of the brachial plexus, carrying the sympathetic innervation to the arm. This particular phenomenon, of autonomic instability associated with neurogenic thoracic outlet compression, frequently leads to referral for consultation with a vascular specialist. This group must be distinguished from those whose symptoms derive from a proximal arterial lesion. Most often, particularly when the symptoms are unilateral, arteriography is the only reliable test to rule out a primary arterial lesion.

None of these patients presenting with arterial compression developed a venous compressive or thrombotic abnormality characteristic of the Paget-Schroetter's syndrome. Nineteen of the patients had a prior evaluation for a rheumatologic or collagen vascular disease. All of these evaluations were negative, although several of the patients had begun corticosteroid therapy.

Six patients underwent initial thrombolytic therapy to restore arterial perfusion, prior to definitive surgical repair. Thrombolytic therapy enabled reversal of acute ischemia, particularly when related to embolic events to the distal circulation. This therapy was followed by anticoagulation in all cases, and facilitated a more meticulous work-up to identify the thromboembolic source. The additional diagnostic opportunity proved to be particularly valuable in two cases of circumflex humeral artery aneurysm with embolization (Figures 8A and 8B).[10,11]

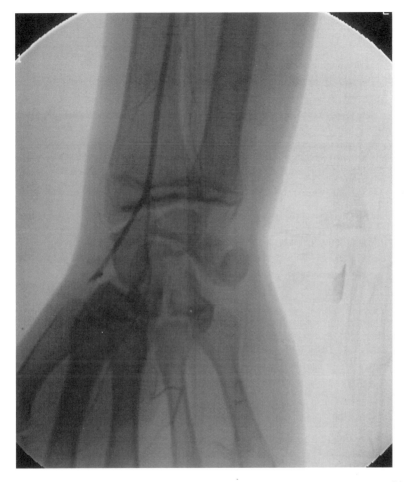

Figure 8A. Severe embolic ischemia from a proximal lesion in a young competitive athlete.

Twenty-two patients underwent transaxillary thoracic outlet decompression that included removal of the first thoracic rib. In 8 patients a cervical rib was also resected from the transaxillary approach. Concomitant arterial reconstruction was required in 11 patients and sympathectomy for ischemic causalgia was undertaken in 7 cases.

No primary obstructive or compressive abnormalities were encountered in the first portion of the subclavian artery. There were 3 patients with abnormalities in the second (retroscalene) portion of the subclavian. Thirteen patients had the abnormality involving the second and third portions of the subclavian, and 4 patients had the compressive or throm-

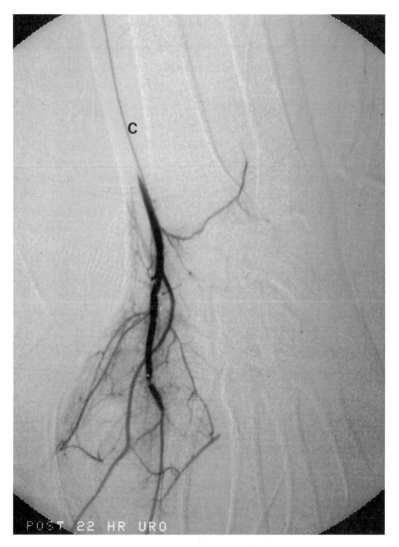

Figure 8B. Catheter-directed thrombolytic therapy prior to definitive repair of the proximal lesion. Preoperative or intraoperative thrombolytic therapy is very useful in cases of upper extremity embolic ischemia. Immediate- and long-term results are enhanced by restoring the arterial vascular bed. C indicates catheter.

botic abnormality confined to the third portion of the subclavian. There were no abnormalities of the first portion of the axillary artery. One patient had occlusion of the second portion of the axillary artery (behind the pectoralis minor tendon), and 2 patients had their arterial lesions in the third portion of the axillary artery. Both of these latter thromboembolic lesions originated at the humeral circumflex trunk. Of the 11 arterial repairs, 9 involved the second and third portions of the subclavian artery. In 4 of these cases, grafts originating in the subclavian terminated at the distal axillary or proximal brachial artery. There were two reconstructions of the axillary segments. One in the second and one in the third segment. This group of patients was under medical surveillance for an average period of 5.1 years.

In reviewing the results of our diagnostic and therapeutic strategies there were no surgical amputations, although one patient auto-amputated through the distal-phalanx of two fingers. There was one PTFE occlusion, corrected by thrombectomy with cumulative secondary patency (to 64 months). There was one embolic occlusion of a graft corrected by a secondary subclavian-carotid graft. Three athletes returned to professional competition. Two of four college athletes returned to intercollegiate competition. After the two secondary procedures, no patient had recurrent symptoms, at a mean follow-up of 61 months.

Both the clinical and radiographic presentation as well as the therapeutic considerations seem to be specific for the segment of the axillary or subclavian artery involved in the compressive abnormality. The following cases illustrate the salient diagnostic and clinical features. Each case is typical for a specific site of occlusion along the subclavian-axillary artery system.

Case 1 is that of a 38-year-old postal worker, which illustrates the consequence of compressive arterial injury, with thrombosis and retrograde propagation toward the innominate bifurcation.[5,13] After decompression of the thoracic outlet via transaxillary first rib resection, arterial continuity was reconstructed with a reversed saphenous vein graft from innominate bifurcation to the distal axillary artery. Placement of the graft in the anatomic location avoids the poor anatomic configuration of having the vein graft cross the clavicle. This would be prone to compression by something as simple as a brassiere strap, seat belt, or a mailbag shoulder strap. The graft remains patent, with normal segmental pressures and Duplex surveillance at 31 months postoperation (Figure 9).

Case 2 is that of a 51-year-old former ice skating champion and current coach and performer. Figure 10A illustrates the typical aneurysmal formation in the second and third portion of the subclavian artery, associated with a cervical rib. Figure 10B illustrates the occlusion that occurs when the arm is abducted and indicates the site of the compressive abnormality. The aneurysm is in reality more characteristic of an area of post-

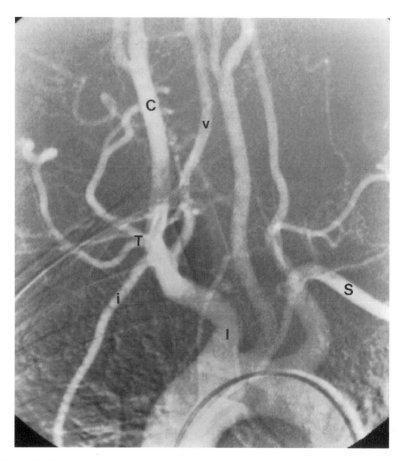

Figure 9. Occlusion of right subclavian artery, from compression in the third segment, with retrograde clot propagation to the bifurcation of the innominate artery. C indicates right common carotid; v, right vertebral; T, thyrocervical trunk; i, internal mammary; I, innominate; S, left subclavian.

stenotic dilatation. Occasionally laminated thrombus may obscure the aneurysmal dilatation. MRI can identify this area, if there is any question about the site or extent of the arterial abnormality. This lesion was repaired by transaxillary first rib resection and anatomic reconstruction using an interposition vein graft. The aneurysm in the MRI (seen in Figure 1A) was repaired by similar thoracic outlet decompression and primary re-anastomosis. Frequently, with removal of the first rib and cervical rib, the previously elevated subclavian artery has as a result considerable length, free of bony displacement. Consequently, resection and primary anastomosis is often possible.

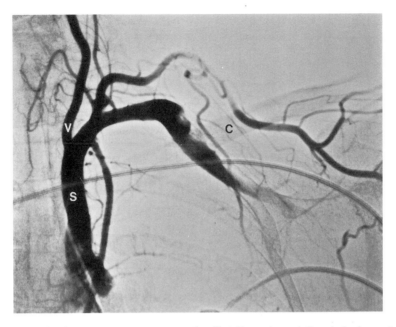

Figure 10A. Aneurysm or post-stentotic dilatation where left subclavian artery crosses a left cervical rib. S indicates subclavian artery; V, vertebral artery; C, clavicle.

Case 3 involves the mid-portion of the axillary artery, where it passes under the pectoralis minor tendon at the lateral aspect of the thoracic outlet. In this 28-year-old professional tennis player, rapid and sudden onset of arm fatigue was the only presenting symptom. The occlusion occurs in a typical location, beneath the pectoralis minor tendon as it inserts on the coracoid process.[14] To preserve the power of the overhand serve, the interposition vein graft was placed subcutaneously and continues to function without problem beyond 114 months. This procedure represented a departure from our customary intention, which was to place the graft in the anatomic position (Figures 11A through 11C).

Case 4 represents a characteristic arterial injury described in volleyball players and most recently in a major league baseball pitcher.[15] Although successfully treated with urokinase, the site of embolization was not initially identified. Emboli are evident in the distal vessels. However, neutral and stress views of the axillosubclavian artery segment reveal no site of compression or injury (Figure 12).

When restudied several weeks later (after the course of lytic therapy for the hand emboli and ischemia), the typical embolizing aneurysm of the posterior humeral circumflex artery was identified (Figures 13A and

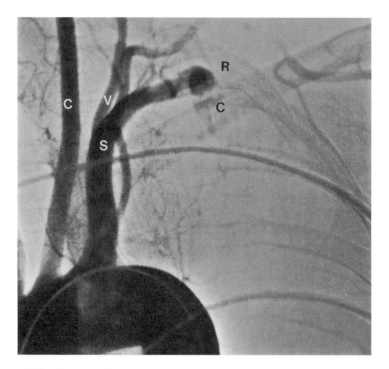

Figure 10B. Same patient as in Figure 10A with arm in the abducted position (out to side). Note the marked difference in appearance in the two positions, and the typical thoracic outlet compression-occlusion in "stress" position. (C indicates left common carotid; S, subclavian; V, vertebral; C, clavicle; R, cervical rib.) Subclavian artery is coursing over cervical rib and under clavicle.

13B).[16] The humeral head is supplied by the anterior branch of the common humeral circumflex and its occlusion or sacrifice is thought to lead to aseptic necrosis. This lesion was corrected, by excising the aneurysm and ligating the residual posterior humeral circumflex. Because the aneurysm involved the distal portion of the common humeral circumflex as well, this artery was repaired and bypassed to the anterior humeral circumflex with a cephalic vein graft. The patient returned to competitive play in 8 weeks.

We have differed from the transaxillary surgical approach utilized by Durham et al.[6] Our technique of placing the incision along the lateral border of the pectoralis major muscle at its humeral insertion serves to orient the exposure directly over the quadrilateral space. The common humeral circumflex and its accompanying axillary nerve are easily identified and dissected from the surrounding tissue.

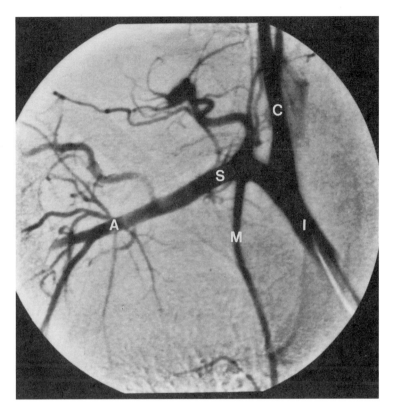

Figure 11A. Innominate arteriogram showing normal subclavian artery, and occlusion of the second segment of the axillary artery (beneath the pectoralis minor tendon). This is a primary compressive lesion at the site, and not the consequence of embolization. C indicates common carotid artery; I, innominate artery; S, subclavian artery; M, internal mammary artery; A, first segment of axillary artery.

Venous compression was not identified in this group of patients, even though we have had extensive experience with the Paget-Schroetter variant of thoracic outlet compression syndrome.[17]

Although cervical rib is most often thought to be the most common identified anomaly in arterial injury at the thoracic outlet, it was present in only 8 (35%) of our cases. Additionally, only 1 patient had arterial thrombosis as a possible result of a chronologically remote clavicular fracture. This emphasizes the importance of soft tissue abnormalities in the etiology of these ischemic compressive injuries, also pointed out by Durham et al.[6]

The most characteristic finding in this group of patients is the unilaterality of ischemic, or Raynaud's symptoms. Absent pulses, abnormal

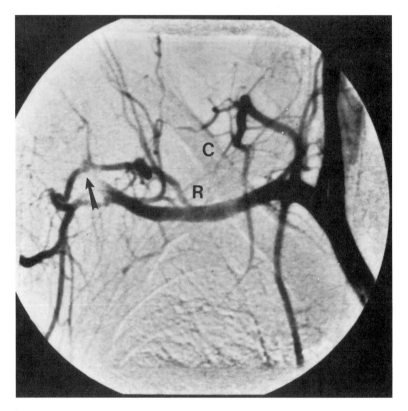

Figure 11B. Angiogram repeated with arm abducted. The radiologist is performing a complete examination to rule out the possibility of a more proximal lesion. Subclavian lesions are occasionally seen only when the arm is placed in the abducted position. The arrow indicates the position of the pectoralis minor tendon, as it courses to insert on the coracoid process. C indicates clavicle; R, first thoracic rib.

Doppler segmental pressures, and abnormalities of digital plethysmography all helped substantiate the diagnosis. Arteriography is invaluable for identification of the site of compressive injury and is essential for proper therapy, particularly if arterial bypass or reconstruction is indicated.

Summary

Recognition of the cumulative trauma arterial injuries in the region of the thoracic outlet requires a high index of suspicion, particularly when

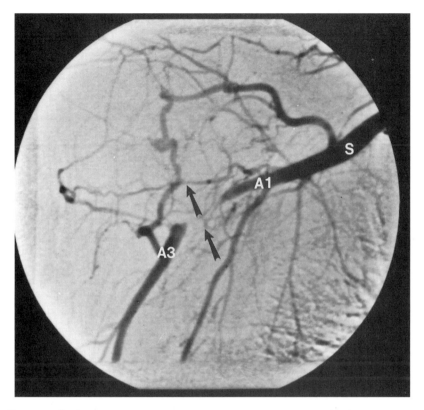

Figure 11C. The area of compressive occlusion and associated collateral vessels is best seen on this axillosubclavian arteriogram. The position of the pectoralis minor is indicated by the arrows. A1 indicates first portion of axillary artery; A3, third portion of axillary artery; S, subclavian artery.

faced with a patient with unilateral ischemic symptoms. The most common pitfall is ascribing these symptoms to a systemic collagen vascular, autoimmune, or vasospastic disorder. The apparent insidious onset of the ischemic events, in the absence of a striking history of trauma, is as characteristic as it is confusing. Nevertheless, the clinical evaluation is very helpful, particularly pulse assessment and auscultation for bruits in the neutral and the thoracic outlet stress positions. Segmental Doppler pressures and digital plethysmography, in neutral and stress positions, represent the most reliable noninvasive test assessments. Angiography in the neutral and in the abducted externally rotated position is essential, to avoid overlooking the occasionally subtle changes in the axillosubclavian

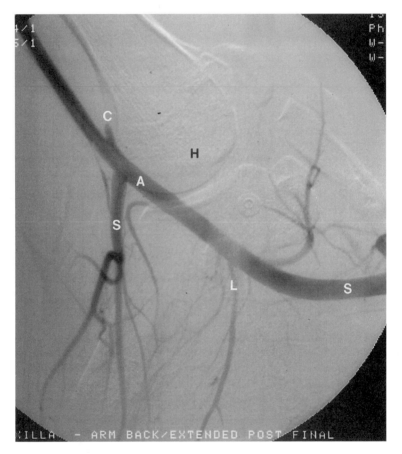

Figure 12. Axillosubclavian arteriogram in the stress position. The angiogram was interpreted as being entirely normal. No embolizing lesion was identified in this young patient with multiple emboli in the radial, ulnar, and digital arteries. No abnormality was recognized in the humeral circumflex artery. S indicates subclavian; L, lateral thoracic; A, axillary; S, subscapular; C, stump of common humeral circumflex; H, humeral head.

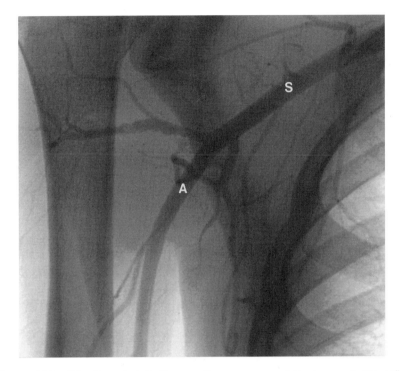

Figure 13A. After thrombolytic therapy the aneurysm of the humeral circumflex artery is evident. S indicates subclavian; A, axillary.

arterial segment. When that segment is uninvolved, the branches, particularly circumflex humeral, must be carefully reviewed.

Effective and durable correction of the axillosubclavian arterial compressive abnormalities requires adequate thoracic outlet decompression, and anatomic vascular reconstruction when necessary. Removal of the first rib is key to adequate decompression in most cases, and can be accomplished via the transaxillary or transcervical approach. Preoperative catheter-directed thrombolytic therapy is very useful, to clear distal emboli that have the potential for compromising the final result. This technique is superior to catheter embolectomy, in these highly vasoreactive upper extremity vessels. Dealing with the initial ischemia in this manner, then proceeding with elective decompression and arterial repair, remains a very effective strategy in our setting (Figures 8A and 8B).

Failed prior procedures that we have seen in our vascular consultative service were most often a consequence of inaccurate diagnosis, failure to identify and correct the proximal embolizing arterial lesion, or inadequate

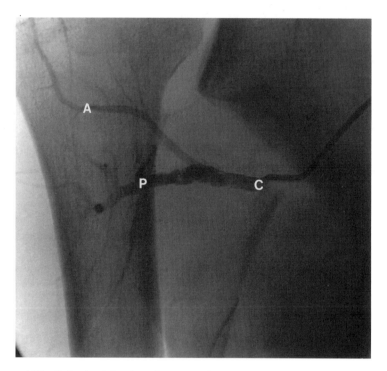

Figure 13B. Selective injection of common humeral circumflex, showing the aneurysm involving the common humeral bifurcation and the posterior branch. This was repaired with excision and an interposition vein graft. C indicates common humeral circumflex artery; A, anterior division; P, posterior division.

decompression. Unilateral Raynaud's symptoms require meticulous investigation for arterial compression at the thoracic outlet with careful interpretation of subtle angiographic findings.

References

1. Telford ED, Stopford JSB: The vascular compression of cervical rib. *Br J Surg* 18:557, 1931.
2. Falconer MA, Weddell G: Costoclavicular compression of the subclavian artery and vein: Relation to the scalenus anticus syndrome. *Lancet* 2:539–544, 1943.
3. Coote H: Exostosis of the left transverse process of the seventh cervical vertebrae, surrounded by blood vessels and nerves, successful removal. *Lancet* 1: 360–361, 1861.
4. Robb CG, Standeven A: Arterial occlusion complicating thoracic outlet compression syndrome. *Br Med J* 2:709–19, 1958.

5. Cormier JM, Amrane M, Ward A, et al: Arterial complications of the thoracic outlet syndrome: Fifty-five operative cases. *J Vasc Surg* 9:778–87, 1989.
6. Durham JR, Yao JST, Pearce WH, et al: Arterial injuries in the thoracic outlet syndrome. *J Vasc Surg* 21:57–70, 1995.
7. Makhoul RG, Machleder HI: Developmental anomalies at the thoracic outlet: An analysis of 200 consecutive cases. *J Vasc Surg* 16:534–45, 1992.
8. Kieffer E, Jeudenis P, Benhamou M, et al: Complications arterielles du syndrome de la traversee thoraco-brachiale. Traitement cirurgical de 38 cases. *Chirurgie* 109:714–22, 1983.
9. Nehler MR, Taylor LM, Moneta GL, Porter JM: Upper extremity ischemia from subclavian artery aneurysm caused by bony abnormalities of the thoracic outlet. *Arch Surg* 132:527–532, 1997.
10. Gelabert HA, Machleder HI: Diagnosis and management of arterial compression at the thoracic outlet. *Ann Vasc Surg* 11:359–366, 1997.
11. Michaels JA, Torrie EPH, Galland RB: The treatment of upper limb vascular occlusions using intraarterial thrombolysis. *Eur J Vasc Surg* 7:744–746, 1993.
12. Fields WS, Lemak NA, Ben-Menachem Y: Thoracic outlet syndrome: Review and reference to stroke in a major league pitcher. *AJNR* 7:73–78, 1986.
13. Machleder HI: Thoracic outlet compression syndrome: New concepts from a century of discovery. *Cardiovasc Surg* 2:137–45, 1994.
14. Finkelstein JA, Johnston KW: Thrombosis of the axillary artery secondary to compression by the pectoralis minor muscle. *Ann Vasc Surg* 7:287–90, 1993.
15. Reekers JA, den Hartog BMG, Kuyper CF, et al: Traumatic aneurysm of the posterior circumflex humeral artery: A volleyball player's disease? *J Vasc Interv Radiol* 4:405–408, 1993.
16. Nijhuis HA, Muller-Wiefel H: Occlusion of the brachial artery by thrombus dislodged from a traumatic aneurysm of the anterior humeral circumflex artery. *J Vasc Surg* 13:408–411, 1991.
17. Machleder HI: Evaluation of a new treatment strategy for Paget-Schroetter's syndrome. *J Vasc Surg* 17:305–17, 1993.

10

Venous Compression at the Thoracic Outlet

Herbert I. Machleder, MD

The Paget-Schroetter Variant of Thoracic Outlet Compression

Spontaneous or effort-related thrombosis of the axillosubclavian vein is a disabling thoracic outlet disorder affecting young, otherwise healthy individuals. The first two cases were published independently over 100 years ago by Paget in England and Von Schroetter in Germany. In 1949, Hughes[1] analyzed 320 cases of spontaneous upper-extremity venous thrombosis collected from the medical literature, and recognized that this represented a unique disorder by naming the entity the Paget-Schroetter's syndrome.

At the time of Hughes' report, the primary therapy was surgical thrombectomy in an attempt to restore normal upper extremity venous hemodynamics. In fact, despite increasing recognition of early rethrombosis, primary surgical therapy remained the standard approach until the early 1980s when techniques for local catheter-directed thrombolytic therapy were popularized (Figures 1A through 1C).

A number of authors had studied and reported on the natural history of the disorder, providing a yardstick against which therapeutic advances could be measured. Untreated patients with Paget-Schroetter's syndrome can be expected to have varying degrees of disability as a consequence of chronic venous hypertension and/or recurrent episodes of venous thrombosis. This disability incidence ranges from a low of 25% reported by Linblad from Sweden, 40% reported by Gloviczki from the Mayo Clinic, to 47% reported by Donayre and 74% by Tilney.[2,3] In addition, there is a small incidence of pulmonary embolism.[4] Upper extremity venous throm-

---

From Machleder HI, (ed): *Vascular Disorders of the Upper Extremity*. Third Revised Edition. Futura Publishing Company, Inc., Armonk, NY, © 1998.

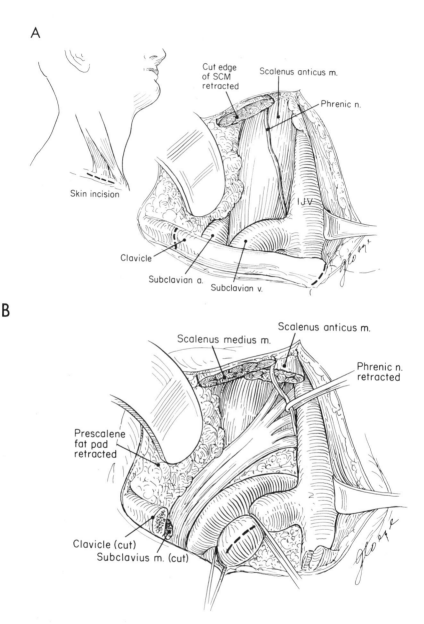

Figure 1. A, B, C: Technique of subclavian venous thrombectomy, used frequently prior to the successful development of catheter directed thrombolytic therapy. (Reproduced from Machleder HI: *Current Problems in Surgery: Vaso-occlusive Disorders of the Upper Extremity.* Volume 25. Year Book Medical Publishers Inc., 1988.)

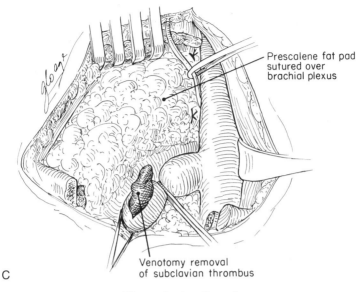

Prescalene fat pad
sutured over
brachial plexus

Venotomy removal
of subclavian thrombus

C

Figure 1. *(continued)*

bosis is estimated to account for 11 cases/100,000 hospital admissions, or approximately 2% of deep venous thrombosis.[5,6]

The underlying cause of Paget-Schroetter's syndrome is now recognized to be a mechanical abnormality at the costoclavicular portion of the axillosubclavian vein, with superimposed thrombosis resulting in the complexity of the clinical manifestations. The acute thrombosis is almost invariably in an area of chronic compression and stricture of the axillosubclavian vein at the thoracic outlet. The vein is compressed between a hypertrophied scalene or subclavius tendon and the first rib. A large exostosis is often found at the costoclavicular junction (Figures 2A through 2C).

Presenting History and Physical Signs

Patients who are very often tradesmen or competitive athletes suddenly notice severe and uniform swelling of one upper extremity. This usually occurs in the absence of any recognizable trauma. In addition to edema, the arm will have a slight rubor or cyanosis, often erroneously suggesting a cellulitis but without fever or any other systemic signs or symptoms. The patient may notice prominence of the upper extremity veins or be aware of collateral veins appearing around the shoulder or

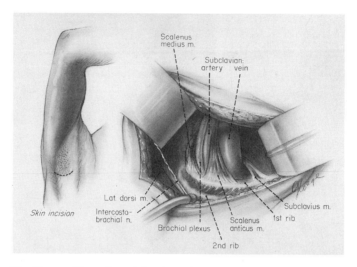

Figure 2A. Transaxillary view of the thoracic outlet. Note the relation of the neuro-vascular structures, first thoracic rib, and subclavius tendon. The subclavian vein traverses the costoclavicular space between the anterior scalene muscle and subclavius tendon.

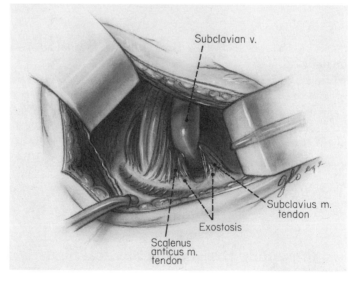

Figure 2B. Typical abnormality seen in the Paget-Schroetter's syndrome of primary axillosubclavian vein thrombosis. In tradesmen, athletes, and others who use the upper extremity in a vigorous manner, there is often hypertrophy of the subclavius muscle and development of an exostosis at the tendinous insertion at junction of first rib and sternum. There is additionally an associated hypertrophy of the anterior scalene and its insertion in Lisfranc's tubercle. Note the abnormality as seen from this transaxillary approach, and compare that with the radiological appearances of the vein seen elsewhere in this chapter (Figures 4C, 11E).

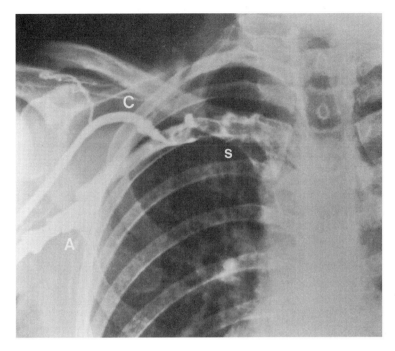

Figure 2C. Very early subclavian thrombus formation in a patient with Paget-Schroetter syndrome. Note dye outlining thrombus in the thoracic outlet portion of the vein. s indicates subclavian vein; C, cephalic vein; A, axillary vein.

lateral pectoral region. Ordinarily there is minimal pain except in the axilla where pain and tenderness may occur over the course of the axillary vein.

If untreated, the swelling will often resolve in a few days to several weeks and the patient will be remarkably asymptomatic at rest. Symptoms of swelling, tightness, heaviness, and easy fatigue, occasionally associated with vasomotor changes of pallor and sweating, will occur with various levels of upper extremity activity. These symptoms are particularly exacerbated in warm weather or other situation stimulating vasodilation in the upper trunk and arms.

A group of 50 consecutive patients studied at UCLA provides an accurate description of the contemporary demographic characteristics in this disorder. There were 31 men with a mean age of 24 years and a range of 14 to 50 years, and 19 women with a mean age of 38 and a range of 23 to 51 years. The women as a group are significantly older ($P < 0.0001$). Forty-seven (94%) of these patients were right-hand dominant and in 33 patients (66%) the dominant hand was the symptomatic side.

All but 1 of the men had been engaged in vigorous physical activity at the time of the episode of swelling and cyanosis, including 10 who were student athletes. Eleven women were engaged in relatively sedentary occupations, while 8 were working in activities involving upper extremity effort. This included 3 who were student athletes. (The student athletes included 5 weight lifters; 3 baseball players; 2 swimmers; and 1 each tennis, volleyball, and rowing crew competitors.) As a group then, 38 (76%) of the patients had the episode associated with effort and 12 (24%) were sedentary. As a good characterization of their customary activities, 15 patients were engaged in competitive sports, 18 were laborers, and 17 were white-collar workers.

The physical examination will vary depending on the interval between occurrence and examination. In patients who have had an acute episode of thrombosis, the characteristics outlined above will be readily evident to the examiner. In patients who have an established thrombus with collateral venous development there may be surprisingly few physical findings during the interval periods, and the examiner may need to examine the patient after exercise. A series of push-ups, particularly in a warm room, will often disclose the underlying difference between the two arms. The edema may be quite minimal under these circumstances, although a general duskiness will be evident as well as increased prominence of the collateral veins. With further exercise the patient will often complain of pain in the collateral veins particularly in the supraclavicular, pectoral, or axillary regions. In addition, these veins may be tender. However, the rapid resolution after rest will discount the impression of phlebitis.

It should be recognized that a tradesperson will normally have an 1- to 1.5-cm increase in circumference at the biceps in the dominant compared with the nondominant arm, and a 0.5- to 1-cm asymmetry at the forearm. Measurements, if made, should be done before and after exercise.

Because of extensive and progressive collateral development, the disparity between symptoms and signs will increase with time. However, in most patients, the resistance in the collaterals will be such that symptoms will almost invariably increase with increasing work of the arm.

In a remarkably similar characteristic to patients with other forms of thoracic outlet compression syndrome, these individuals will complain of severe exacerbation when the arm is used in the outstretched or overhead position. This position will lead to rapid fatigue and typical dysesthesias in the C8-T1 dermatomal distribution. Signs of sympathetic hyperreactivity will also be present to a variable degree, although true causalgia is very uncommon in this disorder.

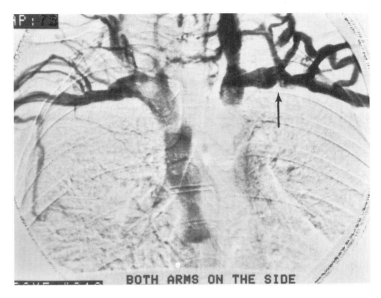

Figure 3A. Bilateral axillosubclavian venogram in a patient having recurrent episodes of upper extremity edema, and a remote episode of axillosubclavian vein thrombosis. With arms in the neutral position (at the side) there is suspicion of some restrictive problem, as evidenced by the extensive supraclavicular collateral vein development. The exact etiology and/or underlying abnormality is obscure although the arrow denotes a possible site of compression or stricture.

Diagnosis

Patients presenting with a swollen arm, without an obvious etiology such as cellulitis, insect bite, trauma, etc., should undergo axillosubclavian venography. Venography is preferentially performed in two supine positions; with the arm at the patient's side and with the humerus at right angles to the chest wall. Unfortunately, duplex ultrasound scanning and magnetic resonance angiography are reported to be inaccurate for venous assessment in the area of the retroclavicular space (Figures 3A and 3B).[7–9]

Thrombolytic and Anticoagulant Therapy

Immediately after verification of the diagnosis, patients should be treated by catheter-directed fibrinolytic therapy into the thrombus, when this is available. Heparin is administered concomitantly and continued until therapeutic anticoagulation with coumadin (warfarin sodium) can

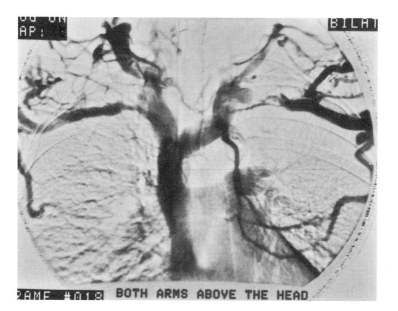

Figure 3B. With arms in the abducted position the compressive abnormality is particularly evident at the left costoclavicular space (thoracic outlet). Note additionally the new appearance of chest collaterals, as the thoracic outlet collaterals are compressed in the abducted position.

be accomplished.[10,11] Although streptokinase had been used successfully in axillosubclavian vein thrombosis, much of the prior reported experience suggested the superiority of urokinase for this disorder: consequently the later drug is generally considered to be the preferred agent (Figures 4A through 4C).[12-14]

This approach is based on the effectiveness of thrombolytic therapy as reported by Zimmerman in 1981.[15] Subsequent case reports by Taylor et al[16] then Perler and Mitchel[17] added surgical treatment of the underlying anatomic abnormality and the use of selective transluminal angioplasty to this new therapeutic design.

In 1989, Kunkle and Machleder[18] reported the results of a definitive, staged, multidisciplinary approach to the problem that had been initiated at UCLA. The results of this approach in a series of 50 consecutive patients was published in 1993[19] (Figures 5 and 6).

To avoid rethrombosis, surgical therapy is delayed after successful thrombolysis and anticoagulation. Drawing from experience with lower extremity venous thrombosis and studies of upper extremity venous endothelium, a 1- to 3-month period of anticoagulation with coumadin is preferable prior to definitive treatment of the underlying structural abnormality.[20] As radiologists have become more skilled with catheter-directed

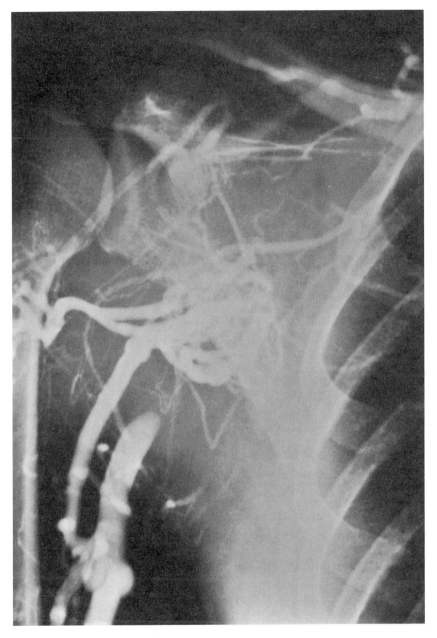

Figure 4A. A right axillary-subclavian venogram via the basilic vein approach in a 24-year-old woman with spontaneous edema and cyanosis of the right hand and arm.

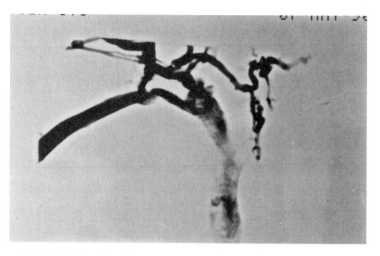

Figure 4B. A digital subtraction venogram is performed, after clot lysis with catheter-directed urokinase. This film, done in the neutral position (with the arm at the side), shows an area of venous compression at the thoracic outlet. Note the prominent collateral veins around the narrowed region.

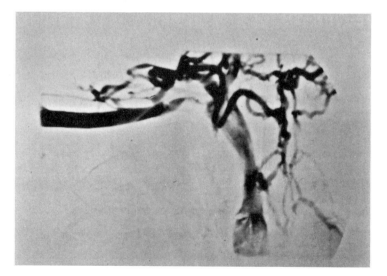

Figure 4C. A venogram obtained with the arm in the outstretched position (abducted) shows high-grade compression at the thoracic outlet compared with the compression demonstrated with the arm in the neutral position. (Reproduced with permission from Machleder HI: Upper extremity venous thrombosis. *Semin Vasc Surg* 3:221, 1990.)

**Management of Suspected Thrombosis
of the Axillosubclavian Vein**

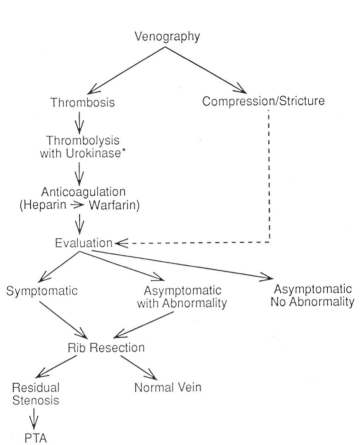

Figure 5. Algorithm for the management of primary axillosubclavian vein thrombosis.

lytic therapy, we have recognized reduced intimal injury to the vein segments and more rapid lysis of the thrombus. Our current practice is to delay definitive surgical correction for 4 weeks, during which time we protect the damaged segment of the axillosubclavian venous segment with therapeutic anticoagulation with coumadin.

Although initial thrombolytic therapy and the staged approach has been gaining wider acceptance, there remain proponents of early surgical thrombectomy as well as initial surgical repair.[21,22] Nevertheless, surgical intervention at the time when the vein is most thrombogenic has consider-

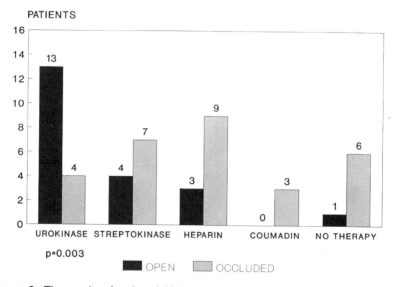

PATIENTS

Figure 6. The results of various initial treatment strategies. Catheter-directed lytic therapy with urokinase seems to give the best results in restoring patency. The age of the thrombus at the time of therapy appears to be the only significant variable affecting successful lysis.

able theoretical disadvantages. This variation on the staged approach remains to be validated by appropriate follow-up studies.[23–25] Several authors have additionally suggested treating the thrombotic process alone without addressing the underlying anatomic abnormality. The rational for this approach is neither supported by these authors' published data nor by our own experience (Figure 7).[26]

It must be appreciated that there are substantial differences between the spontaneous, effort-related axillosubclavian vein thrombosis, and the secondary thrombosis which results from indwelling lines and other iatrogenic trauma. A number of studies have documented these essential differences in pathophysiology and outcome.[27–29] Cases of secondary thrombosis are multifactorial and generalizations regarding therapy are hazardous.[30,31]

Surgical Treatment

Surgical treatment is recommended if: (1) an underlying compressive abnormality is demonstrated venographically after restoration of vein patency or (2) if symptomatic patients with an occluded vein demonstrated obstruction of the venous collaterals with abduction of the arm.

PATIENTS

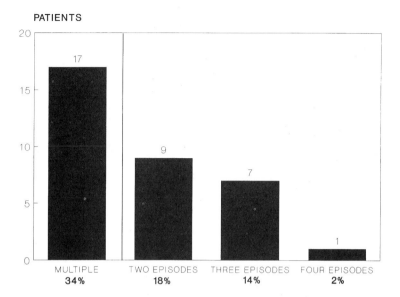

Figure 7. Incidence of venographically documented rethrombosis of the axillosub-clavian vein, when lytic therapy is used as definitive therapy without surgical decompression of the thoracic outlet.

Transaxillary first rib resection is considered the procedure of choice in this situation, based on the extensive literature documenting long-term results, effectiveness of decompression, and the excellent anatomic visualization of the area (Figures 8A and 8B).[32,33]

Postoperative transluminal angioplasty can be used when the subclavian vein does not return to a normal configuration, ie, if a residual stricture is demonstrated on postoperative venogram. The continued presence of collateral venous channels after operation, generally signifies that the stricture is hemodynamically significant.

Recurrent episodes of thrombosis characterize this group of patients, if the underlying anatomic abnormality is not corrected. Prior to definitive therapy, 34% had multiple venographically verified recurrent episodes of thrombosis (Figure 7).

The contralateral vein was studied venographically in 34 patients (68%). Five of these patients (15%) had an episode of thrombosis of the contralateral axillosubclavian vein and 18 (53%) had evidence of 50% or greater diameter compression. The vein was normal in 11 patients and not studied in 16 patients. One patient had a clinically diagnosed and angiographically proven pulmonary embolus associated with the initial thrombotic event.

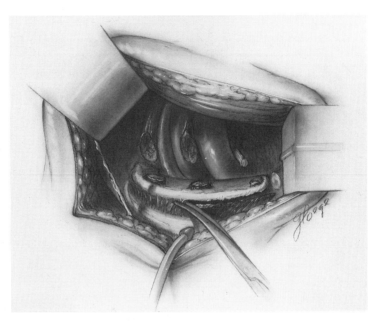

Figure 8A. Removal of the first thoracic rib via the transaxillary approach. The subclavius tendon and the insertion of the anterior and middle scalene muscles has been divided.

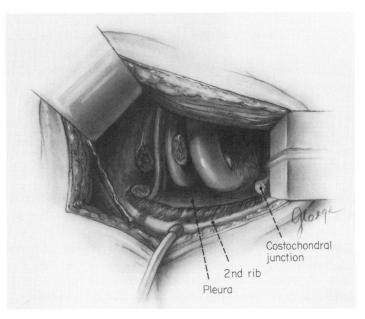

Figure 8B. After removal of the first rib, and lysis of surrounding reactive tissue and adhesions, there is excellent decompression of the axillosubclavian vein.

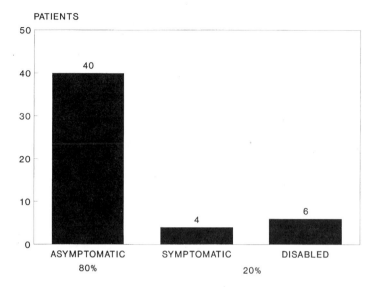

Figure 9. Final clinical result in 50 consecutive patients, treated according to the published algorithm.

Results of Treatment

At the time of final clinical evaluation 88% of the patients had resumed their usual occupations and full activity. Forty patients (80%) were either completely asymptomatic (31) or had minimal symptoms (9). Ten patients (20%) were symptomatic (4 working, but with symptoms, and 6 disabled for their usual occupations). Nine of the 10 symptomatic patients were laborers, and these 9 represented 50% (9/18) of that working group. This was a significantly higher percentage of symptomatic patients than in the athlete or white-collar worker groups (1/32 or 3%, $P = 0.0002$) (Figure 9).

In a final analysis of results, patients who underwent first rib resection had a significantly higher percentage of patent veins at the conclusion of the study than those not treated surgically ($P = 0.05$). The objectives for correcting the underlying disorder are: (1) relief of the venous hypertension; (2) correction of compression of both the axillary-subclavian and the collateral veins; and (3) prevention of further episodes of thrombosis.

These objectives have been achieved with first rib and subclavius tendon resection. After surgical decompression of the costoclavicular space, no patient experienced a recurrent episode of thrombosis. Viewed

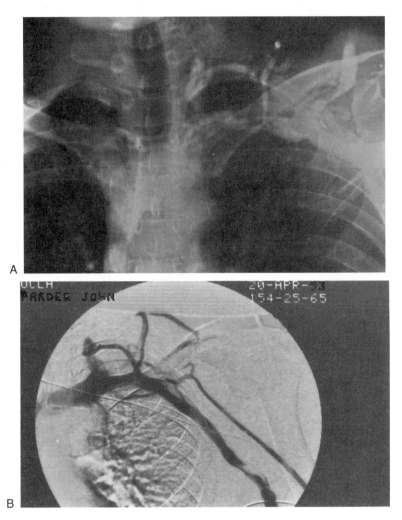

Figure 10. A: Thirty-year-old stone mason with presumably chronic axillosubclavian vein thrombosis. Lytic therapy was unsuccessful. The patient underwent first rib resection to relieve compression of the collateral veins. He subsequently returned to work. **B:** Re-evaluation, including venography, after 3 years shows recanalization of the vein. The caliber is relatively normal. Several collateral veins persist. In contradistinction to previously held beliefs, recanalization occurs fairly regularly and is enhanced by thoracic outlet decompression. Additionally, rethrombosis has not occurred in patients followed long-term after surgical decompression.

from another perspective, 29 of 35 patients (83%) who underwent transaxillary first rib resection were asymptomatic at the conclusion of the study. Twenty-two of these had a patent and normal appearing vein with 13 patients having residual occlusion. The three patients who remained symptomatic postoperatively all had residual venous occlusion.

The most significant determinant of ultimate vein patency was establishment of patency at the outset with medical therapy (P = 0.0003). Nevertheless, recanalization has been observed, even in chronically occluded veins, when the external compression is relieved (Figures 10A and 10B).

In the group of patients who remained symptomatic or disabled, there was a significantly higher incidence of contralateral vein occlusion (P = 0.05), or inability to open the ipsilateral vein by initial medical therapy (P = 0.03). Of 35 patients who underwent first rib resection, 30 (86%) were essentially symptom-free (25 completely, 5 with minimal symptoms) and engaged in unrestricted normal activity. Five patients had residual symptoms and 2 of these remained disabled for their usual occupations.

Angioplasty

Twenty-one patients underwent percutaneous balloon venoplasty. Twelve were done *preoperatively* after successful thrombolytic therapy, with 7 veins occluding immediately after the procedure. The 5 uncomplicated preoperative balloon angioplasties had no effect on the extrinsic compressive abnormality. With long-term follow-up, 3 of the occluded veins had restoration of patency postoperatively, with 4 remaining occluded. The failure of preoperative balloon angioplasty had a significantly adverse association with long-term patency of the vein (P = 0.02). Conversely, in patients with uncomplicated balloon angioplasty after successful thrombolysis, there was no additional benefit in terms of long-term patency over those veins treated with thrombolytic therapy alone (P = 0.99) (Figures 11A through 11E).

Nine angioplasties were attempted *postoperatively* for residual stricture. Of 7 immediately successful cases, 1 required redilation due to an inadequate initial result with an undersized balloon. The remainder were uncomplicated. At long-term venographic follow-up (of the entire group of postoperative venoplasties), 2 remained occluded, and 7 were patent. In this situation, simple balloon angioplasty performed postoperatively, proved to be much more durable than that reported for other venous strictures.[34]

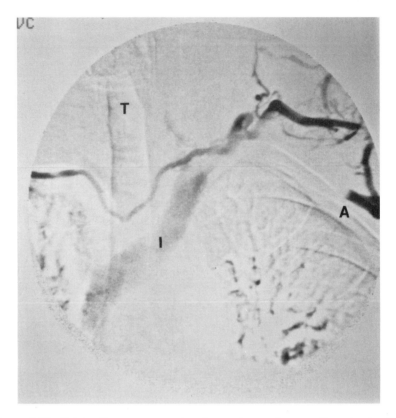

Figure 11A. Subtraction venogram showing acute spontaneous thrombosis of the left axillosubclavian vein. Several collateral veins are already evident. T indicates trachea; I, innominate vein; A, axillary vein.

Stenting

We have avoided using stents in the retroclavicular portion of the axillosubclavian vein. If the first rib and clavicle are intact, then the stent rapidly becomes deformed, fractured and compressed between the bony structures. This becomes evident as soon as the patient begins to use the arm in a relatively normal manner. Even after surgical decompression, the range of movement as well as the musculotendinous elements at the thoracic outlet, lead to almost inevitable stent deformity and thrombosis. This consequence has been well documented by Meier et al, although there has been limited success in stenting strictures due to intrinsic vein damage in arteriovenous dialysis access fistulas.[35,36]

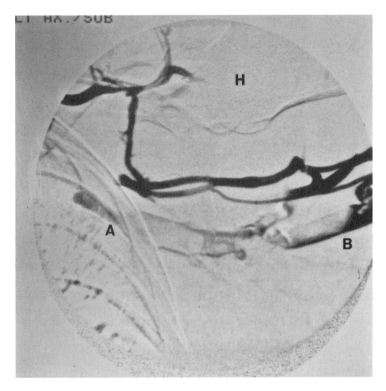

Figure 11B. Thrombus extends into the axillobrachial segment. H indicates humerus; A, axillary vein; B, brachial vein.

Jugular Subclavian Bypass

In cases where there has been irremedial damage to the subclavian vein, and there are persistent symptoms of venous hypertension, a jugular-subclavian bypass can be performed. Durability of this veno-venous bypass is enhanced by construction of a small arteriovenous fistula just distal to the anastomosis.[37,38] Although other reconstructive techniques have been described, the efficacy remains to be established.[39]

Typical Clinical Presentations

Recently, Machleder[40] described a group of 76 consecutive patients presenting to the UCLA Medical Center for treatment of acute spontaneous axillosubclavian vein thrombosis. An analysis of these cases indi-

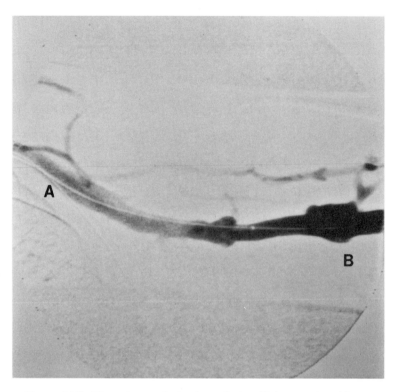

Figure 11C. Thrombus entirely cleared after 12 hours of urokinase.

cates the spectrum of demographic settings, and the range of decisions that need to be individualized for recurring distinctive clinical patterns.

In classifying the major daily activities of this population: 21 were professional or student athletes; 21 were laborers; and 34 were what would be considered white-collar workers. Seven of these patients were engaged in sedentary activity at the onset of thrombosis, and 69 were directly engaged in some vigorous upper extremity activity just prior to the onset of edema and cyanosis. In further characterizing their usual daily activities, 19 would be considered relatively sedentary individuals, with the remaining 57 leading very active lives. Thirty-two were avid recreational athletes. Five were weight lifters and 3 were rowers. There were 2 basketball players, baseball players, skiiers, swimmers, and aerobic exercisers. There was 1 representative of each of the following sports: gynmastics, jogging, cycling, golfing, handball, boxing, soccer, tennis, vollyball, and wrestling.

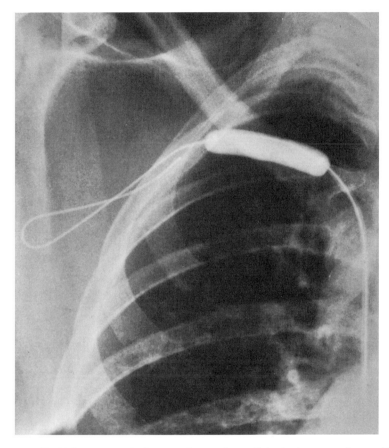

Figure 11D. Using a 1-cm balloon catheter, the radiologist is attempting to dilate the compressed segment, mistakenly thinking that this is a stricture.

Subgroups

Perhaps the most common situation is the young student athlete with sudden swelling of the upper extremity. This group probably demonstrates the most straightfoward therapeutic approach. We have treated 17 student athletes, the average age of the 14 boys being 18 years and the 3 girls, 21 years.

Among the young men there were 4 baseball players, 2 basketball players, 2 rowers, 1 swimmer, and 5 weight lifters. Of the young women 2 were competitive swimmers and 1 rowed crew. The presentation of sudden edema and cyanosis is characteristic, with patients appearing ex-

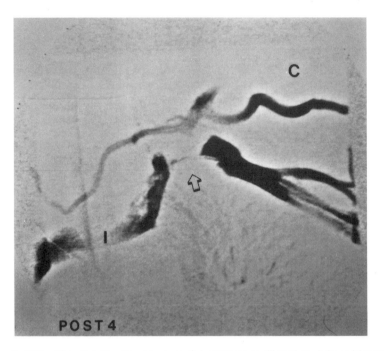

Figure 11E. After the fourth unsuccessful attempt at dilatation, it is evident that although the balloon can be inflated, the elastic recoil of the externally compressing musculotendinous structures cannot be reversed by stretching. The segment rapidly underwent rethrombosis. The disaster is only compounded by the occasional misguided attempt to stent the segment. At the current state of our knowledge about the problem, surgical decompression is the only reliable method to maintain the venous patency and restore normal venous hemodynamics.

peditiously for treatment. Clot lysis is usually prompt, within 24 hours, and the vein appears quite satisfactory in the neutral position. Venography in the stress position demonstrates the site of the compressive abnormality. Surgical repair is usually delayed for 4 weeks while the patient remains on dicumarol.

The Chronic Thrombus

There is a subgroup of individuals, usually somewhat older, who appear to have a chronic thrombus that resists lysis. Initially it was perplexing to us attempting to explain the sudden onset of edema. After studying several patients repetitively during acute exacerbations of edema, it became evident that older individuals can develop chronic fibrosis in the area of compression, often with a small attached chronic thrombus. Collateral venous circulation develops over a period of time and results in only minimal transient symptoms during vigorous activity. These episodes are often overlooked by the patient. On unexpected occasions the area destabilizes and the thrombus propagates, blocking the collateral veins which are often in close proximity to the compressed area. With thrombus propagation, and obstruction of collaterals, the arm becomes edematous and swollen. With rapid sequential studies we have seen spontaneous clot lysis and return to baseline in two patients.

In patients who do not experience spontaneous remission, the initial lytic therapy dissolves the new thrombus, revealing the well-developed collateral veins and the usually very discrete area of chronic thrombus. Unfortunately, these patients remain at risk of recurrent events and we have seen the vein recanalize and respond to transluminal dilatation after surgical decompression. We have observed 30 patients with residual chronic occlusions of the subclavian vein. Four of these patients remained relatively asymptomatic and nondisabled for their usual occupation. We have recommended no further therapy. Nine of these patients continue to be symptomatic and may yet benefit from a surgical approach. We have proceeded with thoracic outlet decompression in 17 patients with residual occlusion. Ten are asymptomatic and unrestricted; 7 remain with residual symptoms.

Stable Occlusion with Recurrent Transient Episodes of Cyanosis and Mild Edema

There are a group of patients that we have followed, who have stable occlusion of the axillosubclavian vein. Some of them complain of very transient episodes of cyanosis, lasting minutes, occasionally followed by swelling lasting for minutes or up to an hour. Initially, these patients were referred for venous bypass or had a venous reconstructive procedure. Based on careful observations, we have come to recognize that these patients have more extensive thoracic outlet compression. Their symptoms reflect autonomic instability, rather than transient venous hypertension. These symptoms derive from sympathetic stimulation from compression of the inferior trunk of the brachial plexus, the source of sympathetic innervation of the arm. Decompression of the thoracic outlet with specific attention to the brachial plexus area, particularly the C8-T1 nerve roots, will relieve these symptoms. Venous reconstruction will usually provide no benefit.

In this regard it is essential to recognize that a significant number of patients with effort thrombosis will have some symptoms based on coincidental arterial or brachial plexus compression. We have found the most useful way of evaluating the neurogenic component to be assessment of somatosensory evoked responses, or by the electromyographic-guided scalene muscle block.

When the anterior scalene muscle is identified by its characteristic electromyographic response using a shielded needle, the muscle can be infiltrated with a small amount of local anesthetic. This avoids a brachial plexus or sympathetic block. In affected patients, there is prompt and profound relief of symptoms and reversal of the provocative tests. Relaxation of the anterior scalene permits the first rib to drop, relieving costoclavicular compression. In addition, there is relief of compression in the interscalene triangle, where the subclavian artery and brachial plexus pass between the anterior and middle scalene muscles.

The Role of Transluminal Angioplasty

We have developed a rule to avoid dilating the vein after successful lytic therapy. One exception to that rule has been in cases of very highgrade stricture associated with the external compression. In these instances, where the postlytic venogram suggests very poor flow across the damaged area, we have dilated the stricture with a 4-mm balloon. This tends to rupture some of the synechia without unduly damaging the remaining intima. Better flow is then evident across the stenosed area during the healing process. We have resorted to this tactic on two occasions.

After surgical decompression we will restudy the vein, usually at about 1 month (Figures 12A and 12B). If a hemodynamically significant stricture remains on cross-sectional area assessment corroborated by residual large collaterals, we will dilate the vein to 1 cm and maintain the patient on 4 additional weeks of anticoagulant protection with dicumarol. We have never stented the area and discourage this practice. Long-term venographic follow-up of our patients has demonstrated the transluminal angioplasty to be durable in this situation. Fourteen (22%) of our patients, who satisfied the above criteria, underwent postoperative transluminal angioplasty (Figures 13A and 13B).

Recurrent Edema and Cyanosis with Exercise, Despite Adequate Decompression and a Normal Appearing Vein on Follow-up Venography

We have encountered this phenomenon in two young patients. After somewhat exasperating follow-up, very careful restudy by venography demonstrated a fine web or diaphragm at the costoclavicular portion of the subclavian vein. This likely represented some residual valve leaflet fusion, barely discernible on conventional venography. There was no evi-

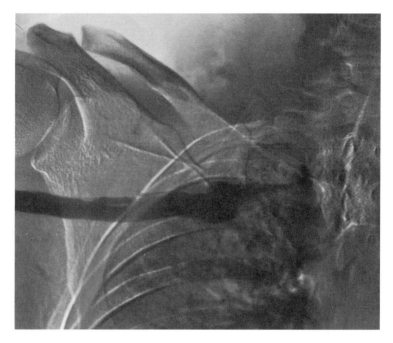

Figure 12A. (Pre-Op): After successful lytic therapy, this completion venogram documents an area of compression at the thoracic outlet, when the arm is in the abducted (elevated) position.

dence of residual compression in the stress position. Inflation of a transluminal balloon revealed the thin diaphragm. This was followed by complete relief of symptoms.

The Dilemma of the Contralateral Vein

Sixty-one percent of our patients studied with bilateral venography, had thrombosis or compression of the contralateral vein. We recommend study of the contralateral vein whenever this is possible. When a patient presents with thrombosis in the nondominant arm we have recommended subsequent elective repair of the contralateral side, when the vein in the dominant arm demonstrates the potential for thrombosis, and the patient is in an occupation that exposes them to further risk. In 41 patients we were able to obtain full bilateral venographic studies. Eleven of these patients had a normal contralateral vein. Twenty patients demonstrated evidence of compression and stricture in the neutral position, and 5 had evidence of hemodynamically significant compression in the stress posi-

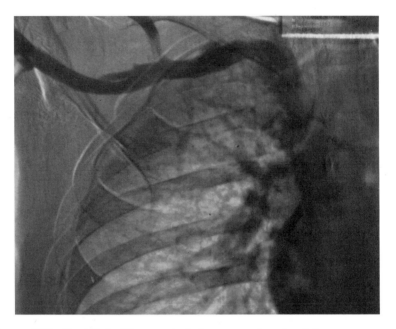

Figure 12B. (Post-Op): After surgical decompression, the follow-up venogram shows no evidence of compression even in the stress position. No further therapy is needed in this case. We would anticipate the patient returning to normal activity, with no further risk of thrombosis.

tion. Five patients underwent occlusion of the contralateral vein during the course of our initial review. Seventy-three percent of the patients studied had a bilateral abnormality and 12% went on to bilateral thrombosis.

Results of Treatment

In reviewing the results of treatment in this group of patients, there were 63 surgical procedures at the thoracic outlet, including 5 patients who were treated bilaterally.

We classified the results into 7 general categories: 4 patients with occluded veins were not treated surgically and remained essentially asymptomatic (5%); 9 patients had chronic occlusion of the subclavian vein, declined surgical correction and remained symptomatic or disabled (12%); 7 patients had chronic venous occlusion, underwent surgical correction but remained symptomatic (9%). A similar group of 10 patients, with chronic subclavian vein occlusion, underwent surgical decompres-

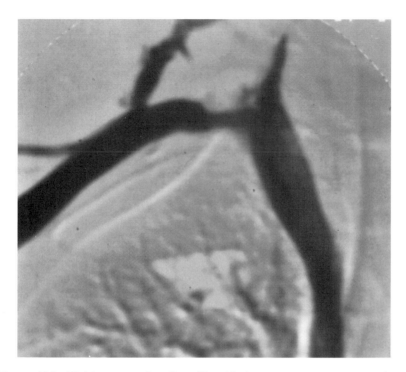

Figure 13A. Right upper extremity axillosublavian venogram, post-resection of the first rib and decompression of the thoracic outlet. Note the residual deformity in the retroclavicular portion of the axillosubclavian venous segment. This abnormality most likely represents fibrosis and stricture of the valve leaflets after an episode of thrombosis. This patient was advised to undergo transluminal balloon venoplasty in the postoperative period.

sion and were essentially asymptomatic when returned to their usual activity (13%).

In 46 patients we were able to restore normal patency. Five of these patients did not have surgical correction and remained patent and asymptomatic (7%). One patient had a patent vein but remained symptomatic postoperatively (1%). Forty patients with restoration of normal patency were asymptomatic and returned to normal activity post-surgical correction (53%). No patient treated surgically experienced an episode of re-thrombosis during the 10 years of follow-up.

Sixty-four of the patients returned to their usual activity without restriction (84%). Seven workers required retraining for a less physically stressful occupation. Five individuals remained disabled for their usual work or accustomed recreational activity.

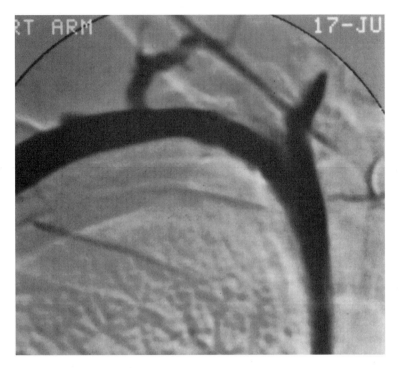

Figure 13B. Yearly follow-up venogram in the the stress position after thoracic outlet decompression and transluminal venoplasty. The anatomic result is durable, and the patient remains symptom-free.

Summary

In the natural history of Paget-Schroetter's syndrome, resumption of normal activity after a period of recuperation (after an episode of thrombosis) frequently leads to symptoms of upper extremity venous hypertension exacerbated by using the arms in the overhead position. This position can be demonstrated venographically to further occlude collateral vessels in the thoracic outlet. A number of patients develop more extensive symptoms of neurogenic thoracic outlet syndrome accompanied by positional numbness and dysesthesias.

Anticoagulation may protect the collateral vessels and interrupt the period of active clot propagation, producing a better functional result than would be expected from the natural history of the thrombotic event (Figure 7). To summarize our experience:

(1) Local urokinase was the most effective means for re-establishing venous patency.

(2) With clot dissolution, the underlying compression of the vein at the thoracic outlet can be demonstrated.

(3) Balloon angioplasty should not be undertaken in the acute setting nor prior to relieving the musculo-tendinous compression.

(4) The acute phlebitic process should resolve under the protection of coumadin for 4 weeks. At that time it can be determined more effectively which patients require additional therapy.

(5) Removal of the first rib will decompress the axillosubclavian vein and the thoracic outlet collaterals, permitting the vein to regain its normal configuration (particularly in younger patients with more acute onset of compression).

(6) Postoperative transluminal balloon venoplasty can be used in those patients with more chronic compression where the vein has become stenotic. Improvement of the luminal configuration has been accomplished without the necessity for venous recon-structive procedures.

Patients with Paget-Schroetter's syndrome have a symptom complex that often reflects more extensive neurovascular compression at the thoracic outlet than that which might result from venous hypertension alone. Although thrombolytic therapy can restore patency of the axillosubclavian vein, first rib resection is necessary to relieve the external compression. This procedure was very effective in patients who had restoration of subclavian vein patency, and to a lesser degree in those with residual occlusion.

Based on 76 patients, treated consecutively over a 10-year period, it remains evident that an algorithm directed toward treating the acute event then correcting the underlying anatomic abnormality yields excellent results at very low risk.

References

1. Hughes ESR: Venous obstruction in the upper extremity (Paget-Schroetter's syndrome). *Int Abstr Surg* 88:89–127, 1949.
2. Tilney NL, Griffiths HJG, Edwards EA: Natural history of major venous thrombosis of the upper extremity. *Arch Surg* 101:792–96, 1970.
3. Linblad B, Bornmyer S, Kullendorff B, Bergqvist D: Venous haemodynamics of the upper extremity after subclavian vein thrombosis. *Vasa* 19:218–222, 1990.
4. Harley DP, White RA, Nelson RJ, Mehringer CM; Pulmonary embolism secondary to venous thrombosis of the arm. *Am J Surg* 147:221–224, 1984.
5. Hurlbert SN, Rutherford RB: Primary subclavian-axillary vein thrombosis. *Ann Vasc Surg* 9:217–223, 1995.
6. Ricotta JJ, Dalsing MC, Ouriel K, et al: Research and clinical issues in chronic venous disease. *Cardiovasc Surg* 5:343–349, 1997.

7. Haire WD, Lynch TG, Lieberman RP, et al: Utility of duplex ultrasound in the diagnosis of asymptomatic catheter-induced subclavian vein thrombosis. *J Ultrasound Med* 10:493–96, 1991.

8. Haire WD, Lynch TG, Lund GB, et al: Limitations of magnetic resonance imaging and ultrasound-directed (duplex) scanning in the diagnosis of subclavian vein thrombosis. *J Vasc Surg* 13:391–97, 1997.

9. Baxter GM, Kincaid W, Jeffrey RF, et al: Comparison of colour Doppler ultrasound with venography in the diagnosis of axillary and subclavian vein thrombosis. *Br J Radiol* 64:777–81, 1991.

10. Machleder HI: Upper extremity venous thrombosis. *Semin Vasc Surg* 3:219–26, 1990.

11. AbuRahma AF, Short YS, White JF III, Boland JP: Treatment alternatives for axillary-subclavian vein thrombosis: Long-term follow-up. *Cardiovasc Surg* 4: 783–787, 1996.

12. Druy EM, Trout HH 3rd, Giordano JM, Hix WR: Lytic therapy in the treatment of axillary and subclavian vein thrombosis. *J Vasc Surg* 2:821–27, 1985.

13. Steed DL, Teodori MF, Peitzman AB, et al: Streptokinase in the treatment of subclavian vein thrombosis. *J Vasc Surg* 4:28–32, 1986.

14. Landercasper J, Gall W, Fischer M, et al: Thrombolytic therapy of axillary-subclavian venous thrombosis. *Arch Surg* 122:1072–75, 1987.

15. Zimmerman R, Morl H, Harenberg J, et al: Urokinase therapy of subclavian-axillary vein thrombosis. *Klin Wochenschr* 59:851–56, 1981.

16. Taylor LM, McAllister WR, Dennis DL, Porter JM: Thrombolytic therapy followed by first rib resection for spontaneous ("effort") subclavian vein thrombosis. *Am J Surg* 149:644–47,1985.

17. Perler BA, Mitchel SE: Percutaneous transluminal angioplasty and transaxillary first rib resection; A multidisciplinary approach to the thoracic outlet compression syndrome. *Am Surg* 52:485–87, 1986.

18. Kunkel JM, Machleder HI: Treatment of Paget-Schroetter syndrome: A staged, multidisciplinary approach. *Arch Surg* 124:1153–58, 1989.

19. Machleder HI: Evaluation of a new therapeutic strategy for treatment of Paget-Schroetter syndrome: Axillary-subclavian vein thrombosis. *J Vasc Surg* 17: 305–17, 1993.

20. Sundqvist SB, Hedner U, Kullenberg HKE, Bergentz S: Deep venous thrombosis of the arm: A study of coagulation and fibrinolysis. *Acta Chir Scand* 138: 313–9, 1972.

21. Deweese JA: Results of surgical treatment of axillary-subclavian venous thrombosis. In: Bergan JJ, Yao JST, eds. *Venous Disorders*. Philadelphia: W.B. Saunders; 1991, pp. 421–33.

22. Aziz S, Straehley CJ, Whelan TJ: Effort-related axillo-subclavian thrombosis. A new theory of pathogenesis and a plea for direct surgical intervention. *Am J Surg* 152:57–61, 1986.

23. Molina JE: Surgery for effort thrombosis of the subclavian vein. *J Thorac Cardiovasc Surg* 103:341–46, 1992.

24. Urschel HC, Razzuk MA; Improved management of the Paget-Schroetter syndrome secondary to thoracic outlet compression. *Ann Thorac Surg* 52:1217–21, 1991.

25. Rutherford RB, Hurlbert SN: Primary subclavian-axillary vein thrombosis: consensus and commentary. *Cardiovasc Surg* 4:420–423, 1996.

26. Wilson JJ, Zahn CA, Newman H: Fibrinolytic therapy for idiopathic subclavian-axillary vein thrombosis. *Am J Surg* 159:208–11, 1990.

27. Donayre CE, White GH, Mehringer SM, Wilson SE: Pathogenesis determines late morbidity of axillo-subclavian vein thrombosis. *Am J Surg* 152:179–84, 1986.

28. Gloviczki P, Kazmier FJ, Hollier LH: Axillary-subclavian venous occlusion: The morbidity of a nonlethal disease. *J Vasc Surg* 4:333–37, 1986.

29. AbuRahma AF, Sadler D, Stuart P, et al: Conventional versus thrombolytic therapy in spontaneous (effort) axillary-subclavian vein thrombosis. *Am J Surg* 161:459–65, 1991.

30. Burihan E, Poli de Figueiredo LF, Francisco J Jr, Miranda F Jr. Upper-extremity deep venous thrombosis: analysis of 52 cases. *Cardiovasc Surg* 1:19–22, 1993.

31. Hingorani A, Ascher E, Lorenson E, et al: Upper extremity deep venous thrombosis and its impact on morbidity and mortality rates in a hospital-based population. *J Vasc Surg* 26:853–860, 1997.

32. Roos DB: Thoracic outlet syndromes: Update 1987. *Am J Surg* 154:568–73, 1987.

33. Pittam MR, Darke SG: The place of first rib resection in the management of axillary-subclavian vein thrombosis. *Eur J Vasc Surg* 1:5–10, 1987.

34. Lumsden AB, Hughes JD, MacDonald MJ, Ofenloch JC: The thrombosed arteriovenous graft: An endovascular model for vascular surgeons. *Cardiovasc Surg* 5:401–407, 1997.

35. Shoenfeld R, Hermans H, Novick A, et al: Stenting of proximal venous obstructions to maintain hemodialysis access. *J Vasc Surg* 19:532–539, 1994.

36. Meier GH, Pollak JS, Rosenblatt M, et al: Initial experience with venous stents in exertional axillary-subclavian vein thrombosis. *J Vasc Surg* 24:974–983, 1996.

37. Hansen B, Feins R, Detmer DE: Simple extra-anatomic jugular vein bypass for subclavian vein thrombosis. *J Vasc Surg* 2:921–923, 1985.

38. Bell T, Stevens SL, Freeman MB, Goldman MH: Jugular venous bypass for subclavian vein obstruction. *Ann Vasc Surg* 8:390–393, 1994.

39. Sottiurai VS, Lyon R, Ross C, et al: Surgical management of brachioaxillary-subclavian vein occlusion. *Eur J Vasc Endovasc Surg* 11:225–229, 1996.

40. Machleder HI: Thrombolytic therapy and surgery for primary axillosubclavian vein thrombosis: Current approach. *Semin Vasc Surg* 9:46–49, 1996.

11

Surgical Approaches to Primary and Recurrent Thoracic Outlet Compression Syndromes

David B. Roos, MD

The clinical presentations of the thoracic outlet syndromes (TOS) are classified into three major categories: the neurogenic type caused by abnormal compression and irritation of the brachial plexus; the venous type from unusual compression of the subclavian vein passing through the anterior aperture of the thoracic outlet; and the arterial type, usually caused by anomalous bone formation in the thoracic outlet affecting the subclavian artery. The neurological type of TOS is by far the most common, comprising about 95% of all the TOS patient population, whereas the subclavian vein compression syndrome is seen in about 4%, and the primary involvement of a subclavian artery in only about 1% of all TOS patients. The latter two vascular outlet syndromes are dealt with in other chapters, so only the surgical considerations of the neurological form will be presented below.

On a clinical basis, it is important to differentiate the neurogenic symptoms of pain, paresthesia, weakness of specific muscles, and hypesthesia to touch and pin prick, as involving the lower nerves of the brachial plexus, C8 and T1, compared with the upper nerves of the plexus, C5, C6, and C7. The lower plexus involvement is the more common, with patients describing pain in the back of the neck and shoulder, and from

From Machleder HI, (ed): *Vascular Disorders of the Upper Extremity*. Third Revised Edition. Futura Publishing Company, Inc., Armonk, NY, © 1998.

the axilla through the triceps area and inner brachium, inner forearm into the ring and small fingers with numbness, tingling, and coolness of these digits. The examination usually shows weakness of the ulnar innervated interosseous muscles and the triceps muscle, with hypesthesia in the ulnar distribution.

The upper plexus involvement is distinctly different with symptoms of pain in the anterior neck from the ear and mandible down through the clavicle and upper chest to the third rib level, back of the neck, suprascapular area, and radiating down the radial nerve distribution of the outer arm, brachioradialis of the forearm, and sometimes reaching the dorsum of the thumb and index finger. The surgical treatment for these two types of TOS is so different, they will be described separately.[1] They should be performed only after careful delineation of the specific nerves involved rather than performing "shotgun" operations of releasing all five nerves of the plexus routinely. This latter approach, which unfortunately is commonly followed, may subject the patients to a major operation that is not clearly indicated by clinical evaluation, and, thereby, exposing them to unnecessary risks, and later scar formation causing severe recurrent symptoms from an operation that was not required.

Technique of Transaxillary First Rib Resection

For the more common symptoms of lower plexus involvement with predominantly ulnar nerve distribution, the safest and most complete decompression is achieved by transaxillary resection of the first rib and all anomalous fibromuscular bands that are always encountered in the outlet that cause the compression and irritation of the lower plexus, and possibly the subclavian artery and vein as well, in carefully chosen patients.[2]

After intubation, the patient is turned and secured in a lateral decubitus position, then slightly tilted back toward the surgeon, who stands behind the patient. The second assistant stands cephalad to the surgeon to control and elevate the upper extremity and shoulder to provide exposure through the axillary tunnel. He abducts the brachium 90° from the thorax, and holds the forearm in a double wrist lock (Figure 1), which provides the most comfortable and effective grip to elevate the shoulder intermittently during the procedure. This assistant should stand on at least two stepstools so that the patient's forearm is held at the assistant's waist level, so he may stand straight, which offers the best mechanical advantage to support and raise the shoulder and arm without tiring the assistant's back and arms. The surgeon must instruct the assistant to elevate the shoulder slowly and intermittently, avoiding sudden or prolonged stretching of the brachial plexus. He must avoid grasping the upper arm circumferentially with both hands and thrusting the arm upward, as this grip will

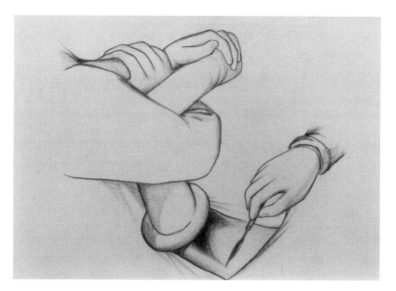

Figure 1. The double wrist lock by the second assistant holding the arm for exposure through the axillary tunnel is illustrated along with the transverse incision in the lower axilla between the edges of latissimus dorsi and pectoralis major muscles.

press the major nerves of the patient's arm against the humerus, causing postoperative arm pain and quickly tire the assistant.

With the arm elevated 90° from the thorax, the incision is placed over the third rib, below the hairline in the lower aspect of the axilla, not in the axillary apex, to avoid troublesome fat, lymph nodes, and numerous small vessels and nerves of the axillary contents. The transverse incision is made from the anterior edge of the latissimus dorsi muscle to the posterior edge of the pectoralis major muscle. In women, the exact location is achieved by pushing the shoulder joint and breast toward each other to demonstrate the axillomammary crease over the third rib. In average-sized patients, 8-cm length is adequate, but in larger patients, 10 cm may be required. In men, the axillomammary crease cannot be demonstrated, but the same location is determined by forcefully raising the arm toward the ceiling and marking the break in the skin over the rib cage where it turns upward to cover the axilla. At the break, a small mark is made, the shoulder lowered, and the standard incision performed. The skin edges are held open throughout the procedure with self-retaining retractors (ie, Gelpis). The first assistant stands across the table from the surgeon to provide exposure with retractors during the procedure. The incision is deepened down to the rib cage before angling up to form the axillary tunnel to the thoracic outlet to avoid encountering the excess fat in the axilla that impairs exposure through the tunnel.

The first structure encountered is the thoracoepigastric vein, sometimes accompanied by the small lateral thoracic artery, in the mid-axillary line. These vessels are clamped, divided, and tied before proceeding to develop the axillary tunnel through the areolar tissue between the rib cage below and the axillary vessels in the roof of the tunnel.

The second structure that crosses the axillary tunnel vertically is the intercostal brachial cutaneous nerve, which usually arises from the second intercostal space, but sometimes an accessory intercostal brachial cutaneous nerve may arise from the third intercostal space. An attempt should be made to preserve these nerves, but if they are overstretched, and visibly injured, it is best to divide them, which will result in numbness of the axilla and inner brachium. The numbness is far more acceptable to the patient than causalgic burning hypersensitivity of the skin of the lateral chest wall, axilla, and inner brachium that results from an overstretched or frayed sensory nerve.

By blunt finger dissection, the surgeon develops the axillary tunnel to the first rib. The third structure crossing the tunnel is the supreme thoracic artery and vein passing from the major axillary vessels to the first intercostal space. These should be anticipated to avoid troublesome bleeding, dissected free, clamped, divided, and tied before proceeding further into the thoracic outlet above the first rib. The thoracic outlet is separated from the axilla by a cul-de-sac of fascia, which must be opened carefully by finger dissection or spreading with long scissors, but never cutting with the scissors, to avoid injury to the subclavian artery and vein just beyond the fascia. Exposure is expanded by finger dissection along the first rib posteriorly, and in front of the anterior scalene muscle to free the subclavian vein in the anterior aperture, and the subclavian artery and brachial plexus in the posterior aperture behind the anterior scalene muscle. Usually the major vessels, T1 nerve, and lower trunk of the brachial plexus can readily be freed from light attachments to the upper surface of the first rib by finger dissection, but if the area is scarred, they must be separated from the periosteum by scissor dissection with extremely meticulous technique.

To open the tunnel and thoracic outlet, the first assistant uses a right angle retractor, such as the Heaney, preferably with a fiberoptic light attached. It is best to avoid a curved retractor, such as a Deaver, as the curved tip may gouge into important structures without being seen by the surgeons. A fiberoptic suction (Vital-Vue) provides bright light combined with suction in the depths of the thoracic outlet throughout the procedure. The surgeon must frequently monitor the tightness of the T1 nerve of the brachial plexus to minimize the stretch of the nerve which could result in a neuropraxic injury, as the second assistant holding and elevating the arm cannot determine the amount of tension being created when he is providing deep exposure at the base of the neck. He must also be reminded

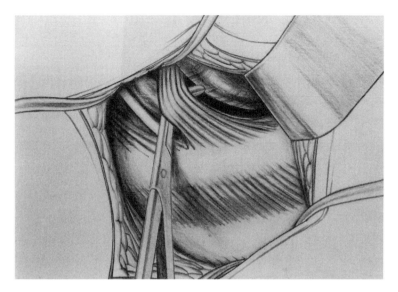

Figure 2. This illustration depicts the anterior scalene muscle being hooked by a right angle hemostat to separate it from the subclavian vein shown to the right of the muscle, and the subclavian artery and brachial plexus shown to the left of this muscle. The muscle is divided at its attachment to the first rib.

to release the pull of the shoulder girdle frequently to avoid prolonged tension on the lower nerves of the plexus.

The long thoracic nerve usually can be visualized in the back of the axillary tunnel, lying over the outer surface of the posterior scalene muscle that attaches to the second rib. Usually it is safely out of harm's way, but occasionally it will be found in an aberrant position passing toward the mid-axillary line, which may subject it to injury if this variation is not appreciated by the surgeon. It can readily be identified with the battery nerve stimulator, and then must be carefully avoided throughout the procedure to prevent a winged scapula.

The anterior scalene muscle is then exposed and hooked with a right angle hemostat to separate it from the artery and vein, and divided at its attachment to the first rib (Figure 2). The subclavius tendon anterior to the vein is separated from fat by scissor dissection, and carefully divided to release pressure on top of the vein from this muscle and to provide further depth for resection of the anterior end of the first rib. The middle scalene muscle, and intercostal muscle between first and second rib are then released from the attachments to the rib with an Overholt #1 raspatory with careful visualization and protection of the T1 nerve. This is accomplished by light traction of the nerve with a suction tip or, preferably, the long-handled metal spatula specifically designed for protecting

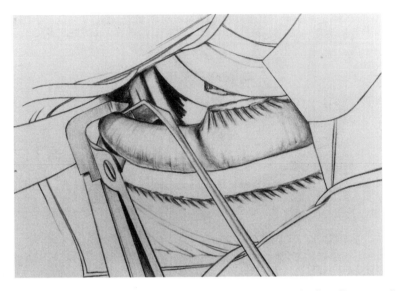

Figure 3. The right-angled rib shear is placed as far back on the first rib as possible to divide the rib posteriorly as the metal nerve shield retractor protects the C8 and T1 nerves of the plexus from slipping into the jaws of the rib shears. The divided anterior scalene muscle is shown to the right of the nerve retractor.

the nerve and the vein. The intercostal muscle is divided at the lateral edge of the first rib and Sibson's fascia is released from the inner edge of the rib with the hook of the raspatory, dropping the pleura to second rib level.

The first rib is then resected with a right-angle rib shear specifically designed for this purpose. The metal spatula, or suction tip is again used to keep the T1 nerve from slipping into the jaws of the rib shear as it divides the bone near the transverse process (Figure 3). The rib is then resected anteriorly near the costal cartilage with a 60° rib shear, with careful protection of the vein with the right angle retractor or metal spatula. The anterior stump is shortened to the costocartilage and left smooth in front of the vein. The posterior stump is shortened with rongeurs so it is well behind and somewhat above the T1 nerve, which, again, must be clearly visualized and carefully protected when using the rongeurs. The posterior stump must be left smooth without spicules or a sharp corner that might stab into the T1 nerve. It is sealed with bone wax to reduce bleeding and scar formation from the marrow cavity. The T1 nerve is then carefully visualized and any remaining fibrous tissue that may cross or form a sling under the nerve is resected.

To reduce the risk of scar forming from the stump that may entrap the T1 nerve and cause severe recurrent symptoms later, the lower divided end of middle scalene muscle is drawn down with a right-angle hemostat and sutured over the stump of first rib behind the T1 nerve with a figure-of-eight absorbable suture to fibromuscular tissue under the neck of the rib. At times, this muscle may be too soft and friable to hold the suture and the reattachment cannot be performed. A scalenus minimus muscle is commonly found between the subclavian artery and T1 nerve. It should be fully resected. A type 8 anomaly of muscle tissue passing from the anterior scalene muscle anteriorly under the vein and attaching to the costocartilage also is a common finding. This should be separated from the vein with a hemostat and fully resected to release all compression mechanisms affecting the vein. This is the anomaly that may cause the effort-vein thrombosis or Paget-Schroetter's syndrome of the subclavian vein. Similarly, if there is a fibrous sling of the anterior scalene passing posteriorly under the artery, it must be separated from the artery with extreme care and fully resected to release the subclavian vessels and lower plexus completely from these common anomalies that are found in carefully selected surgical patients with lower plexus and venous symptoms.[3]

To help protect the T1 nerve and lower trunk of the plexus from scar formation from the surgical bed and the posterior stump of rib, I now routinely form a 4-inch pedicle of fat from the roof of the axillary tunnel, invert the tip of the pedicle, which originates in the subcutaneous tissue of the upper edge of the incision, on the central base for blood supply, and suture the tip behind the T1 nerve, preferably covering the posterior stump of rib, using absorbable suture. The fat is then spread under the nerve and sutured to tissue under the artery to provide a soft fat cushion for the T1 nerve and lower trunk of the plexus to lie in from the neural foramen to the axilla, interposing normal fat tissue between the nerves, the posterior stump, and the surgical bed of the rib resection. Hemostasis is carefully secured, and the wound is irrigated with antibiotic solution to test the integrity of the pleura. A suction drain is placed at the base of the neck, brought out over second rib, and passed through the lateral tissue of the chest wall with the trocar. If a tear in the pleura has developed, the tip of this drain is passed directly through the hole part way down the mediastinum as a chest tube under the fat pedicle. The shortened outer end of the drain is sutured to the skin, and a small suction device is applied.

Closure

The shoulder is lowered, the subcutaneous tissue of the axilla is closed with continuous absorbable suture, the skin closed with a continuous absorbable subcuticular suture, and a gauze dressing is applied.

If a cervical rib is present, the middle scalene muscle engulfing the rib, and the intercostal muscle between cervical and first rib, are released from attachments to the cervical rib with the raspatory. The cervical rib is then resected with the same instruments as used for resecting the posterior first rib, again with clear visualization and meticulous protection of the C8 and T1 nerves with the suction tip or, preferably, the spatula retractor. The stump of cervical rib is shortened with rongeurs as far back as the first rib stump and left smooth without spicules.

Technique of Complete Anterior Scalenectomy

If the patient has clearly defined severe symptoms of upper brachial plexus involvement of the C5, C6, and C7 nerves, as described previously, with special tenderness of these nerves on palpation and light percussion, both tested from behind the patient, and with the patient's head tilted to the opposite shoulder, consideration should be given to thorough decompression of these nerves if reasonable conservative measures have failed.[1]

With the patient under general anesthesia in the supine position, the head of the table is elevated, the patient's head turned to the opposite side, and the neck extended. A 5-cm oblique incision is made one fingerwidth above the top of the clavicle in the natural skin crease and developed through the platysma muscle. Longer incisions are unnecessary, more disfiguring, and may cause annoying numbness of the anterior shoulder and infraclavicular area from injury to the cervical sensory nerves. The incision extends from the lateral edge of the sternal head of the sternocleidomastoid muscle to the external jugular vein, which is preserved (Figure 4). The skin edges are held open with a self-retaining retractor. The clavicular head of sternocleidomastoid and the omohyoid muscles are divided, the prescalene fat is dissected off of the jugular vein, and reflected laterally behind an army retractor. The phrenic nerve is immediately identified and carefully avoided throughout the procedure without being tagged or retracted. The transverse cervical artery and vein usually cross the lower portion of the anterior scalene muscle directly overlying the phrenic nerve. These vessels must be clamped, divided, and tied to allow exposure and resection of the anterior scalene muscle. On the left side, the thoracic duct may be prominent in some patients and should be carefully avoided. If it is directly in the way of removal of the anterior scalene muscle, it should be clamped, divided, and tied with fine suture. Any lymphatic leaks must be thoroughly controlled, preferably by oversewing with fine absorbable suture before closing the incision to avoid a troublesome lymphocele.

An important unusual anomaly of the brachial plexus should be anticipated by the surgeon when first exposing the anterior scalene muscle.

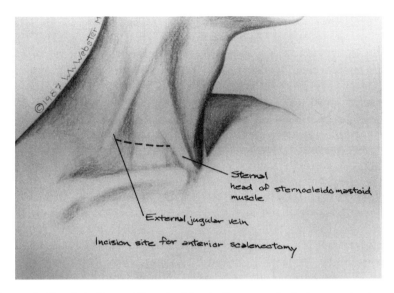

Sternal head of sternocleidomastoid muscle

External jugular vein

Incision site for anterior scalenectomy

Figure 4. The 5- to 6-cm oblique incision in the supraclavicular area is shown in this illustration. It extends from the external jugular vein to the lateral edge of the sternal head of sternocleidomastoid muscle, and is located 1 to 2 fingerwidths above the clavicle when the head is turned to the opposite side.

The C5 nerve of the plexus may be congenitally displaced from its usual position behind the anterior scalene muscle and lie on the anterior surface of this muscle just lateral to the phrenic nerve. The upper portion of this scalene muscle may pass between the C5 and C6 nerves, as well as between C6 and C7 nerves to join with the middle scalene muscle behind the nerves. If this anomaly is not anticipated and recognized, the displaced C5 nerve and upper trunk of the plexus may be seriously injured.[1]

The anterior scalene muscle is dissected from under the phrenic nerve with care. If the patient has just undergone transaxillary first rib resection, the lower end of this muscle that was divided from the rib is drawn up into the neck wound, grasped with a hemostat, and elevated as all muscle fiber attachments to the epineurium of the brachial plexus nerves are dissected free up to the transverse processes of the vertebrae where the muscle originates (Figure 5). If the patient's symptoms and examination indicate upper plexus involvement only with no lower plexus ulnar pattern (a less common presentation), supraclavicular scalenectomy may be indicated without transaxillary rib resection. The anterior scalene muscle then is divided through its middle third, and each divided section of muscle is removed separately. This muscle must be handled with great care, especially as it is passed under the phrenic nerve to dissect and remove the upper portion of the muscle to avoid phrenic injury.

A small artery is commonly found arising from the arch of the subclavian artery that passes posteriorly between C7 and C8 nerves. This vessel is clamped, divided, and tied to provide unimpeded access to complete the dissection of the middle and lower trunks of the brachial plexus. The subclavian artery itself often is found much higher in the neck than expected, and as shown in standard anatomic textbooks. It may be two, even three fingerwidths above the clavicle in a surprisingly and dangerously high position that the surgeon must anticipate and identify early in the procedure, and protect it with great care. Even a slight tear or nick in this vessel causes alarming blood loss, and it is a difficult artery to repair as the walls seem so much softer than other vessels its size. The subclavian vein usually seems to be tucked well under the clavicle in the expected position. All five nerves of the brachial plexus must be completely cleared of the abnormal scalene muscle tissue always found in patients with upper plexus symptoms. Each nerve is tested with a battery nerve stimulator for appropriate muscle contraction. For unknown reasons, the T1 nerve frequently fails to fire with the stimulator even though the nerve appears normal and functions well postoperatively.

After all these techniques are accomplished, the prescalene fat is lengthened and tailored to fit loosely over the bare, exposed anterior as-

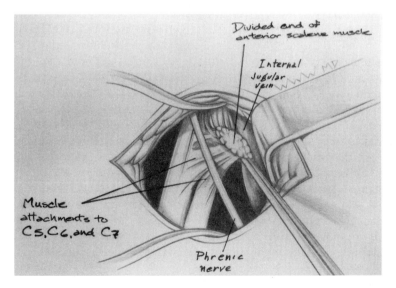

Figure 5. This illustration depicts the divided anterior scalene muscle being dissected from the prominent muscle fiber attachment to the epineurium of the C6 and C7 nerves of the right brachial plexus. The phrenic nerve crosses the surgical field and must be treated with great care to avoid a phrenic nerve palsy with a paralyzed diaphragm.

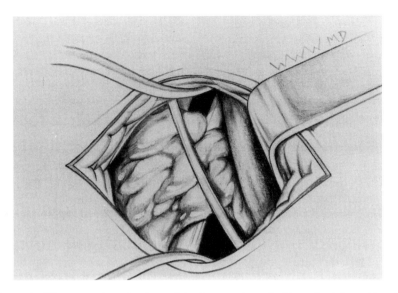

Figure 6. The prescalene fat that originally was dissected from the internal jugular vein and preserved, is layed over the bare, exposed anterior surfaces of all the nerves of the brachial plexus, after complete neurolysis, as depicted above. It is passed under the phrenic nerve to support the nerve that crosses the large empty fossa left by removing the entire anterior scalene muscle. The fat pad is sutured under the internal jugular vein and behind the subclavian artery to cover the exposed brachial plexus with normal soft fat as a cushion for protection of the nerves and to help reduce scar tissue formation involving the plexus after scalenectomy.

pect of the brachial plexus. It is split to form a small tongue of fat above the phrenic nerve to be sutured to the medial aspect of the neck over the proximal part of the C5 and C6 nerves with the majority of the fat pad passed under the phrenic nerve to support the nerve crossing the large empty fossa left by the resected anterior scalene muscle. The fat is then sutured to neutral tissue in the medial aspect of the neck with fine suture to form a soft fat cushion to protect the brachial plexus and to reduce scar formation over the bare nerves that may result from uncovered nerves beneath the skin (Figure 6).

Closure

The wound is irrigated with antibiotic solution, the patient's head is straightened, and put in slight cervical flexion. The divided ends of the clavicular head of sternocleidomastoid muscle are reapproximated with figure-of-eight permanent sutures. The platysma muscle is closed with continuous absorbable suture, and the skin edges approximated with continuous absorbable subcuticular suture. Collodion is used to seal the incision as the only dressing, or a gauze dressing may be applied. If the patient is found, on careful clinical evaluation, to have clear evidence of both upper and lower plexus neurogenic TOS, which is not unusual, the transaxillary decompression of the lower nerves is followed by the supraclavicular decompression of the upper nerves under the same anesthesia.

Postoperative Care

The patient's postoperative pain is felt predominantly in the periscapular region from the transaxillary rib resection, and in the supraclavicular region from the scalenectomy. A heating pad applied to the back of the shoulder is quite comforting for the periscapular pain, and an ice pack in the supraclavicular area is soothing and helps reduce swelling. These operations are quite painful, especially for patients who have suffered severe pain without relief from conservative measures for many months. Therefore, special attention should be made to offer as complete pain relief as possible with whatever drugs may be required, especially for the first few weeks postoperatively. The suction drain in the axilla usually may be removed the day after surgery if drainage is minimal. The patient is encouraged to rest the arm on a pillow, both in the lying and sitting positions, and to wear a sling to support the arm and avoid the heavy weight of the shoulder and arm causing drag on the very sensitive brachial plexus. The sling is allowed for a couple of weeks, if the patient is advised to straighten the elbow, and abduct the arm 180° at the shoulder twice a day to prevent stiffness of these joints from immobilization. Additionally, many patients are benefitted by muscle relaxant drugs and a bedtime sedative to try to establish an early, relatively sound sleep pattern with maximum comfort that these patients have been deprived of for many months. Active pulmonary care and early ambulation are important. They may shower and wash directly over the incision 2 to 3 days postoperatively. The criteria for being dismissed from the hospital are 24 hours of being nearly afebrile; an acceptable, if not perfect, postoperative chest x-ray; reasonable pain control; and adequate eating, sleeping, and bathroom function. Structured professional physical therapy is strictly avoided, as most therapists in their empathy to hasten the patient'vs recovery, provide much too vigorous exercises and massage that predictably severely aggravate the pain and muscle spasms that surgery is attempting to relieve. Patients are advised to use heat applications, hot showers, and deep soaking tub baths regularly, and to use the appropriate medication to achieve maximum reasonable comfort for light activity, normal eating, sleeping, and muscle relaxation of the shoulder and neck structures. The only exercises necessary are strong hand gripping several times a day, straightening the elbow, and abducting the shoulder twice a day, and walking outdoors, as much as possible, to build strength, regain appetite, and well being.

The interval that patients are ready to return to their regular job varies considerably with different employment, and the patients themselves. For light desk work, most patients require about 6 weeks of convalescence. For moderate office work with keyboarding with the hands outstretched, reaching, and filing, 2 to 3 months may be required, but for more vigorous arm activities, such as supermarket checkers, hairdressers, and construction workers, 3 to 4 months of convalescence may be required. If the patients are returned to their specific vocation prematurely, persistent or recurrent painful muscle spasms in the shoulder and arm will occur, and may negate any benefits of the surgical procedure.

Recurrent TOS Symptoms

Surgery around the brachial plexus is prone to produce scar tissue during the healing stage, which affects the patient more than surgery in most other parts of the body due to fibrotic attachment and entrapment affecting the highly sensitive nerves of the brachial plexus. There are no known ways of completely avoiding scar tissue formation postoperatively, but some conditions may be associated with excessive fibrosis. These include hematoma or deep infection of the surgical wound, and possibly vigorous motion, strain, and exercise of the surgical areas in the early healing stages. However, the neurogenic recurrence of symptoms seen in these patients usually occurs in the absence of these factors, and apparently indicates a propensity of some patients to form much more scar tissue during the healing stages than the average person. In my own series, about 6% of the transaxillary first rib procedures have resulted in scar tissue recurrence severe enough to require reoperation, but 19% of the supraclavicular scalenectomies have suffered recurrence of the original problem from fibrotic entrapment of the nerves. Because of this discrepancy, I feel the supraclavicular approach should be carefully avoided whenever possible, except for compelling symptoms and clinical findings of severe upper plexus involvement. Patients with equivocal or mild upper plexus symptoms should not be subjected to supraclavicular neurolysis, as they would be exposed to relatively high incidence of recurrence, that is reported to be 50% in one university series, from severe scar tissue entrapment of the plexus requiring reoperation.

If the patient felt good relief of the pain in the neck, shoulder, arm, and hand with the numbness, tingling, coldness, and weakness following the previously described operations, those results indicate the diagnosis was correct and the choice of operation was appropriate. After a variable period of time, however, some patients will feel recurrence of the same type of symptoms they had before surgery, which can be a distressing development. This may occur spontaneously or after new trauma. Light, never strenuous, physical therapy, anti-inflammatory and muscle relaxant medication are offered, along with encouragement as they become quite anxious, even frightened. If the symptoms progress despite these conservative measures, and they display significant tenderness in the supraclavicular area and aggravation of symptoms by reaching outward or sideways and tilting the neck to the opposite side, almost certainly they have developed scar tissue involving the nerves of the brachial plexus. Although the pathophysiology of the scar tissue entrapment is different from the original anatomic anomalies, the symptomatic results are remarkably similar. If reasonable amount of time and appropriate conservative treatment fails to resolve the recurrent symptoms, surgical neurolysis of the scarring of the nerves offers the only chance of improvement.

If the symptoms and tests indicate the lower plexus involvement with ulnar nerve symptoms down the inner arm towards the ring and small fingers as the predominant pattern, transaxillary exploration with neurolysis of the T1 nerve and lower trunk of the plexus offers the best chance of relief, as scar tissue binding these nerves in the thoracic outlet bed of resected first rib will always be found. This surgery entails much higher risk of potential life-threatening hemorrhage from injury to the subclavian vessels, or serious neurological complications from injury to the T1 or long thoracic nerve than the original operation performed through normal tissue.[5] It carries such a high risk that it should be performed only by surgeons quite knowledgeable in the anatomy and experienced in the techniques of transaxillary rib resection and neurolysis, who are technically prepared to handle severe complications, such as sudden life-threatening hemorrhage, and have the appropriate special instruments for this type of surgery.

My preferred technique, which differs from other authors,[6,7] is to use the original transaxillary incision, perform an apical pleurectomy, which greatly increases the safety and exposure for dealing with the T1 nerve and lower trunk of the brachial plexus caught in dense scar tissue, and safer protection of the subclavian vessels. After complete neurolysis of the T1 nerve to the neural foramen, shortening the posterior stump of rib if it is found to be longer than 1 cm from the transverse process, and freeing the subclavian artery to the mediastinum, a 4-inch axillary fat pedicle is again formed and placed behind and under the T1 nerve, as described for the original operation. The subclavian vein is not dissected free as patients rarely have venous congestion symptoms with scar tissue recurrence, and to work on the thin-walled vein entails extreme risk of tearing the vein and scar tissue, where control and repair are extremely difficult.

If a patient has recurrent symptoms typical of upper plexus involvement, supraclavicular exploration through the same incision is performed with complete neurolysis of all five nerves of the plexus. Usually the entire plexus is found to be covered with a sheet of white fibrous scar, and on opening the sheet, each individual nerve is found encircled with a sleeve of scar. On opening each sleeve, the nerve trapped inside usually appears surprisingly normal with smooth, shiny cream-colored epineurium, and may stimulate well, but only after each is freed from all scar entrapment from the neural foramen to the clavicle. The phrenic nerve often is found displaced along the medial wall of the cervical exposure after the anterior scalene muscle has been removed previously, and, again, it is carefully avoided without dissection or traction. After completing the neurolysis and freeing each nerve, the prescalene fat, again, is prepared and placed over the anterior surface of the brachial plexus, or it may be split vertically with a posterior leaf placed behind the plexus and the anterior leaf placed in front of the plexus to sandwich the plexus in normal fat.

As with any operation, the first procedure has the best chance of the most improvement, but a follow-up operation for recurrence still has a reasonable chance of significant, if not total, relief in about 70% of the cases in experienced hands with a serious complication rate of about 1%.

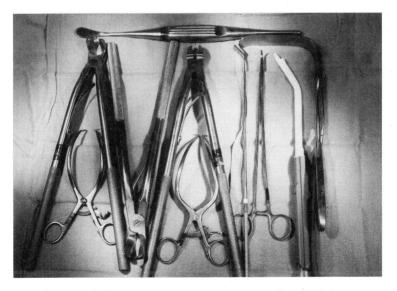

Figure 7. The special instruments designed for transaxillary first rib resection are shown in this photograph with the two rib shears to the left, the two Gelpi skin edge retractors in the center and left, and the square-jawed box rongeur in the center of the picture. To the right of center are the thin-handled nerve shield retractor, the long right angle hemostat, the Vital-Vue fiberoptic suction tip, and the fiberoptic right angle Heaney retractor to the far right. The specially designed raspatory (periosteal elevator) with the Overholt #1 hook on the right end and the Matson round tip to the left is at the top of the picture.

All of these operations should be performed only by surgeons with training and experience in the complexities of TOS surgery. They must be well versed in the details of the anatomy and congenital variations of the contents of the thoracic outlet, use competent assistance, and preferably the special lighting and instruments developed for these intricate procedures (Figure 7) in order to minimize serious complications that may potentially be catastrophic. However, if the stringent requirements of accurate diagnosis, proper choice of operations, performed with meticulous technique by well-prepared, experienced surgeons, many patients with severe, even disabling TOS, may still obtain substantial relief that allows them to resume a much happier, more comfortable, and productive life.

References

1. Roos DB: The place for scalenectomy and first rib resection in thoracic outlet syndrome. *Surgery* 92:1077–1088, 1982.
2. Roos DB: Transaxillary approach for first rib resection to relieve thoracic outlet syndrome. *Ann Surg* 163:354–358, 1966.
3. Roos DB: Congenital anomalies associated with thoracic outlet syndrome: Anatomy, symptoms, diagnosis, and treatment. *Am J Surg* 132:771–778, 1976.
4. Quarfordt PG, Ehrenfeld WK, Stoney RJ: Supraclavicular radical scalenectomy and transaxillary first rib resection for thoracic outlet syndrome. *Am J Surg* 148:111–116, 1984.
5. Sessions RT: Recurrent thoracic outlet syndrome: Causes and treatment. *South Med J* 75:453–461, 1982.
6. Machleder HI, Moll FL: Reoperations for thoracic outlet compression syndrome and vascular disorders of the upper extremity. In: Trout HH, Gcordano JM, DePalma RG, eds: *Reoperative Vascular Surgery*. New York: Marcel Dekker; 1987, pp. 325–351.
7. Urschel HC Jr, Razzuk MA, Albers JA, et al: Reoperation for recurrent thoracic outlet syndrome. *Ann Thorac Surg* 21:19–25, 1976.

12

The Management
of Neuropathic Pain

Jacob P. Schwarz, BA and
Allan J. Belzberg, BSc, MD

Introduction

The International Association for the Study of Pain defines pain as "an unpleasant sensory and emotional experience associated with actual or potential tissue damage or described in terms of such damage."[1] Pain remains the most common symptom for which a patient seeks out medical care. Over the past three decades, great strides have been made in understanding the biology of pain. It is often stated to medical students that if one can understand the visual system, they can master much of the nervous system. A more compelling argument can be made for understanding the pain system, for not only does this encompass a complex sensory experience, but also involves an emotional component. It should not be surprising that when dealing with complex or chronic pain problems, a multidisciplinary approach is often required.

Pain sensations derive from activity generated in nociceptors, undifferentiated terminals of myelinated a-delta and unmyelinated c fibers in sensory nerves.[2] These fibers are capable of discriminating between harmful and nonharmful stimuli applied to the nerve and its surrounding tissue. When nociceptors are stimulated by high-threshold mechanical or thermal stimuli, they respond by increasing their rate of activity. It is this increased rate of firing among nociceptors that the nervous system interprets as pain. There is modulation of the pain signal at multiple locations as it projects from the peripheral nervous system receptors to the spinal cord and on upward in the central nervous system. The most impor-

From Machleder HI, (ed): *Vascular Disorders of the Upper Extremity*. Third Revised Edition. Futura Publishing Company, Inc., Armonk, NY, © 1998.

tant goal of pain therapy, is to eliminate nociceptive activity, and subsequently eliminate the sensation of pain that persists after injury. When this cannot be achieved, various techniques are used to modulate the activity in the projection system.

A simple classification of pain includes, but is not limited to somatic, visceral, neuropathic, and sympathetically maintained pain. Somatic and visceral pain are elicited by injury to tissue. In most cases these pains are self-limited and relieved by healing of the tissue, inactivity, or is a self-limited cramping pain that goes away with time. The focus of this chapter is neuropathic and sympathetically maintained pain. Examples of neuropathic pain often seen by the vascular surgeon are post-thoracotomy pain, thoracic outlet, and post-herpetic neuralgia. Neuropathic pain is not considered a normal response to stimuli. Rather, it results from direct injurious stimuli to a nerve and often persists long after the stimulus has been removed. It is commonly described as a burning or stabbing pain that may be constitutive or occur in paroxysmal episodes known as lancinating or "lightning" pain.

Nerve Injury and Pain

Occasionally, injury may induce a nerve, that would otherwise be quiescent, to become spontaneously active.[3] If an injured nociceptor develops ongoing spontaneous activity, neuropathic pain may ensue even after the original stimulus has been removed. Nerve injury can further contribute to chronic pain by inducing ectopic generators. A few fibers can become ectopically excitable such that stimulation along the fiber, away from the receptor in the periphery, elicits an action potential.[4] This is thought to be due to an overexpression of sodium channels in the nerve membrane. When this occurs, the nerve is easily excited by either exogenous or endogenous stimuli. In theses circumstances, palpation of the nerve can result in a discharge and a paresthesia sensation (Tinel's sign) or a painful response (dysesthesia). Continued motion of the extremity with mechanical stimulation of the nerve may result in repeated discharge and pain.

Influences of the Nerve Injure Milieu

After some soft tissue injuries, a nerve may become entrapped in the desmoplastic response of the tissue. The fibrotic reaction that occurs in response to injury and healing can lead to compression or tethering of the nerve resulting in pressure and traction forces on the nerve.[5] As the nerve becomes entrapped, it loses its ability to glide with motion of the extremity. As a consequence, movement of the extremity results in excessive traction on the nerve and activates the nervi nervorum resulting in local tenderness. Given the frequency of this symptom, entrapment is likely a common mechanism by which injury causes chronic pain.

When a nerve is entrapped, axonal transport can be slowed or blocked. This leads to the local accumulation sodium channels as demonstrated by a Tinel's sign. When local tenderness and Tinel's sign are both present, a compelling case for nerve entrapment can be made. Confirmation of entrapment can be accomplished using electrophysiological studies. Evidence of entrapment includes focal slowing of nerve conduction, and in advanced stages, axonal loss with muscle denervation.[6] It is important to emphasize, however, that negative results do not indicate that focal nerve entrapment can be excluded.

An example of local entrapment may be thoracic outlet occurring after whiplash type injuries. If there is trauma to the anterior scalene muscle with bleeding, the underlying plexus elements may lose some mobility and become entrapped at the edge of the muscle and or under an elevated first rib. This would account for local tenderness, local Tinel's sign, and increased symptoms with movement of the extremity. If the nerve then becomes ectopically excitable, the patient will experience sensations in the area innervated by the plexus element, likely the hand.

Neuropathic Pain

Patients complaining of neuropathic pain symptoms often describe two components of the pain. The first is pain felt in the area innervated by the nerve. For example, injury to the ulnar nerve can lead to burning pain in the fourth and fifth fingers of the hand, the dermatomes subserved by the ulnar nerve. The second component is pain felt along the anatomic course of the nerve and is thought to represent sensitivity of the nervi nervorum innervating the nerve. An example is pain along the forearm with injury to the ulnar nerve at the elbow.

An integral component of neuropathic pain is that pain may be evoked by normally innocuous stimuli signifying the presence of hyperalgesia and/or allodynia.[7–9] A nociceptive response elicited by an otherwise innocuous stimulus is known as allodynia and may reflect the sensitization of a nociceptor by mechanisms in the peripheral or central nervous system. An example of allodynia is when light touch of skin close to a sun burn is reported as painful. Allodynia should be differentiated from hyperalgesia, which is hypersensitivity of a nerve. When this condition arises, the nerve responds with greater amplitude to a given stimuli.

Hyperalgesia can conceivably give rise to allodynia. Wide dynamic response (WDR) cells are located in the dorsal horn and project to the spinal-thalamic tract signaling pain sensations. Nociceptor fibers from the periphery synapse on WDR cells as do touch fibers, however, normally only the nociceptor synapse is active. In response to prolonged input from a nociceptor neuron, the WDR cell "winds up" and becomes sensitized such that the touch fiber synapse becomes active. The WDR cell will now signal pain to an otherwise innocuous touch stimulus (central sensitization). Pain elicited by central or peripheral sensitization will occur in tissue innervated by damaged nerve (primary hyperalgesia), but it may also spread far outside this area (secondary hyperalgesia).

As an illustration, consider a patient who suffers a burn to a small area on the hand. The nociceptors located in the burned skin become sensitized (peripheral sensitization) secondary to local inflammation resulting in increased response to a given stimulus (primary hyperalgesia). Eventually, light stroking of the burned skin results in pain (allodynia) because of the ongoing drive on the WDR cells (central sensitization). Eventually, stroking the skin close to, but outside the area of burn will also cause pain (secondary hyperalgesia).

Neuromas

When a nerve is severed, the axons in the proximal end remain in continuity with their cell body in the dorsal root ganglion or anterior spinal cord. In the distal nerve, the axons have been disconnected from their cell body and undergo wallerian degeneration. The axons in the proximal nerve will send out sprouts in an attempt to re-innervate the distal portion of the nerve and re-establish connection with the end terminals. A neuroma is a densely packed cluster of regenerative sprouts that forms when the continuity of the nerve is interrupted and regeneration is blocked by fibrous scar tissue or the distal part of the nerve is removed from the region by trauma.

Sodium channels can be overexpressed in the axons forming the neuroma leading to mechanical sensitivity and pain.[10] As described above, the milieu the neuroma finds itself in may greatly influence the degree of resulting pain. Excessive scar formation, external pressure from prosthesis, and chronic inflammation from poor wound healing can all lead to chronic pain. If there is persistent pain, hyperalgesia can develop such that even the stimulus from a shirt sleeve lying on an amputation stump has been known to cause intractable pain in patients with neuromas. A neuroma that forms after limb amputation will refer pain to the original distribution of the nerve, leading to phantom pain.

Surgical management of the nerve of amputation neuromas involves division of the nerve proximal to the neuroma. The proximal end is then turned and protected by deeply seating it in muscle or bone. Although a new neuroma will form, it will hopefully not be subject to repeated motion at a joint or to mechanical pressure.

Lesions in Continuity

A nerve may be injured in such a way that a neuroma in continuity forms. This occurs when only some axons are severed in a nerve while others remain intact. Sprouting from damaged axons occurs forming a neuroma within the nerve. In this condition the scarring occurs both within and outside the nerve.

Management of a neuroma in continuity requires a determination of the loss versus remaining function of the nerve. An internal neurolysis can be performed, separating the fascicles and testing them individually to determine which are functional.[11] Removal of both internal and external scar is done, and finally, nerve graft repair of the damaged fascicles is entertained. The outcome of surgery for this type of lesion is marginal especially when treating pain rather than loss of function.

Palliative Measures for Pain Control

Techniques for management of pain have been traditionally separated into treatment of acute pain, cancer pain, and chronic nonmalignant pain. It was initially thought that certain medications were appropriate for only certain types of pain, however, this has become less clear. For example, use of opioids to manage chronic nonmalignant pain was frowned upon because of potential for addiction and lack of efficacy in pain relief. This class of drug has more recently been demonstrated to be highly beneficial for neuropathic pain and nonmalignant pain syndromes including chronic back pain.[12] The risk of psychological addiction is exceeding low.

Neuropathic pain is a common example of chronic nonmalignant pain that has been favorably responsive to medications such as antidepressants and anticonvulsants.[13] These drugs may be used as a first-line therapeutic regime and often lower the necessary dose of a primary analgesic. The goal of therapy is to bring pain symptoms into an acceptable range for the patient. This is best attempted by a trial of each drug, titrating the dose up until symptoms are controlled or unacceptable side effects arise. While complete remission is unlikely, by using a combination of medications it is often possible to bring symptoms within a tolerable range of pain. A typical end point is a drop of 50% in the visual analogue pain score.

Antidepressants

Tricyclic antidepressants have been studied in various pain syndromes and have been shown to be beneficial in a number of conditions including neuropathic pain and peripheral neuropathy.[14] While depression is likely to play a role in the perception of pain, the efficacy of these drugs has been established at doses too small and at a time interval too short to be attributable to alterations of mood. Amitriptyline is commonly tried because of a combination of pain relief and sedating effects. By taking the medication at night, patients benefit from a good night's sleep, something often lacking in these patients. Initial dose is 10 to 25 mg with a 10- to 25-mg increase each 7 days to 150 mg per day. The secondary amine desipramine has also proved to be beneficial.[15] It is less likely to produce sedation and hypotension, and therefore, may be prescribed for patients who wish to avoid sedation. Regardless of the tricyclic antidepressant of choice, it is important to remember that the analgesic properties may take a week or more to have an affect on symptoms.

Use of selective serotonin re-uptake inhibitors in the treatment of chronic neuropathic pain has met with controversy. Fluoxetine has been demonstrated to be of no benefit; however, paroxetine has proven beneficial.[14]

Anticonvulsants

Pain that is paroxysmal and lancinating might be generated by ectopically excitable sites on the injured nerve. This situation has been likened to epilepsy in the brain, but occurring in the peripheral nervous system. The use of an anticonvulsant may suppress foci of activity and thus eliminate the pain. Trigeminal neuralgia, pain secondary to spontaneous activity in fifth cranial nerve, has long been known to respond to carbamazapine (Tegretol®). Gabapentin (Neurontin®) has been shown to possess anxiolytic and antinociceptive properties in addition to its effectiveness as an anticonvulsant. Gabapentin also has a favorable safety profile relative to other anticonvulsants and is becoming the anticonvulsant of choice for treatment of neuropathic pain.[16,17]

Opioids

An opioid is any member of the group of analgesics that shares the properties of morphine. Opioids produce analgesia through their activities at opioid receptors in the central and peripheral nervous system. These receptors are know μ, Δ, or κ receptors with the μ receptor providing the most significant analgesic activity. These receptors act with GTP second messenger system to suppress adenylate cyclase activity and hyperpolarize the cells responsible for nociceptive response. Opioid analgesics differ principally in the potency of their agonist activity. Some are pure agonists like morphine, and others like butorphanol are mixed agonist/antagonist. They also have varying half-lives and can be administered as immediate release or delayed release.

The use of opioids for the management of nonmalignant pain has been undergoing a revolution.[18] It has become clear that many types of pain previously not thought to be opioid-sensitive, including various forms of neuropathic pain, are in fact opioid-sensitive. The dosage should be titrated up until pain relief is achieved or unacceptable side effects occur. When used for long-term treatment, a slow-release opioid such as methadone or MS-Contin® is utilized. These allow a more sustained drug level avoiding the peaks and valleys in blood level associated with short-acting drugs. By avoiding the rapid onset of the short-acting opioids, there is less chance of psychological addiction.

Multiple studies have been published in the last decade that have demonstrated usefulness of spinal administration of opioids for malignant and nonmalignant etiologies of pain.[19,20] However, these studies have been uniformly small and nonblinded so that little can be said definitively about the effects of chronic administration. Implantable morphine pumps for spinal administration allow more direct application of the analgesic pharmacopoeia, providing greater potency and efficacy. These pumps, however, should only be used in patients in whom oral administration of opioids has failed either due to unacceptable side effects or lack of efficacy.

The stigma of drug addiction to opioid medication has hampered the use of a very effective pain management drug. It needs to be stressed that although physical dependence to opioids is routine, psychological addiction is uncommon. In general, when opioids are given to control pain, psychological dependence does not result. However, caution should always be exercised when prescribing habit-forming pharmaceuticals to patients with a history of substance abuse or drug dependence. The development of tolerance is a complex clinical issue and should not be confused with abuse.[21] It is now clear that the loss of analgesic effects over time has a differential diagnosis, only one component of which is tolerance. Evidence from a variety of sources suggests that true pharmacological tolerance to the analgesic effects of opioids is an uncommon cause for the need to escalate the opioid dose to maintain analgesic effects.[21]

Electrical Stimulation Modalities

Transcutaneous electrical nerve stimulation

Transcutaneous electrical nerve stimulation (TENS) attempts to control pain through stimulation of peripheral nerve afferents. TENS devices stimulate peripheral nerves with electrical pulses of varying amplitudes and frequencies. It is thought that TENS activates the descending inhibitory pain fibers to induce analgesia or blocks the primary afferent (gait control theory[22]). TENS is most effective in patients suffering from musculoskeletal pain, phantom limb pain, and headache.[23] TENS units are frequently used by physiotherapists taking advantage of the pain relief to allow further mobilization of the affected limb. Another pain syndrome treated by TENS with variable success is post-thoracoscopy pain.[24] TENS typically induces relief of a few days' duration, but its long-term success rate is unclear.

Spinal Cord Stimulation

Spinal cord stimulation (SCS) delivers electrical stimulation to the dorsal columns of the spinal cord by way of electrodes placed in the epidural space. When the electrode is properly placed, the patient feels paresthesia or "buzzing" sensations in the same distribution as the pain often accompanied by reports of decreased pain. SCS is most effective when used in patients for whom there is a clear etiology of pain symptoms and in whom the conventional therapeutic regimens mentioned earlier have failed.[25] Presently, failed back syndrome is the most common indication for its use,[26] but many types of pain syndromes can be treated in this manner.

To be effective, stimulation must be able to reach the peripheral sensory fibers responsible for the painful sensation. As a result, patients with monoradiculopathies, ischemic pain from peripheral vascular disease, and phantom limb pain do very well with spinal cord stimulation. Patients in whom signal conduction to the periphery is compromised, such as those with spinal cord injury, do not benefit from this therapy. A trial of this procedure should be performed in all stimulation candidates to demonstrate that paresthesias can be elicited by spinal stimulation in the distribution of pain.[26] The patient determines if indeed there is pain relief, and if so, permanent implantation of the devise occurs. If the trial fails, it is a simple matter to pull out the epidural electrode. It is more difficult to maintain coverage and pain relief in the upper extremity versus the lower as there is more motion in the cervical spine associated with migration of the electrode.

Dorsal Root Entry Zone Lesion

Avulsions of the brachial or lumbar plexus occur when the nerves of the plexus are sufficiently stretched such that the spinal roots are torn free from the spinal cord. Avulsion is severely traumatic to the dorsal horn of the spinal cord resulting in a local gliotic scar. It has been postulated that the scar induces an epileptic focus in the dorsal horn. If the WDR cells discharge secondary to activity in the scar, severe disabling pain in the affected dermatome occurs. This accounts for certain forms of phantom pain.

When oral medications fail to control the pain of avulsion, consideration is given to surgical intervention. The dorsal root entry zone (DREZ) procedure involves use of a radiofrequency electrode to create a series of lesions in the dorsal horn region of the avulsed roots. A new iatrogenic lesion replaces the old traumatic epileptic focus. The effectiveness of this operation for pain secondary to avulsion injury has been impressive; however, other neuropathic pain syndromes have not fared as well.[27,28]

Physical Therapy

Patients who suffer from chronic pain often benefit from various forms of physical therapy. Pain in a limb can lead to disuse of the extremity with subsequent adhesive capsulitis in the joints. Contractures of ligament and tendons occurs further limiting range of motion. Pain secondary to the musculoskeletal issues can then complicate the picture. An aggressive therapy program will maintain both active and passive range of motion as well as general muscle conditioning. Mobilization of the affected limb has long been considered a cornerstone in the management of reflex sympathetic dystrophy.[29]

Pain and the Sympathetic Nervous System

Pain syndromes can become complex and defy simple pathophysiological explanations. Patients describe extreme burning, dysesthetic pain sensations involving large areas of the body with little relation to any demonstrated soft tissue or nerve injury. Autonomic dysfunction is manifest by temperature and color changes, edema, and trophic changes. Formerly known as reflex sympathetic dystrophy and causalgia, these pain syndromes are now labeled complex regional pain syndrome type I (CRPS-onti I), or if there is a documented nerve injury, type II (CRPS-II).[30]

If the pain is related to activity in the sympathetic nervous system, then the term sympathetically maintained pain (SMP) is used.[31] The *sine qua none* of sympathetic involvement are the following observations: (1) sympathetic block or sympatholysis provides at least transient relief of symptoms, and (2) sympathetic stimulation exacerbates pain.[29] If a patient is treated with guanethidine, which depletes norepinephrine from the sympathetic synapse, or phentolamine, which blocks the α-adrenergic receptors, and his pain subsides, it is reasonable to assume that the sympathetic nervous system had played a part in the maintenance of that pain. Furthermore, if the administration of norepineperine then brings about a return of the controlled pain, the syndrome is certainly consistent with SMP.

CRPS often presents with autonomic dysfunction suggestive of sympathetic involvement, but it is important to assert that SMP cannot be diagnosed by those findings. Signs such as increased temperature or sweating may occur in either the affected or unaffected extremity or not at all in certain cases of SMP. Definitively, SMP is that pain that is resolved by administration of sympathetic blockade and exacerbated by sympathetic agonists with signs of autonomic dysfunction being a frequent but nonspecific finding.

The effect of cooling stimuli and its diagnostic implications may also be confusing. Whereas as many as 50% of patients with sympathetic independent pain may have cooling hyperalgesia, it is extraordinarily unlikely that an SMP patient won't demonstrate this phenomenon, thus presence of cooling hyperalgesia is sensitive but not specific for SMP.

SMP can often be managed by sympathetic ganglion blockade. This might be accomplished by local anesthesia at the level of the sympathetic ganglion, by oral antiadrenergic therapy, or surgical sympathectomy. SMP in the distribution of the hand that failed nonsurgical management is treated by removal of the T2 ganglion either through conventional surgical approaches, or using the more recent techniques of endoscopic ganglionectomy.[32] In cases of lumbar surgical sympathectomy, patients may experience some post-surgical pain in the groin or lower extremity but this is usually self-limited and quickly goes away. Unfortunately, the pain can return and necessitate a contralateral sympathectomy.

Summary

Pain is a complex phenomenon influenced by subjective and emotional factors. This chapter has described several of the elemental syndromes of pain. Somatic and visceral injury can cause protracted pain that is self limited by the extent of injury. In this case, opioids and other analgesics are helpful to keep pain within tolerable limits until recovery can occur. When a nerve is injured, neuropathic pain may result. This form of pain is often out of proportion to the injury and spreads in a distribution greater than that of the affected nerve. Neuropathic pain is generally less responsive to opioids but anticonvulsants such as Gabapentin and antidepressants including amitriptyline, as well as other adjuvant analgesics have been shown to be beneficial. When these therapies fail, electrical stimulation modalities such as TENS or SPS may be of benefit. In patients with pain secondary to scar foci or entrapment, neurotomy or nerve graft operations may be indicated. In the specific case of brachial plexus avulsion, the DREZ operation has been shown to relieve pain. Some forms of pain are mediated in part by the sympathetic nervous system. In these syndromes, pain is often limited to the face and extremities and can be elicited by cooling stimuli. For these patients, treatment with adrenergic agonists like prazosin or phentolamine often provides relief. Where these fail, sympathetic ganglionectomy can often eliminate the sympathetic component of pain.

References

1. Wall PD, Melzack R: *Textbook of Pain*. Third edition. New York: Churchill Livingstone; 1994.
2. Lynn B, Faulstroh K, Pierau F-K: The classification and properties of nociceptive afferent units from the skin of the anaesthetized pig. *Eur J Neurosci* 7: 431–437, 1995.
3. Michaelis M, Devor M, Jänig W: Sympathetic modulation of activity in rat dorsal root ganglion neurons changes over time following peripheral nerve injury. *J Neurophysiol* 76:753–763, 1996.
4. Han HC, Na HS, Yoon YW, Chung JM: Ectopic discharges from injured afferent fibers in a rat model of neuropathic pain. *Soc Neurosci Abst* 20(Suppl. Pt 1 & 2):00–00, 1994.
5. Gelberman RH, Eaton R, Urbaniak JR: Peripheral nerve compression. *J Bone Joint Surg (Am)* 75A:1854–1878, 1993.
6. de Araujo MP: Electrodiagnosis in compression neuropathies of the upper extremities. *Orthop Clin North Am* 27:237–244, 1996.
7. Cervero F, Laird JMA: Mechanisms of allodynia: Interactions between sensitive mechanoreceptors and nociceptors. *Neuroreport* 7:526–528, 1996.
8. Khasar SG, Miao FJP, Levine JD: Inflammation modulates the contribution of receptor-subtypes to bradykinin-induced hyperalgesia in the rat. *Neuroscience* 69:685–690, 1995.
9. Rowbotham MC, Fields HL: The relationship of pain, allodynia and thermal sensation in post-herpetic neuralgia. *Brain* 119:347–354, 1996.
10. England JD, Happel LT, Kline DG, et al: Sodium channel accumulation in humans with painful neuromas. *Neurology* 47:272–276, 1996.
11. Belzberg AJ, Campbell JN: Peripheral nerve repair. *Neurosurgical Operative Atlas* 3(2):119–133, 1993.
12. Reidenberg MM, Portenoy RK: The need for an open mind about the treatment of chronic nonmalignant pain. *Clin Pharmacol Ther* 55:367–369, 1994.
13. Max MB: Towards physiologically based treatment of patients with neuropathic pain. *Pain* 42:131–133, 1990.
14. Max MB, Lynch SA, Muir J, et al: Effects of desipramine, amitriptyline and

fluoxetine on pain in diabetic neuropathy. *N Engl J Med* 326(19):1250–1256, 1992.

15. Kishore-Kumar R, Max MB, Schafer SC, et al: Desipramine relieves postherpetic neuralgia. *Clin Pharmacol Ther* 47:305–312, 1990.
16. Wetzel CH, Connelly JF: Use of gabapentin in pain management. *Ann Pharmacother* 31:1082–1083, 1997.
17. Rosner H, Rubin L, Kestenbaum A: Gabapentin adjunctive therapy in neuropathic pain states. *Clin J Pain* 12:56–58, 1996.
18. Portenoy RK: Opioid therapy for chronic nonmalignant pain: A review of the critical issues. *J Pain Symptom Manage* 11:203–217, 1996.
19. Winkelmüller M, Winkelmüller W: Long-term effects of continuous intrathecal opioid treatment in chronic pain of nonmalignant etiology. *J Neurosurg* 85: 458–467, 1996.
20. Abram SE: Continuous spinal anesthesia for cancer and chronic pain. *Reg Anesth* 18:406–413, 1993.
21. Portenoy RK: Tolerance to opioid analgesics: Clinical aspects. *Cancer Surv* 21: 49–65, 1994.
22. Melzack P, Wall PD: Pain mechanisms: A new theory. *Science* 150(3699): 971–978, 1965.
23. Meyler WJ, de Jongste MJ, Rolf CA: Clinical evaluation of pain treatment with electrostimulation: A study on TENS in patients with different pain syndromes. *Clin J Pain* 10:22–27, 1994.
24. Brodsky JB, Mark JB: Postthoracoscopy pain: Is TENS the answer? [editorial; comment]. *Ann Thorac Surg* 63:608–610, 1997.
25. North RB: Spinal cord stimulation for chronic, intractable pain. In: Schmidek HH, Sweet WH, eds. *Operative Neurosurgical Techniques.* Third edition. Philadelphia, PA: W.B. Saunders; 1995, pp. 1403–1411.
26. North RB, Kidd DH, Lee MS, Piantadosi S: Spinal cord stimulation versus reoperation for the failed back surgery syndrome: A prospective, randomized study design. *Stereotact Funct Neurosurg* 62:267–272, 1995.
27. Carvalho GA, Nikkhah G, Samii M: [Pain management after post-traumatic brachial plexus lesions. Conservative and surgical therapy possibilities]. *Orthopade* 26:621–625, 1997.
28. Young RF: Clinical experience with radiofrequency and laser DREZ lesions. *J Neurosurg* 72:715–720, 1990.
29. Campbell JN, Raja SN, Selig DK, et al: Diagnosis and management of sympathetically maintained pain. In: Fields HL, Liebeskind JC, eds. *Progress in Pain Research and Management.* Volume 1. Seattle: IASP Press; 1994, pp. 85–100.
30. Stanton-Hicks M, Jänig W, Hassenbusch S, et al: Reflex sympathetic dystrophy: Changing concepts and taxonomy. *Pain* 63:127–133, 1995.
31. Belzberg AJ: Sympathetic pain syndromes. *J Orofacial Pain* 8(1):100, 1994.
32. Samuelsson H, Claes G, Drott C: Endoscopic electrocautery of the upper thoracic sympathetic chain: A safe and simple technique for treatment of sympathetically maintained pain. *Eur J Surg* 160(Suppl. 572):55–57, 1994.

Part III

Intrinsic and Acquired Disorders of the Upper Extremity Vessels

13

Small Artery Disease of the Upper Extremity

*Kent Williamson, MD, James M. Edwards, MD,
Lloyd M. Taylor, Jr, MD, Gregory J. Landry, MD,
and John M. Porter, MD*

In this chapter we discuss the diagnosis, classification, and treatment of vasospastic and obstructive diseases of the digital and palmar arteries. Hand and finger ischemia may be episodic without tissue loss as in vasospastic Raynaud's syndrome (RS), or fixed and severe, occasionally including finger gangrene due to small artery obstructive disease. Obstructive hand and finger ischemia is unusual but not rare. In our experience, 5% to 10% of patients presenting with upper extremity ischemic symptoms have hand and finger ischemia or digital gangrene as a result of potentially correctable arterial obstruction at or proximal to the wrist, including such conditions as subclavian artery occlusion or aneurysm formation with or without thoracic outlet arterial compression, trauma including angiographic complications, emboli, or atherosclerosis.[1-3]

A large majority (over 60%) of patients with digital ischemia presenting for medical evaluation suffer from a variety of systemic diseases that include occlusions of palmar and digital arteries. Another large group of patients have episodic hand and finger ischemia caused by vasospasm. They differ from the obstructive group clinically both by the episodic nature of their ischemic episodes and by a conspicuous absence of tissue loss. The appearance of gangrene or significant ulceration always implies fixed arterial obstructive disease.

During the past two decades we have prospectively studied over 1100

From Machleder HI, (ed): *Vascular Disorders of the Upper Extremity.* Third Revised Edition. Futura Publishing Company, Inc., Armonk, NY, © 1998.

patients with vasospastic and/or obstructive upper extremity small artery disease, including over 200 patients with upper extremity digital tissue loss caused by occlusive disease of the palmar and digital arteries.[4-6] These patients have been divided into vasospastic and obstructive subgroups based on clinical history and noninvasive vascular laboratory testing. We recognize that this division is arbitrary and that there is clearly a continuum of disease between these two categories. Most of the information presented in this chapter has been obtained from our experience in the diagnosis and management of these groups of patients.

Raynaud's Syndrome

RS is a condition characterized by episodic attacks of digital artery vasospasm in response to cold stimuli or emotional stress. The hands and fingers are most commonly involved, although the feet and toes may be affected in a small percentage of patients. A classic attack lasts 15 to 45 minutes and consists of pallor of the distal portion of the extremity, followed by cyanosis and rubor on warming. Most patients do not have the classic tricolor changes as described and will complain of cold hands with either pallor or cyanosis. A number of patients experience no visible color change at all, experiencing only episodic attacks of hand and finger coldness. These patients have the same abnormal arteriographic and vascular laboratory tests seen in patients with classic tricolor changes, hence we no longer require tricolor changes to make the diagnosis.

History

Episodic digital ischemia was first described by Maurice Raynaud in 1862.[7] He hypothesized that the condition was due to vasospasm because a majority of his patients had normal radial pulses in association with distal hand ischemia. Hutchinson,[8,9] around the turn of the century, accurately observed that episodic hand ischemia occurred in association with a variety of disease processes and did not represent a single disease entity as suggested by Raynaud. Thus, he suggested the condition be termed a phenomenon and recognized as a frequent accompaniment to a number of disease processes. In 1932, Allen and Brown[10] again emphasized that other diseases were frequently associated with RS. They proposed division of the syndrome into Raynaud's phenomenon, in which the digital changes were associated with systemic disease, and Raynaud's disease, a benign idiopathic form not associated with other disease states. Eventually, other authors accurately observed that many patients who initially appeared to have the idiopathic form clearly manifested an associated disease, commonly an autoimmune disease, years later.[11-13] By the 1970s it was obvious that a large percentage of patients with RS at tertiary medical centers had significant associated diseases.[5,14] Presently, we feel that there is little justification for the division of RS into disease and phenomenon. Instead, we recognize that all patients with RS are at increased risk for the development of an associated disease over their lifetime.

Pathophysiology

The initial pallor of an attack is caused by spasm of the digital arteries and arterioles. After a variable period of time the capillaries and probably the venules dilate in response to both hypoxia and the accumulation of products of anaerobic metabolism. When the arterial spasm relaxes, the initial blood flow into the dilated capillaries rapidly desaturates causing cyanosis. Finally, rubor results from increasing amounts of blood into the dilated capillary bed, and the digits return to normal as the capillaries constrict.

The underlying pathophysiology of RS has been the object of investigation for over a century. Sir Thomas Lewis,[15] in the 1920s, observed that conduction anesthetic block of the digital nerves did not prevent attacks and therefore concluded that the sympathetic nervous system was not involved. He hypothesized a "local vascular fault" as the cause of the hyper-reactivity to cold seen in digital arteries in patients with RS.[15] Indirect measurements of blood flow and pressure in the hands and fingers have shown that patients with RS have considerably decreased flow at room temperature with a striking additional decrease with cooling. At the critical temperature at 18°C to 20°C digital artery closure occurs.[16-18]

Numerous publications as well as our own experience clearly indicate that patients with RS may be divided into two distinct pathophysiological groups: vasospastic and obstructive.[19,20] Patients with vasospastic RS usually have no associated disease and generally correspond to the groups formerly termed Raynaud's disease. Those with obstructive RS always have an associated disease and thus generally constitute the group formerly described as having Raynaud's phenomenon.

Patients with obstructive RS have obstruction of the palmar and digital arteries that produces a significant reduction of resting digital arterial pressure. As a result, a normal arterial vasoconstrictive response to cold causes complete arterial closure. This theory predicts all patients with severe palmar and digital arterial obstruction yielding a decrease in digital arterial pressure will have cold-induced RS; by our observations this is true.

Patients with vasospastic RS do not have significant hand or digital artery obstruction and have normal digital blood pressures at room temperature. Arterial closure in these patients is caused by an increased force of cold-induced vasospasm. A number of studies have suggested altered adrenergic activity in patients with RS. Coffman and Cohen[16] found decreased digital nutritive blood flow in patients with RS which was increased after treatment with the sympathetic blocking drug reserpine. We have also shown a marked decrease in digital artery cold-induced spasm after intra-arterial reserpine treatment.[21] Jamieson and associates[22] suggested that patients with RS may possess abnormal adrenergic receptors that are hypersensitive after cold exposure.

In recent years, knowledge of human adrenergic receptor function has increased markedly with the characterization of the α_1- and α_2-adrenoceptors. α_2-Adrenergic receptors are present as a pure population on human platelets, and are the predominant adrenoreceptor of the distal extremity. They are believed to be the primary receptor type responsible for vasospasm.[23] We have demonstrated that platelet α_2-receptors are elevated in patients with vasospastic RS (Figure 1), and serum of RS patients causes a decrease of measurable α_2-adrenergic receptor levels (Figure 2).[24,25] As yet there is no direct evidence linking elevated platelet to elevated arterial wall α_2-adrenergic receptor levels, but there is evidence in

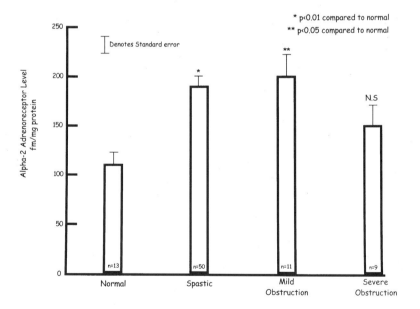

Figure 1. Platelet α_2-adrenoreceptor levels in patients with Raynaud's syndrome. Patients with vasospastic Raynaud's syndrome with or without mild obstruction have α_2-adrenoreceptor levels greater than normals. Patients with obstructive Raynaud's syndrome have levels that are not significantly higher than normals. (Reproduced with permission from from Reference 25.)

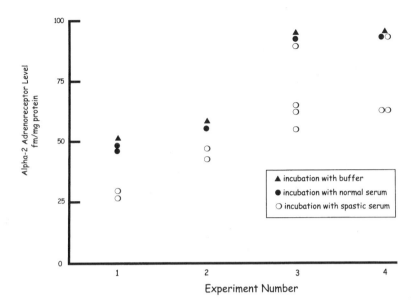

Figure 2. Effect of serum from normal subjects and serum from patients with vasospastic Raynaud's syndrome on normal patients. Incubation of normal platelets with serum from patients with vasospastic Raynaud's syndrome results in a 17% decrease in measurable platelet α_2-adrenoreceptor levels compared to incubation with normal serum ($P < 0.01$). (Reproduced with permission from Reference 25.)

other systems (β-receptors on lymphocytes and atrial wall) that such a relation exists. To explain the decrease in measurable α_2-adrenergic receptor levels seen in the incubation studies we have hypothesized a circulating factor (possibly an antibody) in patients with RS. We suspect that an antireceptor antibody may constitute the primary pathophysiological abnormality in these patients.

Recent work on the etiology of RS suggests that endothelin-1 and calcitonin gene-related peptide play an important role. Levels of endothelin-1 (a potent vasoconstrictor) are found to be three times higher in patients with RS when compared with controls.[26] These levels are also noted to double in both controls and in RS patients during cold exposure.[26] Calcitonin gene-related peptide, a vasodilator, is significantly depleted in patients with RS.[27]

Epidemiology

Neither the prevalence nor incidence of RS in the general population is known with certainty, but several epidemiological studies indicate a prevalence of 20% to 25% in the young adult population in the cool damp climates of Copenhagen, Denmark and Portland, Oregon.[28,29] It is not known whether cool, damp climates increase the incidence of RS, or merely increase the number of people who are symptomatic. We suspect the latter. Females comprise 70% to 90% of most reported patient groups with RS.[30] Typically younger women have vasospastic RS without evidence of associated diseases. Some patients develop an associated disease at a later date. Older males with RS usually have digital artery occlusion, often from arteriosclerosis. Within our database of 1100 patients, 56% were diagnosed with vasospastic and 43% with obstructive RS at initial presentation, while at 10-year follow-up 42% had vasospastic and 58% had obstructive RS.[31]

Certain occupational groups have a high prevalence of RS, especially those associated with the use of vibrating tools. This is becoming increasingly important because of heightened awareness of occupational hazards and resulting liability. The prevalence of vasospasm in chain saw operators and miners using vibrating tools ranges from 40% to 90%, with the higher figures in patients with longer exposures.[19,32] Available evidence indicates a number of individuals with long-term vibration exposure develop ongoing arterial damage which may in certain patients lead to digital artery obstruction. A single report has described an increased prevalence of RS among food workers who work in cold areas, but once again it is impossible to know if the cold exposure were causative or merely facilitative.[33]

Associated Diseases

RS has been observed in combination with many disorders,[4,5,10,13,34,35] and a general classification is shown in Table 1. All or nearly all of the conditions listed in Table 1 may be associated with diffuse obstructive palmar and digital arterial disease. In our experience, patients with obstructive RS with positive serological studies have a 73% liklihood of developing connective tissue disease (CTD), and those with vasospastic RS with positive serological screening have a 48.6% liklihood of CTD. These data are similar at 10 year follow-up.[31] Rates of progression to CTD over 10 years ranges from 2% to 30% depending on serological status and whether patients have spastic or obstructive disease patterns. Patients with positive serological screens and obstructive disease patterns have the highest rates of conversion, with up to 82% in this group developing CTD.[31] The 70% to 80% associated disease rate, with near certainty, does not apply to the minimally symptomatic patient who has never sought medical care. The prevalence of associated disease in minimally symptomatic patients is unknown but is assumed to be low. However, available evidence persuasively indicates that the incidence of associated disease

---

Table 1
Disorders Associated With Raynaud's Syndrome

Immunological and connective tissue disorders
  Scleroderma
  Mixed connective tissue disease
  Systemic lupus erythematosus
  Rheumatoid arthritis
  Dermatomyositis
  Polymyositis
  Hepatitis-B antigen induced vasculitis
  Drug induced vasculitis
  Sjogren's syndrome
  Hypersensitivity angiitis
  Undifferentiated connective tissue disease

Obstructive arterial diseases
  Arteriosclerosis
  Thromboangiitis obliterans
  Thoracic outlet syndrome

Environmental conditions
  Vibration injury
  Direct arterial trauma
  Cold injury

Drug-induced Raynaud's syndrome without vasculitis
  Ergot
  β-blockers
  Cytotoxic drugs
  Birth control pills

Miscellaneous
  Vinyl chloride disease
  Chronic renal failure
  Cold agglutinins
  Cryoglobulinemia
  Neoplasia
  Endocrinological disorders
  Neurological disorders
    1. Central
    2. Peripheral

---

is so high in RS that every physician evaluating a patient with RS should conduct a methodical search for an associated disease as described later in this chapter.

Small Artery Occlusive Diseases

A significant majority of patients with symptomatic peripheral arterial occlusive disease suffer from atherosclerosis of the large arteries sup-

Table 2
Systemic Diseases That May Cause Localized Digital Gangrene

Connective tissue disease and other arteritides
Scleroderma - CRST*
Rheumatoid arthritis*
Sjøgren's syndrome*
Systemic lupus erythematosus*
Polyarteritis nodosa mixed connective tissue disease*
Undifferentiated connective tissue disease*
Wegener's granulomatosis allergic granulomatosis Schonlein-Henoch purpura hypersensitivity
Angiitis*

Myeloproliferative Disorders
Polycythemia rubra vera
Thrombocytosis
Leukemia
Myeloid metaplasia

Immunoglobulin Abnormalities
Mixed cryoglobulinemia
Myeloma or benign monoclonal gammopathy
Macroglobulinemia
Cold agglutinin disease
Tumor produced globulins

Miscellaneous
Systemic malignancy
Disseminated intravascular coagulopathy
Chronic renal failure (calciphylaxis)
Arteriosclerosis*
Buerger's disease*

* Most frequently associated with digital gangrene.

plying the lower extremities. Only about 5% of patients with peripheral ischemia have symptomatic involvement of the upper extremity. In our experience, by far the most frequent cause of upper extremity ischemia is small artery occlusive disease of the palmar and digital arteries, in contrast to lower extremity ischemia that is caused almost exclusively by large vessel occlusion.[36] Fingertip ulceration or localized gangrene may develop in severe cases of upper extremity ischemia.

A partial listing of systemic conditions that may be associated with digital gangrene is shown in Table 2. The recognition that digital gangrene or ulceration may result from intrinsic small artery occlusive disease with normal proximal arteries is often considered only after extensive evaluation finger ischemia fails to reveal proximal arterial obstruction or a cardiac embolic source. A basic principle succinctly states that digital gangrene always implies palmar and digital arterial obstruction. Gangrene is not caused by vasospasm except with toxic doses of certain drugs.

The fact that proximal arterial lesions may serve as a source of distal emboli is widely known; and about 5% of our patients with palmar and digital artery occlusions appear to have these as a result of embolization from either a proximal arterial or cardiac source. In the remainder the small artery occlusive disease occurs as a result of a systemic disease process that does not involve the large arteries proximal to the wrist.

The most frequently associated diseases found in patients with digital gangrene are the autoimmune or CTDs. In our experience these have been present in 43.2% of patients with severe palmar and digital artery occlusive disease. All of the diseases termed CTDs have an associated arteritis, or, in the case of scleroderma, an obliterative arteriopathy that may cause progressive obstruction of the small and medium arteries of the hands and fingers as well as in other similar sized arteries. We presently do not understand the predilection of these arteritides to involve the palmar and digital arteries or the widely variable degree of involvement among different patients with the same underlying disease. In our experience, the autoimmune disease most frequently associated with digital ischemia is scleroderma or the associated CRST syndrome. Virtually all patients with scleroderma develop stenoses or occlusions of the digital arteries.[37] It is important to note that digital ischemia, frequently accompanied by classic RS symptoms, may precede the development of clinical CTD by years.[38]

The CTDs that in our experience have been most frequently associated with digital gangrene are indicated by an asterisk in Table 2. A number of patients will be found who have definite laboratory and clinic evidence of CTD but lack the precise spectrum of findings to place them in a single diagnostic category. These patients are classified as having undifferentiated CTD.[39]

Hypersensitivity angiitis is a term we use to describe a subset of patients we have encountered with digital gangrene resulting from intrinsic small artery occlusive disease. The most striking finding that characterizes this group of patients has been the abrupt onset of severe ischemia at the tips of multiple fingers without any premonitory signs or symptoms.[40] The onset was so abrupt that most patients could recall the exact day symptoms began. These patients are typically young females (mean age, 36 years). Exhaustive immunologic evaluation failed to reveal any consistent abnormalities, while digital angiography in each patient showed massive palmar and digital arterial occlusion. The acute ischemic event resolved with conservative therapy in each case. Long-term follow-up of these patients (up to 15 years) has revealed no development of CTDs nor recurrence of ischemic events in a large majority.[6] Remote arteriograms have shown persistent occlusive disease with the development of collateral digital circulation. Although our designation of this condition as hypersensitivity angiitis in the absence of tissue confirmation remains speculative, its similarity to hypersensitivity angiitis appears to us sufficiently close to warrant use of this classification.

Buerger's disease is another condition that causes widespread digital artery occlusions and finger gangrene. It appears to represent a thrombotic arteriopathy occurring predominately in young male smokers and is characterized by the occurrence of segmental thrombotic occlusions in both the upper and lower extremities, although in general there is a considerable lower extremity preponderance. There are objective clinical criteria available to make the diagnosis of Buerger's disease.[41] These include the onset of distal extremity ischemic symptoms before 45 years of age, absence of embolic source, autoimmune disease, diabetes or hyperlipidemia; healthy proximal arteries; and distal occlusive disease with distinctive plethysmographic, arteriographic, or pathological findings.

Widespread atherosclerosis with involvement of the forearm and palmar arteries is seen occasionally. Detailed autopsy studies by Laws et al[42] showed that arteriosclerotic obstruction of the palmar and digital arteries without severe generalized arteriosclerosis was not found below the age of 50 years. Beyond age 50 years, men were affected earlier than women. The diagnosis is made by finding diffuse palmar and digital occlusive disease in association with typical large artery atherosclerosis.

A small number of patients with digital gangrene will be found to have a malignancy. Digital artery obstruction associated with malignancy has been previously described by us and others.[43,44] In certain patients the malignancy-associated ischemia appears to result from arterial thrombosis while in other patients the mechanism appears that of an inflammatory arteritis.

Patient Presentation

Raynaud's Syndrome

The usual patient with spastic RS is a young woman who describes symptoms that began as a child or teenager. Both hands are affected equally, although the thumbs may be spared. On questioning, some increased sensitivity of the feet and toes can be elicited, with about 10% of the patients complaining primarily of their feet and toes. Obstructive RS seems to have a 1:1 male to female ratio, and most patients are over 40 years of age. The lower extremities are infrequently involved, and there may be only a few involved digits.

Most attacks are produced by cold exposure, with half the patients having occasional attacks in response to fear or anger. The stimulus for an attack may be as mild as walking into an air conditioned room or picking up a cold glass. In addition to color changes, attacks are usually associated with numbness. Severe pain is rare. Most spontaneous indoor attacks will resolve in 5 to 10 minutes. Many if not most attacks precipitated by outdoor cold exposure terminate only when the patient enters a warm area or applies heat to the part.

Digital Gangrene

The term digital gangrene as used in this chapter refers to tissue necrosis occurring usually at the fingertip and varying from black-blue cutaneous gangrene to necrotic ulcerations as seen in Figure 3.

In our experience, two-thirds of patients presenting with digital gangrene are women, with a median age of 46 years. The patients are easily divisible into two groups based on their presentation with an acute or chronic history of finger gangrene. Approximately 40% of patients present within several weeks to a few months of the acute onset of digital ischemia. Most of these patients experienced the precipitous onset of cyanosis and pain involving the distal portions of multiple fingers, followed in days to several weeks by the development of skin necrosis, with a variable amount of tissue loss. Systemic signs and symptoms of CTD are absent in most patients presenting with acute symptoms. Of the patients who present with gangrenous fingertips, about 60% have a chronic history of digital gangrene, often with multiple exacerbations and remissions extending over a period of years. Patients in this group average 5 to 10 years older than those in the acute group. The acutely symptomatic patients as a group are younger, less likely to have preexisting RS, and less likely to use tobacco than members of the chronic group.

Clinical Evaluation

All patients presenting for evaluation of RS or digital ischemia and/ or gangrene should be carefully questioned and examined for signs and symptoms of CTD, specifically arthritis, arthralgia, myalgia, skin rash, alopecia, sclerodactyly, dysphagia, xerostomia, xerophthalmia, telangiectasia, hand swelling, digital skin binding, and oropharyngeal ulceration. A specific inquiry and search should be made for evidence of healed digital tip infarcts and calcinosis cutis. A history of angina pectoris, myocardial infarction, transient ischemic attacks, or findings of diminished peripheral pulses and/or bruits should be carefully sought as an indication of generalized atherosclerosis. Symptoms of carpal tunnel syndrome should be sought as it is present in up to 15% of patients with RS.[4]

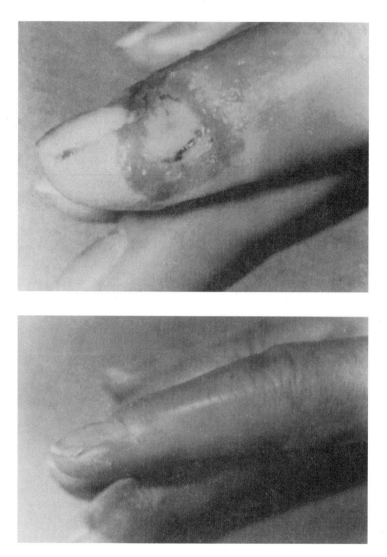

Figure 3. A: A necrotic extraordinarily painful digital ulcer in a 60-year-old female with scleroderma. **B:** Total healing of ulcer after 3 months of conservative therapy.

Other causes of digital artery occlusion should be explored, such as a history of frostbite,[45] repetitive trauma (hypothenar hammer syndrome),[46] accidental intra-arterial drug injection,[47] proximal embolic source,[48] drug ingestion (ergot intoxication),[49] and environmental toxin exposure including heavy metals and vinyl chloride.[50] Physical examination should include palpation for cervical rib and clavicular anomalies. We have found that initial and sequential hand and finger color photographs have been remarkably helpful in objectively documenting the patient's clinical course.

Vascular Laboratory

The noninvasive vascular laboratory is of great utility in the diagnosis of patients with either episodic or obstructive upper extremity ischemia. Digital photoplethysmography is used in association with finger pneumatic cuffs to obtain digital pressures and waveforms, which permits both the detection and quantitation of obstructive digital artery disease.[51] Patients with clinical evidence of vasospasm are further tested with the digital hypothermic challenge test described by Nielsen and associates.[17] In our experience, this has been the most accurate (92%) test for RS.[17] Several other tests are used for the objective diagnosis of RS, including thermal entrainment, which may be as accurate as the digital hypothermic challenge test.[52] However, neither test is widely available. The simple measurement of digital temperature recovery after cold water exposure is very sensitive (100%), but not specific (50%).[4] The objective documentation of digital vasospasm, while often irrelevant in clinical practice, is of great value in industrial compensation cases and for epidemiological screening.

Angiography

Digital photoplethysmography with digital blood pressure determination is as accurate as angiography in the detection of significant digital obstruction, and the finding of a digital blood pressure 10 mm Hg below brachial establishes the diagnosis.[53,54] While the use of the noninvasive vascular laboratory allows the objective evaluation of digital ischemia, it does not eliminate the need for upper extremity arteriography in certain patients. As stated earlier, digital gangrene always implies arterial luminal occlusion and does not result from vasospasm. The purpose of angiography is not to confirm distal arterial obstruction that is obviously present in all these patients, but to rule out a proximal disease process such as subclavian artery stenosis, subclavian aneurysm with or without thoracic outlet syndrome, unexpected pseudoaneurysm, etc., which may be serving as a source of emboli and that may be amenable to surgical repair. If no diagnosis can be made on laboratory data, and particularly if the signs and symptoms are unilateral, the diagnosis of isolated distal small artery occlusive disease can be established with certainty only after proximal arterial disease has been angiographically eliminated. Complete angiography has traditionally constituted an integral portion of the evaluation of patients with digital gangrene, and has required visualization of the arterial circulation from the aortic arch to the fingertips in both hands. These angiograms are best performed by the transfemoral approach using magnification technique for the filming of the hand circulation. An example of the detail obtainable is shown in Figures 4 and 5. The arteriograms may be obtained before and after cold exposure (cryodynamic angiography) and before and after intra-arterial tolazoline if significant vasospasm is seen on the initial films in addition to multiple areas of luminal obstruction. The accurate assessment of digital and palmar arterial spasm requires the delicate placement of a small angiographic catheter into the axillary artery with a minimum of contact with the arterial wall to reduce the incidence of catheter-associated vasospasm. It is essential that the digital temperature be raised to at least 32°C prior to injection to minimize cold-induced vasospasm. An external heating pad and digital disk temperature probe are useful in this regard. A detailed description of our angiographic technique has been published by Rosch et al[21] from this institution. In recent years we have been increasingly willing to forego arteriography in patients with bilateral finger ischemia and a normal upper extremity arterial examination to the wrist. The likelihood of finding bilateral proximal arterial disease in such patients seems quite remote.

Laboratory

The laboratory evaluation of patients with upper extremity ischemia is outlined in Tables 3 and 4. The details and methodology of these tests have been described.[20,55] The use of the additional tests noted in Table 3 is based on the results of the history, physical, and initial laboratory results. As noted above, these tests are performed in a search for a disease process that may be associated with the digital ischemic symptoms. In our recent experience some associated disease has been found in 70% of patients with vasospastic RS and in 100% of patients with fixed palmar and digital arterial occlusions. An accurate assessment of this clinical and laboratory information should allow each patient to be accurately assigned to one of the disease categories listed in Table 2.

Treatment

The treatment for RS remains generally unsatisfactory. There are currently only a few prospective clinical trials that evaluate any of the 40 + treatment modalities available. Thus, our knowledge of the treatment for RS is based primarily on anecdotal experience and retrospective reviews of small patient series.

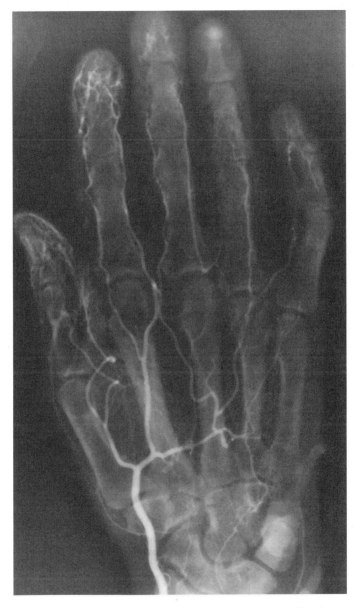

Figure 4. Magnification hand angiography revealing multiple digital artery occlusions.

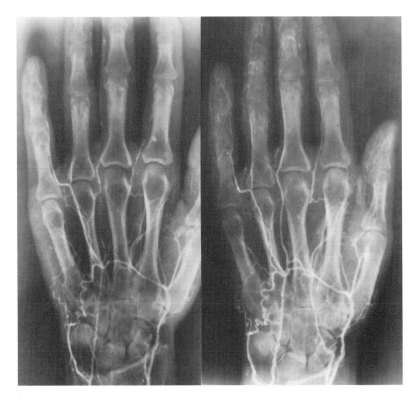

Figure 5. A: The angiogram on the left is that of a 44-year-old male with hypersensitivity angiitis and digital tip gangrene. Extensive arterial occlusion is obvious. **B:** Same patients 3 years later; the patient is asymptomatic with total healing of digital lesions. A striking increase in collateral circulation is present.

The mainstay of treatment for RS remains conservative management. The majority of patients with RS will achieve acceptable relief of symptoms through cold avoidance, wearing gloves and dressing warmly, and avoidance of tobacco. Other conservative techniques include stopping medicines that have been linked to exacerbation of RS, such as ergot alkaloids and β-blockers. Oral contraceptives were once thought to lead to exacerbation of RS, but are now felt to have little or no effect at the doses at which they are given.

A large portion of the treatment options available involve medications. In recent years, many papers have discussed as many as 37 different pharmacological interventions for RS. The following is a list of the most utilized and studied pharmacological intervention for RS.

Table 3
Diagnostic Evaluation of Upper Extremity Ischemia

	Routine	*In Selected Patients*
Laboratory	Complete blood count	
	Urinalysis	
	Sedimentation rate	
	Automated multichemistry	
	Immunologic screen (Table 4)	
Radiographic	Chest film	Barium swallow
	Hand films	Barium enema
	Magnification hand and upper extremity angiography	Intravenous pyelogram
Vascular Laboratory	Finger and toe digital Plethysmography	Digital photoplethysmography after heating and cooling
	Segmental upper and lower limb arterial pressures	Lower extremity pressure measurements
	Digital hypothermic challenge test	
Other	Schirmer's test	Skin biopsy
		Muscle biopsy
		Arterial biopsy
		Oral-mucosal biopsy
		Electromyelogram
		Nerve conductions
		Electrocardiogram

Calcium Channel Blockers

Our first-line medication in the treatment of RS is nifedipine, the most potent vasodilator among calcium channel blockers. Multiple clinical trials have been performed which indicate that as many as two-thirds of patients will demonstrate some improvement, and these tend to be patients with vasospastic RS.[56] In our experience, side effects of headache, edema, pruritis, and lassitude appear in 20% to 50% of patients, causing many of them to discontinue the drug. Most investigators have studied doses ranging from 10 to 20 mg, three times daily, and recent anecdotal experience suggests that one 30-mg dose of extended release calcium channel blocker is associated with fewer side effects.[57] Low-dose sublingual nifedipine (5 mg) has been shown to be an effective agent for prophylaxis in cold-induced vasospasm.[58,59] Other calcium channel blockers have been tested, and among those, diltiazem and felodipine show some benefit while verapamil and nicardipine do not.[31]

Table 4
Immunological Tests

	Test
Essential	Rheumatoid factor (latex particle)
	Antinuclear antibody
Complete	Serum protein electrophoresis
	Cold agglutinins
	VDRL
	Hep-2 ANA
	Anti-native DNA antibody
	Extractable nuclear antigen
	Total hemolytic complement
	Complement-(C3, C4)
	Immunoglobulin electrophoresis
	Cryoglobulins (Cryocrit)
	Cryofibrinogen
	Direct Coomb's tests
	Hepatitis B antibody
	Hepatitis B antigen

Prostaglandins

Prostaglandins and their analogues have been studied closely for their treatment efficacy in Raynaud's patients secondary to their vasodilating and antiplatelet activity. In the investigation of intravenous iloprost (a prostacyclin analogue) in patients with RS and PSS, the mean number of "attacks" were found to decrease by 39.1%. The same study found that 34.8% of patients felt some improvement with iloprost, while only 19.7% of the placebo group reported improvement ($P = 0.011$).[60] In other studies, retrospective analysis showed 58% of patients quoted improvement with iloprost, whereas 43% felt some improvement with other forms of treatment.[31] Iloprost also proved useful in patients who would not respond to other therapies, with up to 50% showing some benefit.[61] Other studies have evaluated the use of intravenous iloprost and its effects Raynaud's episodes and ulcer healing. Intravenous iloprost was found to have some benefit in each of these settings.[60,62] Oral formulation of iloprost has now become available, and studies are being done to determine whether this form is efficacious.[63]

Angiotensin-Converting Enzyme Inhibitors

Although angiotensin-converting enzyme (ACE) inhibitors were once thought to be of some benefit in the treatment of Raynaud's disease, controlled trials have failed to show some benefit.[64] Investigators had theorized that ACE inhibitors lead to relaxation of smooth muscle through the inhibition of angiotensin II and indirect elevation of kinins. We continue to use ACE inhibitors in a few patients who seem to have some subjective improvement, and who do not respond well to calcium channel blockers.

Vasodilators

Several topical and systemic vasodilators have been used in the treatment of RS for many years, however, the only support for their use remains anecdotal. Preparations including nitroglycerin, niacin, and papaverine are still being used despite the lack of objective data. Griseofulvin, an antifungal agent, has also been found to have vasodilating properties that may be useful in the treatment of RS,[65] although the data here are not consistently positive.

Serotonin Antagonists

Ketanserin has been proposed as a treatment for RS in that it is a serotonin antagonist that may offset vasoconstriction and platelet aggregation. Indeed, studies have shown that ketanserin is linked to increased digital temperatures that suggests improved blood flow.[66] Prospective, double-blind trials of ketanserin in the treatment of RS suggests that there is a decreased frequency but not decreased duration of attacks.[67] Ketanserin remains unavailable in the United States.

α-Adrenergic Antagonists

Many α-inhibiting drugs have been evaluated in the treatment of RS. These include methyldopa, priscoline, reserpine, guanethidine, phenoxybenzamine, and prazosin.[4,16] Of these, intravenous reserpine has been one of the most frequently utilized. Our experience with intravenous reserpine, given in a Bier block fashion, has been favorable; but intravenous reserpine is no longer available.[68] β-Adrenergic agonists, such as nylidrin and isoxsuprine, have also been ineffective.[69]

Platelet Inhibitors

Familiar agents such as aspirin, pentoxifylline, and dipyridamole have been hypothesized to be of some benefit in treatment, but none seem to offer any improvement in either anecdotal experience or in clinical trials. Thromboxane inhibitors have also been evaluated and found to have no benefit.[70]

Diet

Recent evidence has suggested that dietary fish oil (ω-3 fatty acid), confers some benefit to patients with vasospastic RS with no associated connective tissue disorders.[71,72] A double-blind, olive oil placebo controlled study evaluated the effect of ω-3 fatty acids on RS and found that patients with RS had an improved ability to tolerate cold water immersion.[71] The exact mechanism of this improvement is unclear, and further research is warranted.

TENS and Behavioral Therapy

The use of transcutaneous electrical nerve stimulation (TENS) has been hypothesized to increase digital blood flow via vasodilation, but controlled trials using finger plethysmography, transcutaneous PO_2, and skin temperature have failed to show benefit.[73] Behavioral therapy, or biofeedback, however, has shown some promise, with reduction in symptoms noted in over 66% of patients.[74] Investigators theorize that biofeedback works by increasing β stimulation.

Surgical Management

Very few patients with RS are surgical candidates. Those who may benefit from surgery typically have obstructive pattern of the disease, and have subclavian, axillary, or brachial arterial obstruction from atherosclerosis, thoracic outlet syndrome, aneurysms, emboli, or trauma. Patients with subclavian artery aneurysm are frequently missed and have good outcomes with autogenous reconstruction.[75] For patients who do not fit in these categories, other more extreme interventions exist that have less impressive results.

Digital Revascularization

A few selected patients may have bypassable disease at the palmar arch,[76] and microvascular bypass may be performed. Situations where such an operation may be of some benefit remain quite rare. Arteriovenous reversal at the wrist has also been attempted,[77] but results remain poor.

Sympathectomy

Cervicothoracic sympathectomy has been used as a treatment for RS for many years, and the most consistent result has been only short-term improvement in symptoms of vasospastic RS.[78] Patients typically feel better for about 6 months then return to baseline. The same cycle is observed when repeat sympathectomy is tried, and the exact etiology of this treatment failure remains unclear. Thoracoscopic sympathectomy has met with similar results.[79–81] Given these dismal results, we do not recommend upper extremity sympathectomy for vasospastic disease.

Lumbar sympathectomy has, however, proven to have durable beneficial effects in more than 90% of patients with lower extremity vasospastic arterial disease. Lumbar sympathectomy therefore should be considered for patients who fit the vasospastic lower extremity arterial disease pattern.[82]

Periarterial Sympathectomy

The technique of periarterial sympathectomy involves disruption of neural input to the arterial wall. This is done by stripping 4 to 5 cm of arterial adventitia just past the bifurcation of the common digital artery.[83] Results from this procedure are limited, but there appears to be some benefit to young patients with purely vasospastic RS; however, as in cervicothoracic sympathectomy, the beneficial effect seems to be short lived. As a result, digital periarterial sympathectomy is not recommended.

Debridement/Amputation

Patients with digital ulceration will occasionally require operative debridement to facilitate healing, but only in rare situations will interphalangeal amputation be indicated. In our case review of over 1100 patients, only 2 have required interphalangeal amputation. Given that most patients with symptomatic digital or palmar artery occlusion have a favorable outcome, the clinician must be sure to avoid premature amputation.[54]

Overview

Occlusive disease of the palmar and digital arteries of the upper extremity can be divided into two categories, obstructive and vasospastic, with the caveat that considerable overlap exists between the two. Both types are traditionally associated with RS, although the pathophysiology of the RS is quite different in the two. Diffuse palmar and digital artery obstruction usually occurs as part of a systemic arteritis. In occasional patients the arterial obstruction results from such unusual conditions as Buerger's disease or digital artery arteriosclerosis. The ischemic lesions that result should be treated conservatively, and this, in conjunction with treatment of the underlying disorder, will lead to healing of ischemic lesions without recurrence in about 90% of patients. We do not recommend thoracic sympathectomy for this disease process.

Vasospastic disease, as represented by RS, in our tertiary referral center, is associated with a systemic autoimmune disease in over 60% of patients. The underlying pathophysiological mechanisms are incompletely understood but seem to result from abnormalities of the sympathetic nervous system and/or digital artery adrenoreceptor function, in which a cold stimulus induces an abnormally forceful contraction of the arterial wall smooth muscle.

Most patients with RS are satisfactorily treated by simple cold and tobacco avoidance. Nifedipine is the drug of choice in the few patients sufficiently symptomatic to require pharmacological treatment. Unfortunately, the combination of poor response and severe side effects results in the drug benefiting only about 30% to 50% of the patients in whom it is used.

References

1. McNamara MF, Takali HS, Yao JST, Bergan JJ: A systematic approach to severe hand ischemia. *Surgery* 83:1, 1978.
2. Dale WA, Lewis MR: Management of ischemia of the hand and fingers. *Surgery* 67:62, 1970.
3. Hardy JD, Conn JH, Fain WR: Nonatherosclerotic occlusive lesions of small arteries. *Surgery* 57:1, 1965.
4. Porter JM, Snider RL, Bardana EJ, et al: The diagnosis and treatment of Raynaud's phenomenon. *Surgery* 77:11, 1975.
5. Porter JM, Bardana EJ, Baur CM, et al: The clinical significance of Raynaud's syndrome. *Surgery* 80:756, 1976.
6. Mills JL, Friedman EI, Taylor LM Jr, Porter LM: Upper extremity disease caused by small artery disease. *Ann Surg* 206:521–528, 1987.
7. Raynaud M: On local asphyxia and symmetrical gangrene of the extremities. Selected Monographs. London, New Sydenham Society, 1888.
8. Hutchinson J: Inherited liability to Raynaud's phenomenon with great proneness to chilblains—gradual increase of liability to paroxysmal local asphyxia-acrosphacelus with scleroderma—cheeks affected. *Arch Surg* 4:312, 1893.
9. Hutchinson J. Raynaud's phenomenon. *Med Press Circ* 123:402, 1901.
10. Allen EV, Brown GE: Raynaud's disease: A critical review of minimal requisites for diagnosis. *Am J Med Sci* 183:187, 1932.
11. Lewis T, Pickering GW: Observations upon maladies in which the blood sup-

ply to digits ceases intermittently or permanently, and upon bilateral gangrene of the digits: Observation relevant to so-called "Raynaud's disease." *Clin Sci* 1:327, 1934.

12. Gifford RW Jr, Hines EA Jr: Raynaud's disease among women and girls. *Circulation* 16:1012, 1957.

13. deTakats G, Fowler EF. Raynaud's phenomenon. *JAMA* 179:99, 1962.

14. Velayos EE, Robinson H, Porciuncula FU, Musi AT: Clinical correlation analysis of 137 patients with Raynaud's phenomenon. *Am J Med Sci* 262:347–356, 1971.

15. Lewis T: Experiments relating to the peripheral mechanism involved in spastic arrest of the circulation in the fingers, a variety of Raynaud's disease. *Heart* 15:7, 1929.

16. Coffman JB, Cohen AS: Total and capillary fingertip blood flow in Raynaud's phenomenon. *N Engl J Med* 285:259, 1971.

17. Nielsen SL, Lassen NA: Measurement of digital blood pressure after local cooling. *J Appl Physiol* 43:907–910, 1977.

18. Hirai M: Cold sensitivity of the hand in arterial occlusive disease. *Surgery* 85: 140, 1979.

19. Taylor W, Pelmear PL: Raynaud's phenomenon of occupational origin: An epidemiological survey. *Acta Chir Scand (Suppl)* 465:27, 1976.

20. Porter JM, Rivers SP, Anderson CJ: Evaluation and management of patients with Raynaud's syndrome. *Am J Surg* 142:183, 1981.

21. Rosch J, Porter JM, Gralino BJ: Cryodynamic hand angiography in the diagnosis and management of Raynaud's syndrome. *Circulation* 55:807, 1977.

22. Jamieson GG, Ludbrook J, Wilson A: Cold hypersensitivity in Raynaud's phenomenon. *Circulation* 44:254, 1971.

23. Motulsky HJ, Insel PA: Adrenergic receptors in man. *N Engl J Med* 307:18, 1982.

24. Keenan EJ, Porter JM: Alpha-2 adrenergic receptors in platelets from patients with Raynaud's syndrome. *Surgery* 94:204, 1983.

25. Edwards JM, Phinney ES, Taylor LM Jr, et al: α-2 adrenergic receptor levels in obstructive and spastic Raynaud's syndrome. *J Vasc Surg* 5:38–45, 1987.

26. Zamora MR, O'Brien RF, Rutherford RB, et al: Serum endothelin-1 concentrations and cold provocation in primary Raynaud's phenomenon. *Lancet* 336: 1144, 1990.

27. Shawket S, Dickerson C, Hazelman B, et al: Selective suprasensitivity to calcitonin gene related peptide in the hands in Raynaud's phenomenon. *Lancet* 2: 1354–1357, 1989.

28. Olsen N, Nielsen SL: Prevalence of primary Raynaud's phenomenon in young females. *Scand J Clin Lab Invest* 37:761, 1978.

29. Porter JM. Unpublished data, 1984.

30. Spittell JA: Raynaud's phenomenon and allied vasospastic conditions. In: Fairbaren JF, Juergens JL, Spittell JA, eds. *Allen-Barker-Hines Peripheral Vascular Disease*. Philadelphia, PA: W.B. Saunders; 1972, pp. 387–419.

31. Landry G, Edwards JM, McClafferty RM, et al: Long-term outcome of Raynaud's syndrome in a prospective analyzed cohort. *J Vasc Surg* 23:76–86, 1996.

32. Chatterjee DS, Petrie A, Taylor W: Prevalence of vibration-induced white finger in fluorspar mines in Weardale. *Br J Indust Med* 35:208, 1978.

33. MacKiewisz A, Piskorz A: Raynaud's phenomenon following long-term re-peated action of great difference of temperature. *J Cardiovasc Surg* 18:151, 1977.

34. Blunt RJ, Porter JM: Raynaud's syndrome. *Semin Arthritis Rheum* 10:282, 19??.

35. Sumner DS, Strandness DE: An abnormal finger pulse associated with cold sensitivity. *Ann Surg* 175:294, 1972.

36. Porter JM, Taylor LM Jr: Limb ischemia caused by small artery disease. *World J Surg* 7:326–333, 1983.

37. Dabich L, Bookstein JJ, Zweifler A, Zarafonetis CJD: Digital arteries in patients with scleroderma. *Arch Intern Med* 130:708, 1972.

38. Johnson ENM, Summerly R, Birnstingle M: Prognosis in Raynaud's phenome-non after sympathectomy. *Br Med J* 1:962–964, 1965.

39. LeRoy EC, Maricq HR, Kahaleh MB: Undifferentiated connective tissue syn-dromes. *Arthritis Rheum* 23:341, 1980.

40. Baur GM, Porter JM, Bardana EJ, et al: Rapid onset of hand ischemia of un-known etiology. *Ann Surg* 186:184, 1977.

41. Mills JL, Taylor LM Jr, Porter JM: Buerger's disease in the modern era. *Am J Surg* 154:123–9, 1987.

42. Laws JW, EL Sallak RA, Scott JT: An arteriographic and histological study of digital arteries. *Br J Radiol* 40:740, 1967.

43. Taylor LM Jr, Hauty MG, Edwards JM, Porter JM: Digital ischemia as a mani-festation of malignancy. *Ann Surg* 206:62–68, 1987.

44. Hawley PR, Johnston AW, Rankin JT: Association between digital ischemia and malignant disease. *Br Med J* 3:208–212, 1967.

45. Martinez A, Golding M, Sawyer P, et al: The specific arterial lesion in mild and severe frostbite: Effects of sympathectomy. *J Cardiovasc Surg* 35:495–501, 1965.

46. Conn JJ Jr, Bergan JJ, Bell JL: Hypothenar hammer syndrome post-traumatic digital ischemia. *Surgery* 68:301–307, 1970.

47. Lindell TD, Porter JM, Langston C: Intra-arterial injections of oral medications: a Complication of drug addiction. *N Engl J Med* 287:1132–1133, 1972.

48. James EC, Khun NT, Fedde CW, et al: Upper limb ischemia resulting from arterial thromboembolism. *Am J Surg* 137:739–744, 1979.

49. Merhoff CG, Porter JM: Ergot intoxication: Historical review and description of unusual clinical manifestations. *Ann Surg* 180:773–779, 1974.

50. Wilson RH, McCormick WE, Tatum CF, Creech JL: Occupational acro-osteo-lysis. *JAMA* 201:83–87, 1967.

51. Gates KN, Tyburczy JA, Zupan T, et al: The non-invasive quantification of digital vasospasm. *Bruit* 8:34–37, 1984.

52. Lafferty K, DeTrafford JC, Roberts VC, Cotton LT: Raynaud's phenomenon and thermal entrainment: An objective test. *Br Med J* 286:90–92, 1983.

53. Holmgren K, Baur GM, Porter JM: The role of digital photo plethysmography in the evaluation of Raynaud's syndrome. *Bruit* 5:19, 1981.

54. McClafferty RB, Edwards JM, Taylor LM Jr, et al: Diagnosis and long-term clinical outcome in patients diagnosed with hand ischemia. *J Vasc Surg* 22:361–9, 1995.

55. Rivers SP, Porter JM: Raynaud's syndrome and upper extremity small artery occlusive disease. In: Wilson SE, Veith FJ, Hobson RW, Williams RA, eds.

Vascular Surgery: Principles and Practice. New York: McGraw-Hill; 1987, pp. 696–710.

56. Smith CD, McKendry RJ: Controlled trial of nifedipine in the treatment of Raynaud's phenomenon. *Lancet* 2:1299, 1982.

57. Stone PH, Autman EJ, Muller JE: Calcium channel blocking agents in the treatment of cardiovascular disorders. Part II. Hemodynamic effects and clinical applications. *Ann Intern Med* 93:886, 1980.

58. Weber A, Bounanaux H: Effects of low dose nifedipine on a cold provocation test in patients with Raynaud's disease. *J Cardiovasc Pharmacol* 15:853–855, 1990.

59. Kahan A Weber S, Amor B, et al: Nifedipine and Raynaud's phenomenon (letter . *Ann Intern Med* 94:546, 1981.

60. Wigly FM, Wise RA, Seibold JR, et al: Intravenous iloprost infusion in patients with Raynaud phenomenon secondary to systemic sclerosis. *Ann Intern Med* 120:199–206, 1994

61. Watson HR, Belcher G: Retrospective comparison of iloprost with other treatments for secondary Raynaud's phenomenon. *Ann Rheum Dis* 50:359–361, 1991.

62. Kyle MU, Belcher G, Hazelman BL: Placebo controlled study showing therapeutic benefit of iloprost in the treatment of Raynaud phenomenon. *J Rheumatol* 19:1403–1406, 1992.

63. Belch JF, Capell HA, Cooke ED: Oral iloprost as a treatment for Raynaud's syndrome: A double blind multicentre placebo controlled study. *Ann Rheum Dis* 54:197–200, 1995.

64. Chancellor VF, Waller DG, Hayward RA, et al: Subjective and objective assessment of enalapril in primary Raynaud's phenomenon. *Br J Clin Pharmacol* 31: 477–480, 1991.

65. Charles CR, Carmick ES. Skin temperature changes in Raynaud's disease after griseofulvin. *Arch Dermatol* 101:331, 1970.

66. Arosio E, Montesi G, Zanmoni M: Efficacy of Ketanserin in the therapy of Raynaud's phenomenon: Thermometric data. *Angiology* 42:408–413, 1996.

67. Coffman JD, Clement DL, Creager MA, et al: International study of Ketanserin in Raynaud's phenomenon. *Am J Med* 87:264–268, 1989.

68. Taylor LM Jr, Rivers SP, Keller FS, et al: Treatment of finger ischemia with Bier block reserpine. *Surg Gynecol Obstet* 154:39–43, 1982.

69. Folich ED, Tarayi RC, Duston HP: Peripheral arterial insufficiency: A complication of beta-adrenergic blocking therapy. *JAMA* 208:2471, 1969.

70. Gresele P, Volpato R, Migliacci R, et al: Thromboxane does not play a significant role in acute, cold-induced vasoconstriction in Raynaud's phenomenon. *Thromb Res* 66:259–264, 1992.

71. DiGiacomo RA, Kremer JM, Shah DM: Fish-oil dietary supplementation in patients with Raynaud's phenomenon: A double, controlled prospective study. *Am J Med* 86:158–164, 1989.

72. McCarthy GM, Kenny D. Dietary fish oil and rheumatic diseases. *Semin Arth Rheumat* 21:368–375, 1992.

73. Mulder P, Dompeling EC, van Slochteren-van der Boor JC, et al: Transcutaneous electrical nerve stimulation (TENS) in Raynaud's phenomenon. *Angiology* 42:414–417, 1991.

74. Freedman RR: Physiological mechanisms of temperature biofeedback. *Biofeedback Self-Regulation* 16:65–115, 1991.
75. Nehler MR, Moneta GL, Taylor LM Jr, et al: Surgical treatment of upper extremity ischemia subclavian artery aneurysm. Presented at the annual meeting of the Western Surgical Association. Nov. 17–20, 1996.
76. Silcott GR, Polich VL: Palmar arch arterial reconstruction for the salvage of ischemic fingers. *Am J Surg* 142:219, 1981.
77. King TA, Marks J, Berrettone BA: Arteriovenous reversal for limb-salvage in unreconstructable upper extremity arterial occlusive disease. *J Vasc Surg* 17: 924–933, 1993.
78. Machleder HI, Wheeler E, Barber WF: Treatment of upper extremity ischemia by cervico-dorsal sympathectomy. *Vasc Surg* 13:399–404, 1979.
79. Claes G, Drotl C, Gotherberg G: Thoracoscopy for autonomic disorders. *Ann Thorac Surg* 56:715–716, 1993.
80. Lowell RC, Gloviczki P, Cherry KJ, et al: Cervicothoracic sympathectomy for Raynaud's syndrome. *Int Angiol* 12:168, 1993.
81. Nicholson ML, Hopkinson BR, Dennis MJS. Endoscopic transthoracic sympathectomy: Successful in hyperhidrosis but can the indications be extended. *Ann R Coll Surg Engl* 76:311–314, 1994.
82. Janoff KA, Phinney ES, Porter JM: Lumbar sympathectomy for lower extremity vasospasm. *Am J Surg* 150:147–152, 1985.
83. Flatt AE: Digital artery sympathectomy. *J Hand Surg* 5:550, 1980.

14

The Axillosubclavian and Brachial Arteries

Herbert I. Machleder, MD

Symptomatic arterial occlusive disease of the upper extremities will comprise approximately 5% of the cases on a large clinical vascular service, and atherosclerosis will be the most common etiologic disease. In cases of acute arterial insufficiency, about 50% will be secondary to embolization, and of the remaining half, 25% will be the result of primary arterial thrombosis and 25% iatrogenic in origin.[1]

Subclavian Artery

Anatomic Considerations

Before considering specific lesions, a review of several anatomic relations will be helpful, particularly as they relate to the pathophysiology of occlusions and details of surgical exposure.

The right subclavian artery is located more anteriorly and superiorly in the neck than is the left, and both are divided into three parts by the overlying anterior scalene muscle. The first part of the subclavian artery, extending to the medial border of the anterior scalene muscle, gives rise to the vertebral and internal mammary arteries as well as the thyrocervical trunk. Throughout its course, the subclavian artery is in intimate relation with both autonomic and somatic nerves: stellate ganglion, vagus, phrenic, recurrent laryngeal, and brachial plexus. On the right side, both the recurrent laryngeal nerve and ansa subclavia loop around the proximal portion of the artery. The second portion of the subclavian artery lies deep to the anterior scalene, with the lateral border of the first rib considered

From Machleder HI, (ed): *Vascular Disorders of the Upper Extremity*. Third Revised Edition. Futura Publishing Company, Inc., Armonk, NY, © 1998.

the surgical boundary marking the termination of the subclavian and the beginning of the axillary artery. The axillary artery is divided into three parts by the pectoralis minor muscle, which crosses the vessel at its mid-portion. The first branch is usually the superior thoracic artery that traverses the axillary space to the intercostal muscle between the first and second ribs. This artery is encountered and divided during the transaxillary approach to the thoracic outlet. The thoracoacromial, lateral thoracic, humeral circumflex, and subscapular arteries are the major trunks arising from the axillary artery, with the brachial artery beginning at the lateral border of the teres major muscle.

Occlusions and Steal Syndrome

The majority of patients with proximal subclavian artery occlusion will be asymptomatic and the condition identified only when a weaker radial pulse is palpable on the affected side, or an asymmetry of brachial blood pressures is detected during routine evaluation. Diagnosis is usually made on physical examination by measuring bilateral brachial artery pressures using pneumatic cuff, and stethoscope or Doppler flow detector. Further work-up of the specific lesion is generally unwarranted if the patient is asymptomatic.

In the symptomatic clinical situation the constellation of observations is termed the subclavian steal syndrome, with the vertebral artery serving as an important collateral vessel reconstituting perfusion in the distal subclavian artery. The syndrome can be demonstrated angiographically by detecting flow reversal in the vertebral artery.[2,3] It is found more commonly in men, and occurs more often on the left side than on the right.[4] The occlusive disease is generally a consequence of atherosclerosis, although it has been described after trauma to the brachiocephalic vessels. It is enigmatic that although symptoms are three times more common with lesions in the left subclavian, autopsy data demonstrate equal distribution of subclavian occlusive disease between right and left sides.[5]

This type of subclavian artery occlusion is always proximal to the origin of the vertebral artery. The resulting pressure differential between the intracerebral circulation and the relatively low-pressure brachial circulation, distal to the occlusion, causes reversal of flow in the vertebral artery, which derives its blood from the basilar artery and from the circle of Willis. This reversal of flow in the vertebral artery has been demonstrated to increase with arm exercise, or with postischemic reactive hyperemia in the involved extremity.[6,7] Initially it was thought that the reversal of flow in the vertebral artery was, in effect, stealing blood from the cerebral circulation. It was later recognized that under physiological circumstances this would be a most unusual phenomenon in the presence of an uncompromised anterior circulation. In fact, reduction of blood flow to the brain by this siphoning effect would become manifest only if some restricting lesion reduced the ability of the normal cardiac output to augment carotid artery flow in the presence of this increased distribution requirement to the arm.

When the classic syndrome is present, however, the patient develops signs and symptoms of vertebrobasilar insufficiency after vigorous arm exercise. This is more likely to occur when the side involved has a dominant or major vertebral artery and the contralateral side is either atretic or absent.

In patients who are symptomatic with subclavian steal syndrome, approximately 30% present with neurological symptoms alone, primarily those of vertebrobasilar insufficiency. In this group, there is a high incidence of associated anterior circulation lesions, such as stenosis of the internal carotid artery at its origin. About 10% of patients present with only arm symptoms, predominantly cramping, easy fatigue, and paresthesias. Approximately 60% will have evidence of both cerebral and upper extremity ischemic symptoms. In a third of those patients who are symptomatic, exercise will aggravate the symptoms.

The classic sign on physical examination is an asymmetry (right compared to left) of the brachial blood pressure usually of at least 20 mm Hg. Several recent reviews have documented the presence of this abnormality confined to the left side in more than 85% of symptomatic cases. Occasionally an innominate artery occlusion may be associated with subclavian steal on the right side. This circumstance is likely to be more symptomatic than obstruction of the subclavian, and in general, the presence of cerebral and upper extremity symptoms on the right side is more apt to be secondary to innominate than subclavian artery occlusion.[8]

Symptomatic patients with arm fatigue will most often have a differential (right to left) brachial pressure between 40 and 50 mm Hg, whereas those with predominantly cerebral symptoms will have pressure differentials in the range of 20 to 40 mm Hg. The lower differential pressures in the later case are often a reflection of a larger ipsilateral vertebral artery with considerable retrograde flow to the arm. The occurrence of posterior cerebral or hemispheric cerebrovascular symptoms, as mentioned previously, is more common than arm symptoms and more likely to occur in the presence of a concomitant hemodynamically significant ipsilateral carotid stenosis.[9]

The occasional ischemic arm symptoms manifest by Raynaud's phenomenon, or cramping arm pain with exercise, are most often found when there is an additional segmental lesion distal to the vertebral artery, or when the vertebral artery is atretic or occluded.

The presence of associated or tandem obstructive stenosis is central to the presenting pattern of symptoms, particularly with the proximal brachiocephalic lesions. Although transient vertebrobasilar insufficiency is encountered, cerebral infarction is unusual with proximal subclavian obstruction unless there are associated cerebrovascular lesions.[10]

Closed trauma to the upper thorax will occasionally lead to intimal disruption of the subclavian artery with either early or late thrombosis. Even in the presence of intact radial pulses, this lesion should be considered likely if there is: mediastinal widening on chest x-ray, clavicular or first rib fracture, a Horner's syndrome, or ipsilateral vocal cord paralysis. Angiography is very useful in establishing the presence of a posttraumatic-subclavian abnormality. Open, gunshot, or knife wounds to the subclavian present a particular surgical challenge that will vary depending on the side of injury.

Congenital Anomalies

Although there are a number of anomalies of the aortic arch and brachiocephalic vessels, few have important clinical significance. The typical congenital anomaly presenting with clinical manifestations is a malposition of the subclavian artery.[11,12] An aberrant left subclavian artery arising from the right side of the aortic arch often causes symptoms of esophageal obstruction as it passes behind the esophagus, forming a constricting ring between the anomalous vessel and the normally placed brachiocephalic arch. Occasionally, a left subclavian artery arising from the right side of the aortic arch develops aneurysmal dilatation prior to its presenting symptoms of dysphagia.[13] This aneurysmal dilatation is often identified on chest roentgenogram or esophagram. For the most part, vascular rings are the result of a retroesophageal position of an aberrant vessel (usually subclavian) that compresses the esophagus against the normally located anterior vessels.[14] The diagnosis is most often made within the first 4 years of life and, usually within the first year. The symptoms may be secondary to esophageal compression or to severe associated neuromuscular lesions. The symptoms tend to become less prominent with growth of the child.[15]

Surgical Correction

Recent advances in surgical therapy emphasize the extra-anatomic approach to surgical repair of proximal subclavian lesions because even in contemporary reports, transthoracic repair of brachiocephalic vessels

EXTRA-ANATOMIC BYPASS
Brachiocephalic Occlusive Disease

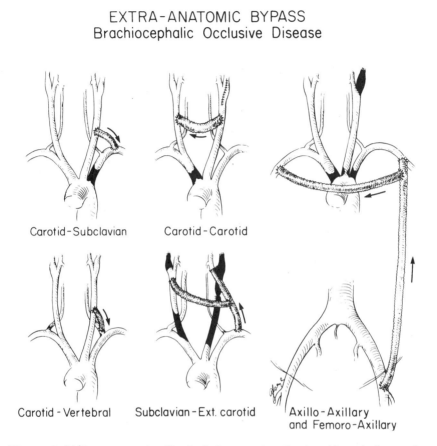

Carotid-Subclavian   Carotid-Carotid

Carotid-Vertebral   Subclavian-Ext. carotid   Axillo-Axillary
and Femoro-Axillary

Figure 1. Various reconstructive techniques using the brachiocephalic vessls. (Reproduced with permission from Machleder HI: Vaso-occlusive disorders of the upper extremity. *Curr Probl Surg* 25(1):1–67, 1988.)

carries about a 15% mortality (Figure 1).[16] Procedures most commonly used to correct this abnormality include: carotid subclavian bypass with vein or prosthetic material, direct subclavian-carotid anastomosis by subclavian transposition, and vertebral-carotid anastomosis (Figure 2).[17] The occasional stroke that accompanies mobilization and clamping of the carotid or vertebral vessels has led to use of an extra-anatomic approach; axillo-axillary artery bypass to restore upper extremity and vertebral circulation from the contralateral subclavian-axillary circulation.[18,19] Ligation of the vertebral artery to prevent retrograde flow may relieve symptoms temporarily, but this procedure is associated with a significant incidence of symptomatic recurrence as collateral vessels from vertebral to subclavian artery gradually develop. Subclavian and innominate endar-

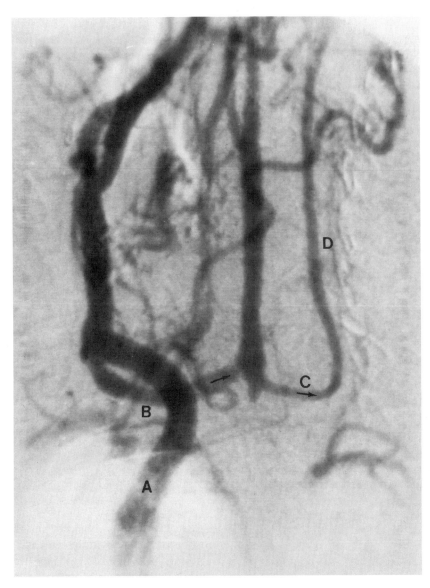

Figure 2. Complex reconstructive procedure for a patient with symptomatic left subclavian steal and a single patent vessel arising from the aortic arch (the right carotid). **A**: right common carotid. **B**: carotid-carotid vein graft. **C**: vertebral-carotid transposition. **D**: left vertebral artery. (Reproduced with permission from Machleder HI: Vaso-occlusive disorders of the upper extremity. *Curr Probl Surg* 25(1):1–67, 1988.)

terectomy have been reported in several series but this represents an unnecessarily hazardous operation in most cases. We have renewed our interest in axillo-axillary bypass grafting as a very effective secondary procedure in complex reoperative cases. Chang et al[21] have recently reviewed a large series of this procedure.[20]

Surgical Exposure

Direct exposure of the innominate artery or proximal right subclavian artery can be accomplished through a median sternotomy that can be limited to the upper mediastinum by entering the third intercostal space and creating a trapdoor type of exposure. Upward extension of the incision into the supraclavicular area enables more distal exposure of the subclavian artery. The transclavicular approach, by excising the middle third of the clavicle, affords excellent exposure of the mid-portion of right or left subclavian artery with minimal morbidity. Exposure of the origin of the left subclavian is best performed through a left fifth interspace posterolateral thoracotomy, although anterior thoracotomy can also give acceptable exposure (Figure 3). The recurrent laryngeal nerve will be

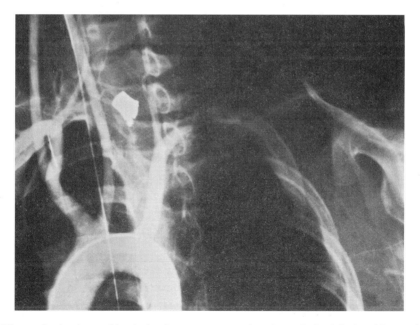

Figure 3. Angiographic study of a young man shot through the left shoulder, and presenting with an ischemic left arm and expanding pulsatile mass in the left supraclavicular fossa. Reconstruction was facilitated by clamping the subclavian through a small left anterior thoracotomy and repairing the vessel after removal of the medial third of the clavicle.

found in close proximity to the left subclavian artery as the nerve returns to the cervical region.[22,23] Although penetrating injury or trauma to the brachiocephalic vessels requires transthoracic or transmediastinal exposure, occlusive disease rarely requires these approaches.[24,25] Useful endovascular techniques have recently been reported for the brachiocephalic vessels.[25a]

Thoracic Outlet

The compressive abnormalities at the thoracic outlet represent a uniquely challenging group of disorders, and are dealt with in detail in Chapter 9. Although other categories of injury can occur, a thorough knowledge of the thoracic outlet area ensures a reasoned approach, even though the surgeon may not have previously encountered a similar lesion.[26,27,27a]

Although most subclavian aneurysms occur in association with the thoracic outlet compression syndrome, there are increasing cases seen in association with military and urban trauma.[28,29]

Axillary Artery

The axillary artery is surrounded by the three cords of the brachial plexus, which are named anterior, lateral, and medial in their relation to this vessel. Vascular repairs in this area must protect these cords. Reconstruction should be of autogenous tissue to avoid fibrous reaction that occasionally will involve the brachial plexus leading to a painful causalgia-like picture (Figures 4 through 6).

Arteritis

Takayasu's arteritis and giant cell arteritis often involve the subclavian and proximal axillary vessels. Although the histological picture and anatomic pattern of involvement is very similar, there are several important clinical distinctions. Takayasu's arteritis starts as a systemic illness with generalized symptoms of fever, malaise, myalgias, and arthralgias as well as abdominal pain and weight loss. During the acute or subacute illness, which can last several weeks, there may be anemia and elevation of erythrocyte sedimentation rate. Typically the patient is a young woman presenting with the vascular occlusive stage of the disease in the second or third decade of age. A panarteritis develops that affects the adventitia and the vasa vasorum, secondarily affecting the media. There can be inti-

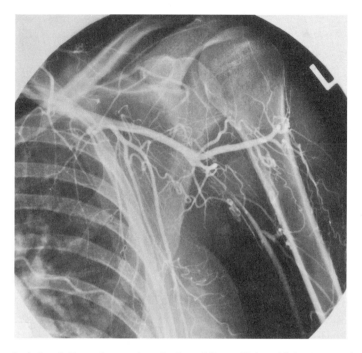

Figure 4. Intimal dissection and occlusion of the axillobrachial artery at the level of the brachial plexus cords. This lesion is best repaired by reverse vein grafting, care being taken to avoid entrapment of brachial plexus elements.

mal proliferation that leads to stenosis and occlusion. Fragmentation of the elastic layers can also lead to aneurysm development. Four patterns of large vessel involvement have been postulated. Type I involves the aortic arch and major brachiocephalic branches; type II involves primarily the descending thoracic and abdominal aorta; type III involves both thoracic and abdominal aorta and branches; and type IV includes involvement of the pulmonary artery (Figures 7A, 7B, and 7C).

Giant cell arteritis also has a predilection for women and Caucasians but is usually found after the fifth decade of age. Constitutional symptoms usually include headache, fever, weight loss, and malaise with myalgias and arthralgias described as polymyalgia rheumatica. Although involvement of the upper extremity vessels is common (Figure 8), involvement of the ophthalmic and posterior ciliary artery is the most urgent problem, because transient and even permanent loss of vision can occur secondary to ischemic optic neuritis. The erythrocyte sedimentation rate is almost invariably elevated and can be followed to monitor therapy. A normochromic normocytic anemia is commonly documented as are other serum abnormalities: elevated immunoglobulins, α_3-globulin, fibrinogen, C-re-

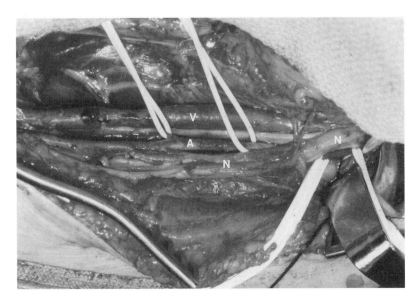

Figure 5. Operative exposure (of Figure 4) showing axillobrachial vein (V), Occluded axillobrachial artery (A) and elements of the brachial plexus (N).

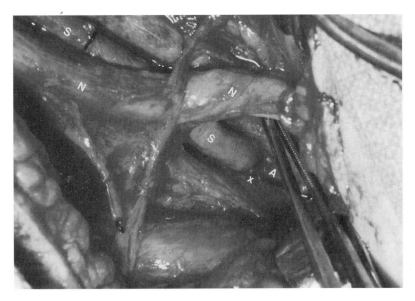

Figure 6. Closer view of Figure 5 after surgical repair (N indicates elements of brachial plexus; S, saphenous vein graft; A, proximal artery; "x," anastomosis).

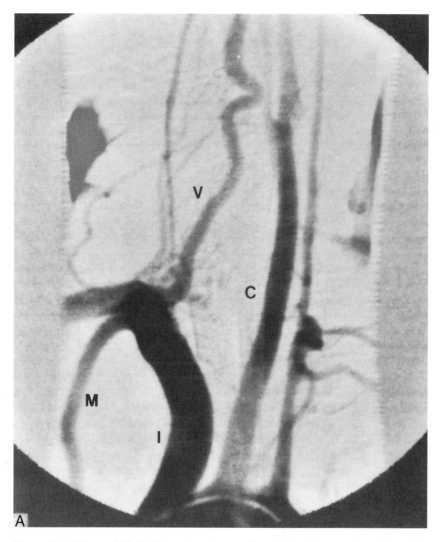

Figure 7: A through C: Aortic arch angiogram in a male college student. Extensive brachiocephalic occlusive disease is characteristic of Takayasu's arteritis. Patient was asymptomatic but brachial pressure asymmetry was noticed on college entrance physical examination. I indicates innominate; M, internal mammary; V, vertebral; C, carotid; S, subclavian; B, brachial.

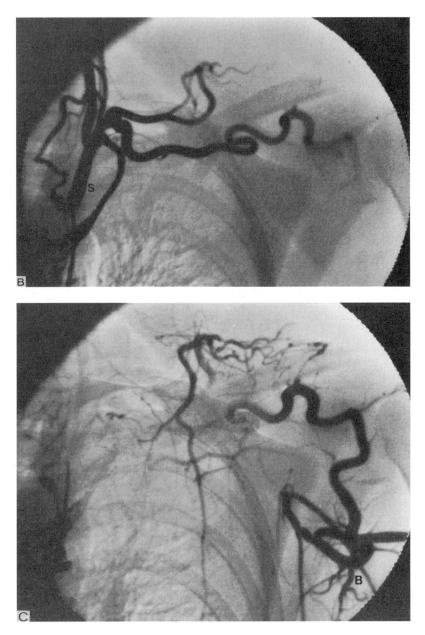

Figure 7: (continued)

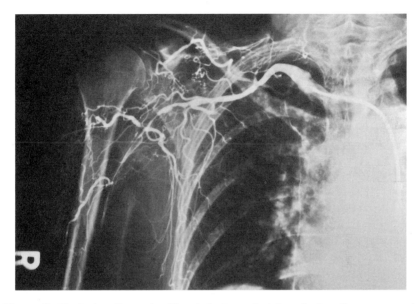

Figure 8. Typical pattern of axillosubclavian arterial occlusive disease seen in giant cell arteritis. (Reproduced from Machleder HI: Vascular disease of the upper extremity and the thoracic outlet syndrome. In: Moore WE, ed. *Vascular Surgery*, 2nd edition. Orlando: Grune & Stratton, 1986.)

active protein and α_1-antitrypsin. The alkaline phosphatase is often elevated, but rarely reflective of severe liver involvement. In contradistinction to Takayasu's arteritis, which has a variable response to corticosteroids, giant cell arteritis is dramatically improved with corticosteroid therapy. After initiation with corticosteroids, symptoms diminish within the first few days and normalization of the sedimentation rate occurs within several weeks. Treatment is started with 40 to 60 mg of prednisone daily and can be tapered after the sedimentation rate has returned to normal (usually within 4 weeks). A maintenance dose of prednisone between 5- to 12.5-mg daily is utilized and can be altered to an every other day regimen in about 50% of patients without evidence of disease recrudescence. Therapy is usually continued for 1 to 2 years to avoid the frequent relapse that is seen with lesser periods of treatment. If upper extremity ischemic symptoms persist, vascular reconstruction can be undertaken when the acute inflammatory stage of the disease has been controlled. Early repairs, prior to control with corticosteroids, are very prone to thrombosis and failure. Diagnosis by temporal artery biopsy is often definitive.

Irradiation Injury

Irradiation injury to the axillary and subclavian vessels occurs on occasion after radiation therapy to the axilla and supraclavicular areas after treatment for carcinoma of the breast with axillary node metastases. These patients will often present with severe ischemic symptoms that may be obscured by lymphedema or suspected radiation neuritis involving the brachial plexus. Three patterns or stages of injury have been suggested. Within the first 5 years after therapy there may be intimal damage that results in mural thrombosis and embolization. Within 10 years of irradiation, fibrotic stenosis leading to occlusion has been demonstrated. Because of dense perivascular fibrosis these patients are best treated with bypass grafting. After a latent period of 20 years, periarterial fibrosis may be complicated by development of atherosclerosis in the irradiated segment of artery without involvement of other more common sites of predilection.[30]

Although we have on occasion endarterectomized a carotid artery with these types of changes, the frequent finding of periarterial fibrosis favors the use of bypass grafting. Radiation skin changes over the area of arterial occlusion also favors the use of bypass grafting through a remote site.

Iatrogenic Injury

Percutaneous cannulation of the axillary or subclavian artery rarely results in thrombosis. When it does occur, the extensive arterial collaterals around the shoulder usually prevent ischemic symptoms from developing. When axillary bypass is necessary our preference is to interpose a graft of saphenous vein (Figure 6). The tissue reaction to this graft is less likely to compromise elements of the brachial plexus that are frequently affected by formation of scar tissue around prosthetic materials.

Injury to the brachial plexus may arise during attempts to cannulate the axillary or subclavian artery: either directly by needle puncture or infusion of contrast medium into the nerve sheath, or indirectly by compression of these structures by a hematoma, which results in neurological deficit. Dysesthesias developing in the median nerve distribution after axillary artery catheterization usually represent the effects of an expanding hematoma in the axillary sheath. Prompt exploration, evacuation of the hematoma, and suture closure of the puncture site usually limits the nerve damage.

Although the direct surgical approach over the hematoma is satisfactory, control of the axillary or subclavian artery may be achieved with two incisions: one in the infraclavicular area, and one in the axilla. The condition of the vessel will dictate the need for an interposition graft or primary arterial repair. `

The upper extremity vessels are now commonly used for revascularization of the extracranial cerebral circulation as well as revascularization

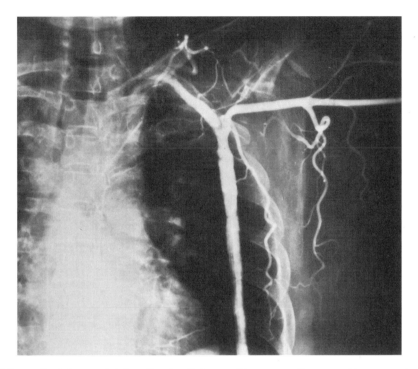

Figure 9. A frequent deformity of axillofemoral bypass grafts caused by excessive tension on graft. Junction of the Y-shaped deformity is a common site for thrombo-embolism.

of the lower extremities. Carotid-subclavian grafts and axillofemoral by-pass grafts have provided valuable extra-anatomic bypass procedures for reconstructive arterial surgery. Nevertheless, these procedures have re-sulted in complications causing ischemia in the upper extremities (Figure 9).[31] Pseudoaneurysm, which leads to upper extremity ischemia can com-plicate axillofemoral bypass grafting. Kempczinski and Penn[32] reported four patients who sustained five upper extremity complications after axil-lobifemoral grafting. These included injuries to the brachial plexus and axillary artery thrombosis, as well as arterial steal. They delineated the following precautions: proper positioning of the patient to prevent hyper-abduction of the shoulder, adequate exposure of the axillary artery during dissection, and gentle handling of the nerve trunks. They also emphasized meticulous technique during construction of the proximal anastomosis and avoidance of undue tension on the graft. Careful preoperative assess-ment of the axillary subclavian artery as a potential donor vessel is essen-tial. Recently, McLafferty et al[31] reviewed additional categories of prob-lems arising from axillofemoral bypass grafting.

Other more unusual cases of complications arising from utilization of the upper extremity vessels in revascularization procedures have been reported. Ligation of the subclavian artery in children for pulmonary artery anastomosis will occasionally lead to ischemia and gangrene. Two cases were reported from the 23-year experience of the Hospital for Sick Children in Toronto.[34] When this infrequent complication is encountered, revascularization is mandatory to avoid serious upper extremity complications. The use of an internal mammary artery graft in the presence of subclavian stenosis can be quite hazardous. In a report by Brown,[35] this circumstance led to myocardial ischemia and infarction, eventually resulting in the patient's death. This complication was related to a "steal" from the coronary circulation to the left upper extremity.

Traumatic Occlusion

Severe ischemia can result from sudden occlusion of the axillary artery after traumatic dislocation of the shoulder or even manual reduction of the dislocation. Injury to major collateral vessels such as the subscapular artery and the humeral circumflex arteries probably accounts for the severity of the ischemia in this condition as opposed to other causes of axillary artery occlusion. In these instances, exposure of the axillary artery by dividing the insertion of pectoralis major and minor will expose the area of injury. The point of thrombosis will usually be located at the level of the subscapular artery origin. The intima is seen to be fragmented with thrombotic occlusion of the vessel and in some cases disruption with false aneurysm formation will be encountered.[36] The damaged segment of axillary artery should be excised and repaired by primary anastomosis or interposition vein graft.[37–40]

Embolic Occlusion

A patient presenting with sudden onset of unilateral severe Raynaud's symptoms or digital ischemia should almost always have a three-dimensional echocardiogram as well as arch and upper extremity angiography to rule out a proximal embolizing lesion. In contradistinction to atherosclerotic occlusive disease, which has a decided symptomatic predilection for the left side, the incidence of embolization is evenly distributed.

Pain, coolness, cyanosis, and dysesthesias are common presenting complaints with clots lodging in the distal brachial artery. Approximately 70% of emboli to the axillary and brachial vessels will be of cardiac origin. These emboli can arise from the left atrial appendage, particularly in cases of mitral stenosis or mitral regurgitation in the presence of atrial fibrillation. Mural thrombi arising from the left ventricle, as a consequence of subendocardial infarction or ventricular aneurysm, provide another typical source for these embolic fragments.

Prosthetic valves, and cardiac valves that have been damaged by rheumatic fever, can also be implicated in many primary cardiac emboli to the upper extremities; this is common, and occurs even in older patients. In a series of 65 elderly patients with upper extremity ischemia secondary to embolization, rheumatic heart disease proved to be the underlying cause of thromboembolization in 8 patients, and arteriosclerotic disease in 57.[41] Emboli from a cardiac source are apt to be multiple and appear at various sites at a specific period in time. Embolization from an arterial aneurysm is likely to be recurrent, and repetitive to a discrete site. The diagnosis is relatively straightforward with a triad of symptoms: sudden onset of pain, paresthesias, and pallor accompanied by a loss of radial and/or ulnar pulses. Noninvasive tests are helpful in substantiating the diagnosis, in particular differential brachial pressure measurements as assessed by a Doppler flow detector. In a study by Maggard and Ekstrom,[42] the average mean pressure differential across an occlusion was 33 mm Hg when the occlusion was in the brachiocephalic trunk, and 20 mm Hg when the occlusion was in the subclavian artery. Mean pressure differences have been shown to increase when there are multiple occlusive lesions in the brachial as well as in the more distal radial and ulnar arteries. This is often the case with thromboembolism and it is therefore useful for establishing this fact at the time of initial diagnosis. In general, preexisting stenosis of brachial vessels will produce less of a pressure difference (left compared with right) than total occlusion or acute thrombotic occlusion.

The mortality rate in patients suffering acute upper extremity arterial embolism is approximately 25%, which is primarily attributable to concomitant or subsequent emboli to the renal, cerebrovascular, coronary, and mesenteric distributions. As reported by Romanoff and Floman,[41] the mortality rate in elderly patients is even higher. In their group of 65 patients it remained high during the early postembolectomy period and was also related to cardiac or respiratory failure or other manifestations of the underlying thromboembolic disease process.

The local course of an episode of acute arterial embolization is somewhat variable. Hodgkinson and Tracy[43] reported a high incidence of gangrene associated with embolization proximal to the origin of the brachial artery. In this group of patients, the therapy selected was prompt embolectomy. The early ischemia in patients with coexisting atherosclerotic disease is often followed by more chronic changes. Despite surgical mtervention, nearly 50% of patients in a recent series required some form of upper extremity or digital amputation because of irreversible tissue changes. In fact, 16% of these were major upper extremity amputations. A large group of patients reported from the Soviet Union by Savelyev and colleagues indicated that cardiac disease was the underlying cause of embolization in more than 90% of 256 patients presenting with upper extremity arterial embolization.[44–45] Although 33% had relatively mild ischemia, it was significant enough to result in total or partial paresis, with a compartment syndrome developing in approximately 10% of these patients. The mortality rate in this group was somewhat higher than 20% primarily related to recurrent embolization, to the cerebral, and mesenteric circulations. Therapy for acute upper extremity arterial embolization must be based on the knowledge that recurrent embolization represents the most significant determinant of fatality, and that untreated cases lead to a high incidence of tissue loss and gangrene. These characterizations are true for embolization of arterial as well as cardiac origin. Prompt embolectomy or primary reconstruction, together with long-term anticoagulation, remain the preferred treatment.

Arterial embolectomy is most effectively approached via the antecubital fossa. In the series from the Soviet Union, this resulted in restoration of circulation 90% of the time. The effects of delayed therapy on the ultimate outcome were reviewed by Kofoed and Hansen.[46] Among their patients, 75% who were operated on within 12 hours of the embolic episode achieved excellent revascularization and long-term results. When an operation was performed after 12 hours, only 35% had normal return of pulses. Half had some residual ischemic changes and restriction of function, and the remaining 25% required forearm amputation.

In addition to cardiac sources, emboli can arise in proximal subclavian lesions either from aneurysms, post-stenotic dilatation, or atherosclerotic ulcerations. Thoracic outlet compression syndrome, or blunt trauma to the axillary artery after clavicular fracture or chronic crutch injury can likewise result in aneurysm formation with thrombosis or embolization.[47]

Cerebrovascular symptoms have been reported as a consequence of subclavian artery embolization. When originating from a proximal subclavian lesion, emboli can result in vertebrobasilar insufficiency symptoms, presumably via antegrade flow in the vertebral artery.[48] Thrombotic occlusions from the more distal subclavian artery can propagate in a retrograde fashion and embolize prograde in the right carotid artery causing transient cerebral ischemia or stroke. Retrograde thrombus propagation can also embolize into the vertebrobasilar system on either side. It is surprising that primary atherosclerotic aneurysms of the subclavian artery subsequently present with distal embolization and occlusive symptoms. Occasionally, however, the aneurysm will undergo thrombosis and cause secondary arm ischemia.[49]

Treatment

A patient presenting with acute upper extremity arterial embolization and ischemia is probably best started immediately on continuous intravenous heparin while the diagnostic and therapeutic procedures are scheduled and undertaken. Although intravenous heparin can be discontinued for a short period of time during angiography, it can be maintained during arterial embolectomy. If surgical exploration and embolectomy are chosen as the mode of treatment, systemic thrombolytic therapy should be used cautiously, if at all. Anticoagulation with heparin should continue until the patient has been adequately anticoagulated with Coumadin. There should be a 2- to 3-day overlap of therapy to offset the hypercoagulable state that accompanies the onset of Coumadin therapy. The combination of low molecular-weight dextran (Dextran 40) with papaverine, although useful in incidents of arterial spasm and problems of microcirculation, is not as beneficial in major arterial occlusive problems.

Operative Approach

For most problems, as mentioned for the traumatic cases, the axillary artery can be exposed directly by transection of the pectoralis major and minor tendons, or by exposing the artery in the infraclavicular position by a muscle-splitting incision through the pectoralis major. The brachial artery can then be exposed in the lateral axilla.[50,51]

An aneurysm or lesion with evidence of distal embolization should, in general, be reconstructed with a saphenous vein graft, although the use of an in situ vein has gained proponants.[52] Embolization from mural thrombus or ulcerated atherosclerotic plaque has also been described.[53] Newer endovascular techniques have opened several additional avenues for repair, including the use of thrombolytic therapy and intra-arterial stents.[54]

The approach to the brachial artery may be more variable depending on the location of the bifurcation. Angiography is helpful and will often indicate the advisability of either the antecubital or the medial bicipital approach.

Embolectomy is almost always preferred via the transbrachial arterial route. In performing balloon embolectomy from the brachial approach, #2 and #3 catheters are used. The radial or ulnar position of the catheters can be ascertained by palpating the balloon at the wrist. When the catheter passes consistently into one or the other of the wrist vessels, the brachial bifurcation may require selective operative exposure. Alternatively, using fluoroscopic control, one balloon catheter can be positioned immediately distal to the bifurcation, then inflated. A second catheter is then usually passed easily into the remaining vessel. Recent reports suggest the superiority of a 30° Coude-tipped catheter.[55] If there has been recent propagation of clot into the palmar arch or digital vessels, streptokinase or urokinase infused through the arteriotomy over approximately 30 minutes will result in dramatic clearing of the smaller vessels. Particular care should be exercised when an innominate artery saddle embolus is suspected. This situation may require additional supraclavicular exposure for subclavian and carotid control, as described by Brusett et al.[56]

Fasciotomy may be necessary when revascularizing a severely ischemic arm, although in a large series of embolic occlusions it was rarely considered useful even in the face of significant edema or ischemia. After revascularization, the edema was seen to resolve within 5 to 10 days without specific therapy or adverse sequelae.[57]

Postoperative heparinization followed by Coumadin anticoagulation is extremely important to control the central embolizing source and to protect the areas of intimal damage that result from passage of the embolectomy catheter. Thrombosis in these areas of intimal trauma can be the cause of disaster after an otherwise successful procedure. Nevertheless, with attention to the described techniques, excellent clinical results can be anticipated.[58,59]

Brachial Artery

Trauma

Trauma to the forearm and upper arm presenting with acute ischemia generally carries a poor prognosis and severe disability. The injury typically involves both the artery and the accompanying nerve, with the continued disability generally resulting from the persistent neurological deficit. Although low-velocity missiles and stab wounds often can be managed with lateral arterial repair or end-to-end anastomosis, high-velocity missiles often leave an area of intimal damage adjacent to the area of thrombosis.[60] This damaged area must be resected to avoid recurrent thrombosis during the early postoperative period. Consequently, high-velocity injuries are best repaired with a reversed interposition vein graft after careful debridement of the hemorrhagic and ecchymotic arterial wall.

Arterial injuries frequently accompany closed trauma, and fractures or dislocations present a somewhat more difficult diagnostic and therapeutic challenge.[61] In the presence of an arterial injury to the upper extremity, there will be pain and dysesthesia distal to the site of injury, accompanied by pallor and an absence of pulses or abnormal Allen's test. The arterial injury that accompanies fractures can arise either from contusion of the vessel, compression, or total transection of the vessel. Some injuries have a high incidence of associated vascular damage, which has been of note with displaced supracondylar fractures occurring in childhood.[62]

It is preferable to reduce a fracture as a primary therapeutic maneuver and then to observe the patient for any residual signs of ischemia, providing the arterial pulse returns promptly. If the pulse does not reappear, or if signs and symptoms of ischemia fail to abate rapidly, noninvasive testing is helpful. This should be followed by expeditious arteriographic investigation should persistent ischemic symptoms prevail despite adequate reduction, or Doppler segmental pressures remain abnormal. Vessels that are involved in transitory spasm will usually transmit a relatively normal pressure to forearm and wrist. Occlusion, however, will produce a significant pressure drop in the range of 20 to 30 mm Hg. A pressure drop of this magnitude lasting between 30 minutes and 1 hour should be considered an indication of total arterial occlusion or transection. The consequence of delaying treatment of this type of ischemia in the upper extremity is the typical Volkmann's ischemic contracture. The development of Volkmann's contracture is an insidious event often occurring in the presence of minimal signs of arterial insufficiency. With injuries such as supracondylar fractures in children, the high incidence of ischemic contracture in the late follow-up period mandate an assessment of arterial integrity at the initial examination and subsequent to reduction of the fracture. If the arterial examination is not satisfactory, further diagnostic tests and immediate intervention are indicated.[63]

Brachial Artery Catheterization

Iatrogenic injury is the most common cause of brachial artery occlusion, and coronary angiography results in the most common iatrogenic injury. Since the earliest reports of the entity in 1971, the incidence of iatrogenic brachial artery injury has increased dramatically.[64] Coronary angiography and percutaneous transluminal angioplasty are performed over 100,000 times per year in the United States with the brachial and femoral route used with equal frequency. The brachial route is favored for the manipulation of catheters across tight coronary stenoses and for the secondary dilatation of aortocoronary vein grafts. In 1979 Abrams[65] reviewed 67,204 cases of brachial artery catheterization performed between 1971 and 1974. Nine hundred fifty-eight cases required surgical intervention for brachial artery complications (a complication rate of 1.4%). There were 890 reported cases of thrombosis, 38 cases of hemorrhage and 30 cases of pseudoaneurysms. In a recently reported series from a single institution, 12,158 brachial catheterizations resulted in a complication rate of 0.9% (106 cases required surgical intervention to correct brachial artery injury or thrombosis).[65a]

Ischemic symptoms include Raynaud's phenomenon and cold sensitivity as well as functional disability with hand fatigue, or cramping with exercise. Occasionally, fingertip or more extensive gangrene will be seen

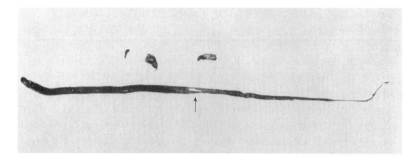

Figure 10. Thrombus removed from a brachial artery after cardiac catheterization. Notice the defect in the clot, through which the catheter had been manipulated. (Reproduced with permission from Machleder HI: Vaso-occlusive disorders of the upper extremity. *Curr Prob;l Surg* 25(1):1–67, 1988.)

where there has been delay in repair and secondary thrombotic occlusion of the palmar and digital vessels. If the radial pulse is weak or absent after brachial catheterization, Doppler segmental pressures should be measured. This provides the best objective means for serial evaluation of the patient if vascular spasm is thought to be the cause of the diminished pulse. The Doppler forearm pressure index, comparing the affected with the normal side, would indicate that patients will develop symptoms of arterial insufficiency at 0.60 and can develop ischemic symptoms and tissue loss at 0.25. From our experience at UCLA, it is evident that the majority of these complications occur in patients with atherosclerotic occlusive disease. The incidence of this injury is increased when there is prolonged catheterization time or a second catheterization via the same artery, multiple catheter changes, brachial artery atherosclerosis, a female gender, or failure to use intraprocedure heparinization. The experience of the operating physician is also a factor, with poor arteriotomy closure often implicated in the subsequent thrombosis (Figure 10).

In our series at UCLA, 26% of patients with diminished radial pulses developed ischemic symptoms during the follow-up period. With conservative treatment, a significant number of patients who are considered asymptomatic in the hospital or during early recuperation will develop symptoms on resumption of normal arm activities. Of those patients with absent radial pulses postcatheterization, 8% developed significant ischemic symptoms with the resumption of normal activity and 25% of patients with absent pulses were occupationally disabled. Patients with postcatheterization brachial artery occlusion should, under most circumstances, undergo surgical exploration because thrombectomy is really the only procedure that is necessary to restore normal circulation. On occasion, short segment resection with either end-to-end anastomosis or interposition of a segment of reversed saphenous vein graft will be necessary.[66] Saphenous vein graft reconstruction is associated with good long-term results and infrequent reports of graft dilatation or stenosis. The basilic vein can also be used and demonstrates excellent long-term results. During exploration for acute thrombosis, streptokinase or urokinase can be instilled into the distal vessel to dissolve residual thrombus. Balloon catheter embolectomy should be performed with particular care in these small very reactive vessels.

Although prosthetic material is satisfactory and might even be preferable for subclavian and proximal axillary artery reconstruction, saphenous veins and cephalic veins have proven to be excellent for arterial bypass grafts in the axillary and brachial positions.[67] Grafts to the more proximal vessels have a better patency rate (83% at 2 years) than grafts below the brachial level (53% at 2 years).[68] Cervicothoracic dorsal sympathectomy should be considered as a primary or adjunct procedure whenever reconstruction is required to the lower brachial or more distal vessels. It should be remembered that systemic as well as focal vascular degenerative disorders can occasionally affect the brachial artery and present with embolization.[69]

Radial and Ulnar

Traumatic occlusion and aneurysmal destruction of the distal radial, ulnar, and digital vessels are the most common causes of hand or digit ischemia not associated with systemic disease.

Ulnar Artery Thrombosis

Ulnar artery thrombosis is more common in males and is a consequence of relatively minor episodes of trauma. The entity termed the hypothenar hammer syndrome has been well documented as a result of repetitive trauma to the palmar surface of the ulnar side of the hand, as when the hand is used in a pounding motion.[70,71] The patients commonly present with Raynaud's symptoms confined, however, to only one upper extremity.

Pain and dysesthesias are frequent, as is cold intolerance. Numbness is usually in the ulnar nerve distribution and patients may have tenderness or even a small aneurysm palpable in Guyon's canal. In this location over the ulnar carpal bones, the artery is exposed to trauma with consequent intimal damage, subintimal hemorrhage, and disruption of the internal elastic lamina.

Diagnosis is usually not difficult and a positive Allen's test result is commonly demonstrable. Digital plethysmography is useful in diagnosis, particularly recorded during compression of the radial artery. The symptoms are a consequence of either ulnar artery occlusion or intimal damage with distal embolism. These changes can be documented by the angiographic appearance of ulnar irregularity or occlusion, with additional embolic occlusions of the digital arteries on the ulnar side of the palmar arch. During arteriographic examination it must be remembered that a small percentage of ulnar arteries will arise proximal to the usual brachial artery bifurcation. Successful treatment has been reported with cervicothoracic sympathectomy as well as direct reconstruction with reversed saphenous vein.[72,73]

In rare instances, arteriosclerotic aneurysms may develop in the hand. Small true aneurysms of the palmar arch vessels can be found in either the thenar or hypothenar eminences that occur in most instances several weeks after significant closed hand injuries. The aneurysmal mass can be easily identified clinically, by the fairly typical symptoms of coolness and paresthesias of the digits exacerbated by exercise. As with trauma to the ulnar artery, treatment comprises resection of the aneurysm and reconstruction of the vessel with a reversed autogenous saphenous vein. Occlusions and aneurysm formation occur far more often in the ulnar artery than in the radial or digital vessels, due to the exposed position of the ulnar artery and its vulnerability to occupational injuries, as previously indicated.[73a,73b]

In acute symptomatic thrombotic events, intra-arterial thrombolysin has been used with some success. After lysis of the clot, the patient begins systemic heparin therapy, after which oral anticoagulants are prescribed, depending on the nature of the thrombotic episode. Kartchner and Wilcox[74] reported this therapy in a series of nine patients who had thrombosis of the palmar arch or digital arteries accompanied by impending gangrene in the hand. These patients were treated by intra-arterial thrombolysin given at an infusion rate of 100,000 units per hour. An excellent result was achieved in eight hands and good results in two additional hands treated in this manner. In general, when the acute thrombotic event is reversed, the underlying lesion must be identified so that definitive therapy can be administered. Resection and reconstruction remain important inasmuch as the incidence of rethrombosis is high.[75]

Iatrogenic Injury

The upper extremities provide access to the vascular system for a variety of diagnostic and therapeutic procedures. The arterial system is often the site of blood sampling for blood gas determinations, arterial pressure monitoring, and access for angiography and cardiac catheterization. Most of the vascular complications occurring in the upper extremity are secondary to these diagnostic procedures. The radial artery is frequently cannulated in the forearm for blood gas sampling or continuous monitoring of systemic blood pressure in a growing number of clinical situations.

Bleeding from the puncture site is an occasional problem, but usually will respond to digital pressure followed by application of a compression bandage. Thrombosis, however, may result in severe disability if there is inadequate collateral blood flow supplied by the ulnar artery.

Before insertion of a cannula into the radial artery, Allen's test should be performed. An abnormal test indicates that the palmar arch is being perfused predominantly by the vessel being compressed, and injury to it may result in severe digital ischemia. Because the radial artery is small and occasionally calcified, successful repair is unlikely, even with microvascular techniques. Allen's test can be supplemented with Doppler studies when test interpretation is unclear. These are important considerations to be made before cannulation of the radial artery; a hand supplied only by the radial artery may develop severe ischemic changes if thrombosis occurs, and amputation may be required despite the best efforts to restore circulation. In a report by Crossland and Neviaser,[76] 10% of patients undergoing this procedure developed complications of ischemia or necrosis in the involved hand. In this series of 60 patients, it was concluded that an adequate circulatory evaluation by Allen's test might have avoided complications inasmuch as most of those who developed problems had evidence of inadequacy of the palmar arch.

In a prospective study of 40 patients. Little et al[77] determined that 22 arteries underwent thrombosis after removal of a percutaneously placed radial artery cannula. In this series, the integrity of the radial artery was examined by using a Doppler flow detector.[77] In another group of 333 radial artery cannulations studied by Davis and Stewart,[78] the frequency of complete occlusion of the vessel was noted to be 30% when assessed 1 day after removing the cannula. At day 8 using a Doppler flow detector and Allen's test, 24% of the vessels were determined to be totally occluded. A multivariate analysis of 13 parameters was done in this group of patients and no important predictive elements were identified. The rate of occlusion with small 20-gauge Teflon cannulas, however, was only 3% and there was a significantly higher occlusion rate in women (37.5%) than in men (27%). This latter difference may reflect the generally smaller vessel diameter relative to the size of the catheter rather than any basic hematologic differences. Although the occlusion rate was surprisingly high, the frequency of major complications was minimal in this group and no permanent sequelae such as gangrene or tissue loss developed.

In a randomized trial conducted in 148 patients, Davis and colleagues[79] prospectively evaluated the thrombotic consequences of four different sized catheters used for percutaneous radial artery cannulation. When 18-gauge polypropylene catheters were used, the incidence of complete occlusion 8 days after decannulation was 34%. There were no instances of occlusion noted when 20-gauge Teflon catheters were used. Another study conducted by Bedford[80] evaluated 108 patients after 24 hours of percutaneous radial or ulnar artery cannulation. Either 18- or 20-gauge catheters were used, and an 8% incidence of radial artery occlusion occurred after cannulation with 20-gauge catheters compared with a 34% incidence when using 18–gauge catheters. Bedford[81] believed that the incidence of arterial occlusion increased linearly as the ratio of the catheter's outer diameter to vessel lumen diameter increased. It is apparent that both the size and material of the cannula are important factors in the occurrence of arterial occlusion, and the increased utilization of small Teflon cannulas will probably reduce the frequency of this complication considerably. Additionally, the catheter should be removed after 12 to 18 hours, particularly if there is evidence of poor local perfusion or hypercoagulability.

Proper performance of Allen's test is important in the accurate assessment of arterial integrity in the hand, and should precede any radial or ulnar artery cannulation. The reader is referred to Chapter 1 on initial evaluation. Hirai and Kawai[82] studied the incidence of false-positive and false-negative results in the Allen's test. Arteriography with independent compression of the radial and ulnar arteries was performed on 44 hands with peripheral arterial disease and the factors responsible for false-positive and false-negative tests were analyzed. Arterial spasm in the uncompressed artery or erroneous compression of both radial and ulnar arteries was a frequent cause for false-positive results in this test. False-negative test results mainly occurred when compression of the arteries was inadequate or missed by inaccurate placement of the examiner's fingers. False-negative results were also obtained in patients who had occlusions in both radial and ulnar arteries. With careful attention to detail and performance of the technique, the Allen's test was then applied to 140 normal hands and 52 hands with arterial occlusion. In comparing these results with arteriographic findings, there were no false-positive results and the test was considered useful not only for diagnosis but for follow-up study, particularly after reconstructive surgery, to assess the patency of the palmar arch and the radial and ulnar arteries.[81]

References

1. James EC, Khuyri NT, Fedde CW, et al: Upper limb ischemia resulting from arterial thromboembolism. *Am J Surg* 137(6):739–744, 1979.
2. Miller-Fisher C: A new vascular syndrome- "The subclavian steal." *N Engl J Med* 265:1912, 1961.

3. Reivich M, Holling E, Roberts B, Toole J: Reversal of blood flow through the vertebral artery and its effect on cerebral circulation. *N Engl J Med* 265:878, 1961.

4. Larrieu AJ, Tyers GF, Williams EH, et al: Subclavian steal syndrome: an update. *South Med J* 72(11):1374–1376, 1979.

5. Schwartz CJ, Mitchell JRA: Atheroma of the carotid and vertebral arterial systems. *Br Med J* 2:1057–1063, 1961.

6. Magaard F, Ekestrom S: The influence of arm ischemia and arm hyperaemia on subclavian and vertebral artery blood flow in patients with occlusive disease of the subclavian artery and the brachiocephalic trunk: A preoperative study. *Scand J Thorac Cardiovasc Surg* 9(3):240–9, 1975.

7. Magaard F, Ryttman A: Regional cerebral blood flow and vertebral angiography at rest and in connection with arm work in patients with the subclavian steal phenomenon. *Scand J Thorac Cardiovasc Surg* 10(1):96–111, 1976.

8. Kempczinski R, Hermann G: The innominate steal syndrome. *J Cardiovasc Surg (Torino)* 5:481–6, 1979.

9. Walker PM, Paley D, Harris KA, et al: What determines the symptoms associated with subclavian artery occlusive disease. *J Vasc Surg* 2:154–157, 1985.

10. Fields WS: Joint study of extracranial arterial occclusion: VII. Subclavian steal: A review of 168 cases. *JAMA* 222:1139–1143, 1972.

11. Akers DL, Fowl RJ, Plettner J, Kempczinski RF: Complications of anomalous origin of the right subclavian artery: Case report and review of the literature. *Ann Vasc Surg* 5:385–388, 1991.

12. Jerois JT, Stevem SL, Freeman MB, Goldman MH: Vertebrobasilar syndrome associated with subclavian origin of the right internal carotid artery. *J Vasc Surg* 21:855–861, 1995.

13. Stoney WS, Alford WC, Burrus GR, Thomas CS, Jr: Aberrant right subclavian artery aneurysm. *Ann Thorac Surg* 19(4):460–7, 1975.

14. Brown DL, Chapman WC, Edwards WH, et al: Dysphagia lusoria. *Am Surg* 59:582–586, 1993.

15. Godtfredsen J, Wennevold A, Efsen F, Lauridsen P: The natural history of vascular ring with clinical manifestations: A follow up study of 11 unoperated cases. *Scand J Thorac Cardiovasc Surg* 11(1):75–7, 1977.

16. Vogt DP, Hertzer NR, O'Hara PJ, Beven EG: Brachiocephalic arterial reconstruction. *Ann Surg* 196:541–552, 1982.

17. Kretschmer G, Teleky B, Marosi L, et al: Obliterations of the proximal subclavian artery: To bypass or to anastomose? *J Cardiovasc Surg* 32:334–339, 1991.

18. Meyers WO, Lawton BR, Ray JF I et al: Axillo-axillary bypass for subclavian steal syndrome. *Arch Surg* 114:394–399, 1979.

19. Welling RE, Cranley JJ, Krause RJ, Hafner CD: Obliterative arterial disease of the upper extremity. *Arch Surg* 116:1593–1596, 1981.

20. Chang JB, Stein TA, Liu JP, Dunn ME: Long-term results with axillo-axillary bypass grafts for symptomatic subclavian artery insufficiency. *J Vasc Surg* 25:173–178, 1977.

21. Mingoli A, Feldhaus RJ, Farma C, et al: Comparative results of carotid-subclavian bypass and axillo-axillary bypass in patients with symptomatic subclavian disease. *Eur J Vasc Surg* 6:26–30, 1992.

22. Halsted W: Ligation of the first portion of the left subclavian artery and excision of a subclavian artery aneurysm. *Bull Johns Hopkins Hosp* 3:93, 1892.

23. Schaff HV, Brawley RK: Operative management of penetrating vascular injuries of the thoracic outlet. *Surgery* 82:182–5, 1977.

24. Bergqvist D, Ericsson BF, Konrad P, Bergentz SE: Arterial surgery of the upper extremity. *World J Surg* 7:786–791, 1983.

25. Rapp, JH, Reilly LM, Goldstone EJ, et al: Ischemia of the upper extremity: Significance of proximal arterial disease. *Am J Surg* 152:122–126, 1986.

25a. Whitbread T, Cleveland TJ, Beard JD, Gaines PA: A combined approach to the treatment of proximal arterial occlusions of the upper limb with endovascular stents. *Eur J Vasc Endovasc Surg* 15:29–35, 1988.

26. Johnson B, Thursby P: Subclavian artery injury caused by a screw in a clavicular compression plate. *Cardiovasc Surg* 4:414–415, 1996.

27. Gelabert HA, Machleder HI: Diagnosis and management of arterial compression at the thoracic outlet. *Ann Vasc Surg* 11(4):359–366, 1997.

27a. Lakshmikumar P, Luchette FA, Romano KS, Ricotta JJ: Upper-extremity arterial injury. *Am Surg* 63:224–227, 1997.

28. Bower TC, Pairolero PC, Hallett JW, et al: Brachiocephalic aneurysm: The case for early recognition and repair. *Ann Vasc Surg* 5:125–132, 1991.

29. Myers SI, Harward RS, Maher DP, et al: Complex upper extremity vascular trauma in an urban population. *J Vasc Surg* 12:305–309, 1990.

30. Butler MJ, Lane RHS, Webster JHH: Irradiation injury to large arteries. *Br J Surg* 67:341–343, 1980.

31. McLafferty RB, Taylor LM, Moneta GL, et al: Upper extremity thromboembolism after axillary-axillary bypass grafting. *Cardiovasc Surg* 4:111–113, 1996.

32. Kempczinski R, Penn I: Upper extremity complications of axillofemoral grafts. *Am J Surg* 136(2):209–11, 1978.

33. McLafferty RB, Taylor LM, Moneta GL, et al: Upper extremity thromboembolism caused by occlusion of axillofemoral grafts. *Am J Surg* 169:492–495, 1995.

34. Geiss D, Williams WG, Lindsay WK, Rowe RD: Upper extremity gangrene: A complication of subclavian artery division. *Ann Thorac Surg* 30(5):487–9, 1980.

35. Brown AH: Coronary steal by internal mammary graft with subclavian stenosis. *J Thorac Cardiovasc Surg* 73(5):690–3, 1977.

36. Henson GF: Vascular complications of shoulder injuries. *J Bone Joint Surg* 38B: 528–531, 1956.

37. McKenzie AD, Sinclair AM: Axillary artery occlusion complicating shoulder dislocation. *Ann Surg* 148:139–141, 1958.

38. Neumayer LA, Bull DA, Hunter GC, et al: Atherosclerotic aneurysms of the axillary artery. *J Cardiovasc Surg* 33:172–177, 1992.

39. Bergqvist D, Ericsson BF, Konrad P, Bergentz SE: Arterial surgery of the upper extremity. *World J Surg* 7:786–791, 1983.

40. Thompson PN, Chang BB, Shah DM, et al: Outcome following blunt vascular trauma of the upper extremity. *Cardiovasc Surg* 1:248–253, 1993.

41. Romanoff H, Floman Y: Peripheral arterial embolectomy in the aged. *J Cardiovasc Surg (Torino)* 17(3):224–9, 1976.

42. Maggard F, Ekestrom S: Preoperative measurements of blood flow and pres-

sure in occlusion and/or stenosis of the subclavian artery and the brachiocephalic trunk. *Scand J Thorac Cardiovasc Surg* 10(1):85–95, 1976.

43. Savelyev VS, Stephanov NV: Comparative evaluation of the methods of treatment of embolism of the main arteries of the arm. *Kardiologiia* 16(6):14–18, 1976.

44. Savelyev VS, Zatevakhin II, Stephanov NVC: Artery embolism of the upper limbs. *J Surg* 81(4):367–75, 1977.

45. Hodgkinson DJ, Tracy GD: Upper limb emboli: A reappraisal. *Aust NZ J Surg* 45(2):139–43, 1975.

46. Kofoed H, Hansen HJ: Arterial embolism in the upper limb. *Acta Chir Scand Suppl* 472:113–115, 1976.

47. Abbott WNI, Darling RC: Axillary artery anewysms secondary to crutch trauma. *Am J Surg* 125:515, 1973.

48. Ricotta JJ, Ouriel K, Green RM, DeWeese JA: Embolic lesions from the subclavian artery causing transient vertebrobasilar insufficiency. *J Vasc Surg* 4: 372–375, 1986.

49. McCollum CH, Da Gama AD, Noon GP, DeBakey ME: Aneurysm of the subclavian artery. *J Cardiovasc Surg* 20:159–163, 1979.

50. Brawley RR, Murray GF, Crisler C: Management of wounds of the innominate, subclavian, and axillary blood vessels. *Surg Gynecol Obstet* 131:1130–1140, 1970.

51. Donovan DL, Sharp WV: Blunt trauma to the axillary artery. *J Vasc Surg* 1: 681–683, 1984.

52. Kniemeyer HW, Sandmann W: In situ and composite in situ vein bypass for upper extremity ischaemia. *Eur J Vasc Surg* 6:41–46, 1992.

53. Sachatello CR, Ernst CB, Griffen WO: The acutely ischemic upper extremity: Selective management. *Surgery* 76:1002–1009, 1974.

54. Ackroyd R, Singh S, Beard JD, Gaines PA: Simultaneous brachial embolectomy and endoluminal stenting of a subclavian artery aneurysm. *Eur J Vasc Endovasc Surg* 10:248–249, 1995.

55. Beckingham IJ, Roberts S, Berridge DC, et al: A simple technique for thromboembolectomy of the upper limb. *Eur J Vasc Surg* 81:367–375, 1977.

56. Brusett KA, Kwasnik EM, Marjani MA: Innominate artery saddle embolus: A pitfall for retrograde brachial embolectomy. *J Vasc Surg* 25:569–571, 1997.

57. Savelyev VS, Sztivakhin II, Stpanov NV: Artery embolism of the upper limbs. *Surgery* 81:367–375, 1977.

58. Brunkwall J, Bergqvist D, Bergentz S: Long-term results of arterial reconstruction of the upper extremity. *Eur J Vasc Surg* 8:47–51, 1994.

59. Mesh CL, McCarthy WJ, Pearce WH, et al: Upper extremity bypass grafting. *Arch Surg* 128:795–802, 1993.

60. Gelberman RH, Blasmgame JP, Fronek A, Dimick MP: Forearm arterial injuries. *J Hand Surg* 4(5):401–8, 1979.

61. Endean ED, Veldenz HC, Schwarcz TH, Hyde GL: Reconstruction of arterial injury in elbow dislocation. *J Vasc Surg* 16:402–406, 1992.

62. Rowell PJ: Arterial occlusion in juvenile humeral supracondylar fracture. *Injury* 75;6(3):254–6, 1975.

63. Holden CE: The pathology and prevention of Volkmann's ischemic contracture. *J Bone Joint Surg* 618(3):296–300, 1979.

64. Machleder HI, Barker WF, Sweeney J: The pulseless arm after brachial artery catheterization. *Lancet* 7747:407–409, 1972.
65. Adams DF, Adams HL: Complications of coronary angiography. *Cardiovasc Res*2:89–96, 1979.
65a.McCollum CH, Mavor E: Brachial artery injury after cardiac catheterization. *J Vasc Surg* 4:355–359, 1986.
66. Gross WS, Flanigan DP, Kraft RO, Stanley JC: Chronic upper extremity arterial insufficiency. *Arch Surg* 113:419–423, 1978.
67. Garrett EH, Morris GC, Howell JF, DeBakey ME: Revascularization of upper extremity with autogenous vein bypass graft. *Arch Surg* 91:751–757, 1965.
68. McCarthy WJ, Flinn WR, Yao JST, et al: Results of bypass grafting for upper limb ischemia. *J Vasc Surg* 3:741–746, 1986.
69. Cheu HW, Mills JL: Digital artery embolization as a result of fibromuscular dysplasia of the brachial artery. *J Vasc Surg* 14:225–228, 1991.
70. Conn J Jr, Bergan JJ, Bell JL: Hypothenar hammer syndrome. *Surgery* 68: 1122–1128, 1970.
71. Koman LA, Urbaniak JR: Ulnar artery insufficiency: A guide to treatment. *J Hand Surg* 6:16–24, 1981.
72. Pineda CJ, Weisman N, Bookstein JJ, et al: Hypothenar hammer syndrome: Form of reversible Raynaud's phenomenon. *Am J Med* 79:651–570, 1985.
73. Nehler MR, Dalman RL, Harris JE, et al: Upper extremity arterial bypass distal to the wrist. *J Vasc Surg* 16:633–642, 1992.
73a.Chetter IC, Kent PJ, Kester RC: The hand arm vibration syndrome. A review. *Cardiovasc Surg* 6:1–9, 1998.
73b.Menon KV, Insall RL, Ignotus PI: Motorcycling and finger ischemia. *Eur J Vasc Endovasc Surg* 14:410–412, 1997.
74. Kartchner MM, Wilcox WC: Thrombolysis of palmar and digital arterial thrombosis by intra-arterial thrombolism. *J Hand Surg* 1(1):67–74, 1976.
75. Von Kuster L, Abt AB: Traumatic aneurysms of the ulnar artery. *Arch Pathol Lab Med* 104(2):75–78, 1980.
76. Crossland SG, Neviaser RJ: Complications of radial artery catheterization. *Hand* 9(3):287–90, 1977.
77. Little JM, Carlk B, Shanks C: Effects of radial artery cannulation. *Med J Aust* 2(21):791–3, 1975.
78. Davis FM, Stewart JM: Radial artery cannulation: A prospective study in patients undergoing cardiothoracic surgery. *Br J Anaesth* 52(1):41–7, 1980.
79. Davis FM, Stewart JM: Radial artery cannulation: A prospective study in patients undergoing cardiothoracic surgery. *Br J Anaesth* 52(1):41–7, 1980.
80. Davis FM: Radial artery cannulation: Influence of catheter size and material on arterial occlusion. *Anaesth Intensive Care* 6(1):49–53, 1978.
81. Bedford RF: Radial arterial function following percutaneous cannulation with 18 and 20 gauge catheters. *Anesthesiology* 47(1):37–9, 1977.
82. Hirai M, Kawai S: False positive and negative results in Allen's test. *J Cardiovasc Surg (Torino)* 21(3):353–60, 1980.

15

Hemangiomas and Vascular Malformations of the Upper Extremity

Patricia E. Burrows, MD and Tal Laor, MD

In this chapter, vascular lesions of the upper extremity are described according to the classification proposed by Mulliken and Glowacki in 1982.[1] This classification divides vascular lesions into two major categories: hemangiomas and vascular malformations. Hemangiomas are benign endothelial cell neoplasms which present in infancy and have characteristic proliferating and involuting phases. Vascular malformations are subclassified according to the channel content and flow characteristics. High-flow vascular malformations include arteriovenous malformations (AVMs) and arteriovenous fistulas (AVFs). Low-flow malformations include capillary, venous, lymphatic, and mixed forms. Each type of lesion will be discussed according to its clinical presentation, diagnostic features, and therapeutic options. Magnetic resonance imaging (MRI) is the best single modality for elucidation of the nature and extent of vascular anomalies. The appropriate imaging sequences include T1-weighted spin echo sequences without and with intravenous contrast medium, T2-weighted sequences (which demonstrate fluid and slow flow vessels), and gradient recalled echo sequences, which can be performed with saturation to show selective venous or arterial flow.[2-7] Gradient sequences also enhance old blood products and phleboliths.

In a recent review of 500 pediatric vascular masses treated at Children's Hospital in Boston, 90% were classified as either hemangiomas or

From Machleder HI, (ed): *Vascular Disorders of the Upper Extremity*. Third Revised Edition. Futura Publishing Company, Inc., Armonk, NY, © 1998.

vascular malformations.[8] Approximately one-half of these lesions were hemangiomas. Most of the remaining 209 vascular malformations were slow flow (venous, lymphatic, or combined). Venous malformations were twice as common in girls as in boys; the other malformations had an even distribution between the genders.

Hemangiomas and vascular malformations form two distinct categories of lesions, with distinct histological, histochemical, and biological differences. Hemangiomas present at or shortly after birth, grow rapidly in infancy by endothelial cell proliferation, apparently driven by growth factors. They undergo gradual spontaneous involution, which typically starts by the end of the first year of life and is complete by 10 years of age in most patients. Vascular malformations, however, are believed to be errors of vascular morphogenesis without increased endothelial cell proliferation. Although most malformations are sporadic, a few hereditary forms have permitted identification of genetic defects (eg, high-flow lesions in Osler-Weber-Rendu syndrome [HHT; hereditary hemorrhagic telangiectasia],[9] and a low-flow form consisting of familial multiple venous malformations[10,11]). The defect in HHT results in a deficiency of elastin in certain vessel types, while the venous malformations appear to involve mural smooth muscle deficiency. Although these defects are assumed to be present at birth, many malformations manifest or become increasingly symptomatic later in life; the factors responsible for progressive symptomatology have not been clearly defined.

Although much excellent literature exists,[12–16] the terminology used in published literature pertaining to vascular lesions has, unfortunately, not been applied uniformly. In particular, the term "hemangioma" has frequently been used in a nonspecific fashion, referring to both the potentially involuting infantile hemangiomas and various forms of vascular malformation, especially venous malformation. As this chapter outlines, each type of vascular lesion has a distinct clinical behavior and appropriate treatment.

Hemangiomas

Hemangiomas are present at birth in 40% of affected infants, often as a faint macular stain that subsequently enlarges rapidly.[17] A small percentage of hemangiomas are fully developed at birth (congenital hemangiomas). Most hemangiomas appear in the first 3 months of life and undergo rapid proliferation, usually plateauing at 9 to 10 months of age. They have a much longer phase of spontaneous involution that is usually complete by 7 to 10 years of age. They most commonly affect the head and neck area; trunk and extremities are infrequent sites. When the skin is involved, it usually is raised and red, with a characteristic strawberry-like appearance. With deep hemangiomas the overlying skin is normal or has a faint bluish hue due to the presence of the draining veins. Adjacent superficial veins may appear mildly dilated. The lesion itself is generally warm and soft, but not compressible. The high-flow nature of the lesion can be determined by "listening" with a Doppler probe. As the hemangioma begins to involute, the color usually fades and the lesion feels softer. Congenital hemangiomas, which are fully developed at birth, typically demonstrate rapid involution, regressing by 1 year of age.

Diagnostic Imaging Features

While most superficial hemangiomas can be diagnosed clinically, those without skin involvement may require imaging. Ultrasound is useful for tissue characterization, demonstrating a focal parenchymal mass and high flow-vessels within and around the mass. MRI is the best single imaging modality to delineate both the tissue character and extent.[3,4] MRI features of hemangiomas include focal, lobulated soft tissue mass with diffuse contrast enhancement, elevated T2 signal, and dilated feeding and draining vessels within and around the focal mass (Figure 1). Magnetic resonance angiography will generally demonstrate some enlarged arteries leading to the mass.

Conventional angiography is not usually necessary, but shows a hypervascular tissue blush, with dilated feeding arteries and draining veins.[18] Hemangiomas must be distinguished from neonatal tumors, especially fibrosarcoma, other soft tissue sarcomas, and neurofibroma. In general, hemangiomas are characterized by discrete margins and homogeneous enhancement and signal characteristics, while sarcomas tend to be less homogeneous.

Treatment

The most common symptom related to upper extremity hemangiomas is ulceration, which occurs in 30% of cases.[15,16] Wet-to-dry dressings, topical antibiotic ointment, and splints are the mainstay of treatment of these complications. Large or severely ulcerated lesions may justify the use of pharmacological treatment such as systemic or intralesional corticosteroids or subcutaneous α-interferon. Rarely, large extremity hemangiomas may be associated with congestive heart failure, requiring arterial

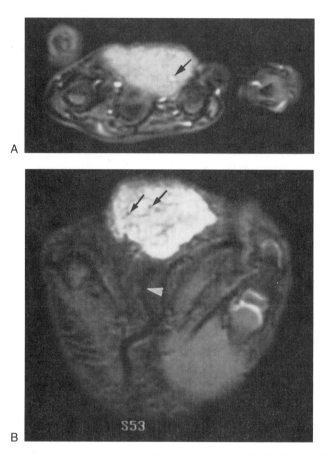

Figure 1. Hemangioma of the left hand in a 3-month-old girl. **A:** T2-weighted axial image demonstrates a hyperintense, well-marginated homogeneous soft tissue mass involving the subcutaneous and muscular layers of the palm. Note the dilated vessels within (arrow) and around the mass indicating increased flow. **B:** T1−weighted gadolinium enhanced, fat suppressed coronal image demonstrates intense homogeneous contrast enhancement. Note the small flow voids (arrows) within the mass and the dilated palmar veins (arrowhead).

embolization or surgical excision. Hypoprothrombinemia, sometimes associated with hypofibrinogenemia, is seen in association with hemangiomatous masses (Kasabach-Merritt phenomenon). The underlying masses are not typical hemangiomas, but have a more aggressive histology, such as Kaposiform hemangio-endothelioma. They often respond poorly to corticosteroids and α-interferon and may warrant more aggressive chemotherapy. Ultimately, most of these lesions appear to regress, with associated improvement in platelet counts.

Vascular Malformations

Capillary Malformations

Capillary malformations or port wine stains consist of abnormal collections of small vascular channels in the dermis. This malformation may be isolated or associated with underlying deep vascular malformations.

Clinical and Imaging Features

The cutaneous capillary malformations may be localized or diffuse, extending over the entire upper extremity and thorax.[16] The skin is usually normal in temperature and pulses are normal in strength. Doppler examination demonstrates no increased arterial flow. Over time, the affected extremity may demonstrate overgrowth.

Imaging studies are generally normal in isolated capillary malformations, although there may be some increased thickness of the subcutaneous fat, and prominent venous channels may be seen (Figure 2).

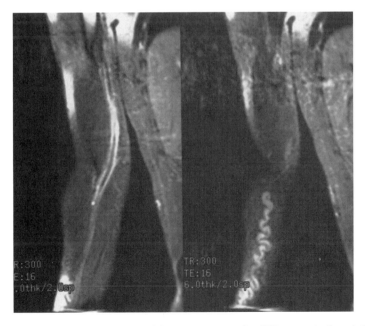

Figure 2. Capillary malformation of the upper extremity. Diffuse port wine stain. T1-weighted MRI, with fat suppression and intravenous contrast, shows an enlarged tortuous superficial vein, but no soft tissue mass or other signal abnormality.

Treatment

Pulsed dye laser is effective in fading some port wine stains.

Venous Malformations

Clinical Features

Venous malformation is the most common symptomatic vascular malformation affecting the extremities. Seventy-five percent of venous malformations in the Children's Hospital registry were evident at birth.[8] These malformations can be further subdivided as spongy masses and diffuse dilatations and varicosities of the major conducting veins. Spongy venous malformations can be localized, affecting the skin or muscle, localized but multiple throughout the extremity, or diffuse. They grow commensurately with the child, but, in females, may become larger or more symptomatic during periods of hormonal change, such as puberty and pregnancy. Males apparently demonstrate no symptomatic change at puberty.

Symptoms consist of swelling and pain. The pain can be attributed to intralesional thrombosis or to focal swelling with compression of muscle or nerves. Diffuse venous malformations tend to manifest as heaviness, with swelling on dependency and pain with activity. Extensive venous malformations are associated with diminished neuromuscular function. Patients with large venous malformations frequently demonstrate disseminated intravascular coagulation or localized intravascular coagulation state due to intralesional thrombosis and thrombolysis. Coagulation studies in these patients demonstrate mild abnormalities of the PT and PTT, with depressed fibrinogen levels. The usually mild clotting dysfunction can be severely aggravated during surgical procedures.

Physical findings depend on the extent and location of the venous malformation. Skin involvement is usually evident as blue or purple-blue discoloration, sometimes with telangiectasia. The affected area tends to distend with dependency or with the application of a tourniquet. Elevation of the upper extremity with release of the tourniquet generally results in evacuation of the blood. Phleboliths and thrombi may be palpable. Skin temperature and pulses are normal. Doppler evaluation does not demonstrate increased flow.

Imaging Findings

Conventional radiographs and computed tomography (CT) may demonstrate lamellated rounded calcifications or phleboliths (Figure 3).

Bones are often slender, with prominent trabeculations and decreased cortical thickness. Ultrasound may show compressible anechoic spaces with or without venous flow. Often, the venous flow can be best demonstrated on release of compression by the transducer. MRI clearly demarcates the lesions that appear as septated hyperintense collections on T2-weighted sequences, with enhancement on postcontrast T1-weighted se-

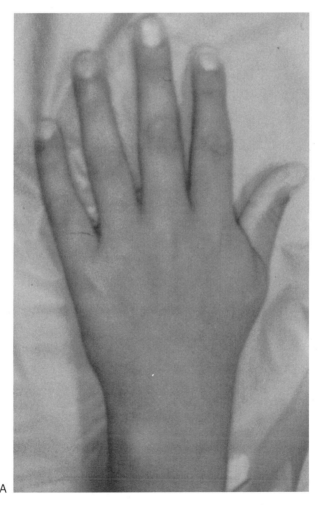

A

Figure 3. Intramuscular venous malformation involving the thenar eminence. The patient had previously undergone surgical resection of part of the lesion, with subsequent recurrence. **A:** Clinical photograph demonstrating soft tissue swelling between the thumb and index finger, associated with mild contracture.

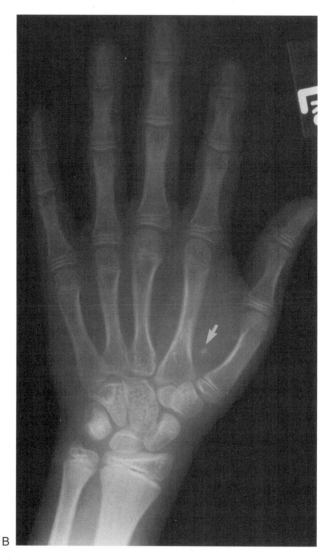

B

Figure 3. *(continued)* **B**: Plain radiograph demonstrates phleboliths (arrow) in the first webspace.

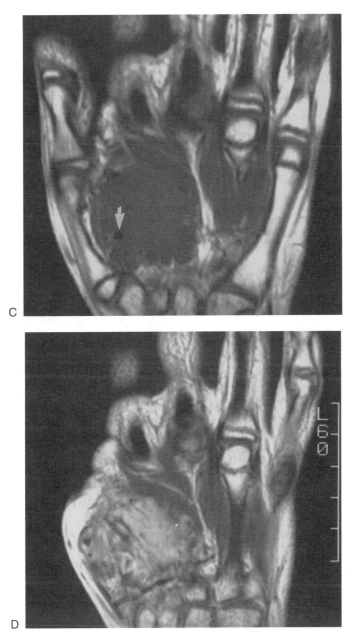

Figure 3. *(continued)* **C**: Coronal T1-weighted MRI without gadolinium demonstrates an intramuscular soft tissue mass, isointense to surrounding muscle, with a signal void corresponding to a phlebolith (arrow). **D**: T1-weighted coronal MRI with intravenous gadolinium demonstrates inhomogeneous enhancement of the mass.

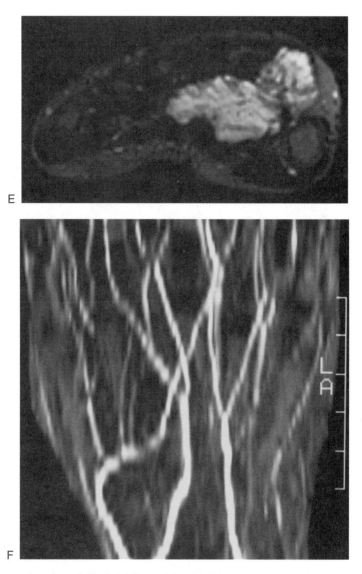

Figure 3. *(continued)* **E:** Axial T2-weighted MRI demonstrates the hyperintense soft tissue mass with longitudinally arranged septations, corresponding to slow flow vascular channels between muscle fibers. **F:** Magnetic resonance angiography demonstrates normal arteries and veins with no abnormally enlarged branches.

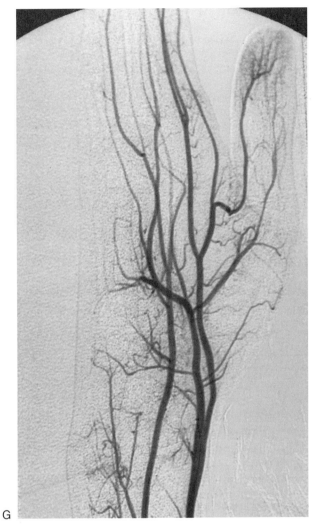

G

Figure 3. *(continued)* **G**: Brachial arteriogram, digital subtraction technique of the left hand demonstrates normal arterial anatomy with no arteriovenous shunting.

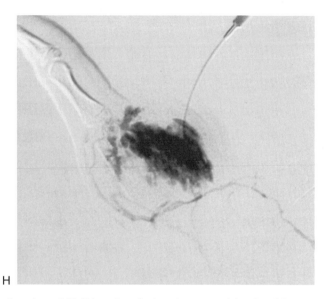

H

Figure 3. *(continued)* **H:** Direct intralesional contrast injection (digital subtraction technique) during a second session of sclerotherapy demonstrates the longitudinal vascular spaces arranged between muscle fibers, and draining into normal appearing vein. After the contrast injection, the venous spaces were injected with absolute ethanol.

quences (Figures 3 and 4).[3,4,19] Signal voids usually represent phleboliths or thrombi, rather than supplying arteries. Gradient imaging shows no increased flow. Magnetic resonance venography frequently reveals dilation or other anomalies of the major venous trunks.[6] Selective arteriography may demonstrate contrast puddling within sinusoidal spaces and abnormal veins, but is not usually necessary.[18] Direct injection of contrast medium with angiographic imaging, is a better technique to opacify the lesion, and shows collections of interconnecting channels, or varicosities (Figures 3 and 4).[19,20]

Treatment

Conservative treatment consists of the use of aspirin for relief of thrombotic pain, in conjunction with tailored elastic compression gloves and sleeves to control swelling.[16] Symptomatic venous malformations can be reduced in size by direct injection of sclerosant drugs. This is generally performed in an angiography suite. Contrast injection is made directly into the venous malformation and recorded serially with digital subtraction angiography, to demonstrate the morphology and extent of the mal-

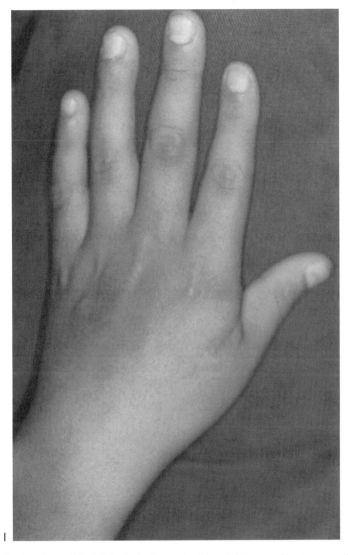

Figure 3. *(continued)* **I:** Clinical photograph of the left hand after two sessions of ethanol sclerotherapy demonstrates regression of the soft tissue mass. The patient still has an abduction contracture.

formation as well as the venous outflow. The venous outflow can be obstructed by application of tourniquets. Sclerosing agents including 100% ethanol, sodium tetradecyl, and Ethibloc can then be opacified and injected with fluoroscopic control.[19-22] The drug causes thrombosis with sclerosis the vessel walls, ultimately leading to fibrosis of the lesion. Unfortunately, recanalization occurs frequently, so sclerotherapy is usually performed more than once. The most frequent complications include skin necrosis (mainly in the presence of skin involvement with the malformation), and neuropathy (with ethanol). Ethanol has also been associated with acute cardiovascular complications in a small percentage of patients. This fact, plus the pain on injection, mandate the use of general anesthesia during ethanol sclerotherapy. Other sclerosants, such as sodium tetradecyl and Ethibloc can be injected under local anesthesia and sedation. An-

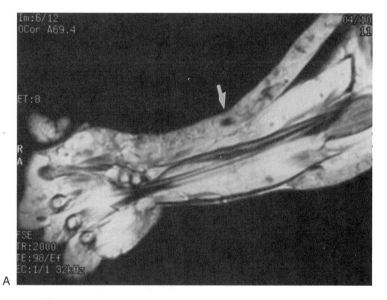

A

Figure 4. Diffuse venous malformation of the upper extremity in a 15-year-old boy with compressible soft tissue swelling of the entire upper extremity, worse on dependency and moderate hand and arm weakness. He also demonstrated a mild coagulopathy consistent with disseminated intravascular coagulation. This patient was managed with a compression glove, sleeve, and vest. A series of sclerotherapy sessions using ethanol and sodium tetradecyl reduced some of the soft tissue bulk and the weight of the extremity. **A:** T2–weighted MRI of the forearm and hand demonstrates involvement of all the tissue layers, including bone, with venous malformation (bright signal). Signal voids (arrow) represent phleboliths or thrombi. Note the remarkable deficiency of muscle mass accounting for the weakness. **B through E:** Direct injections of contrast medium into different portions of the venous malformation of the hand demonstrate large confluent venous phases (C), and dilated, dysplastic veins with areas of stenosis.

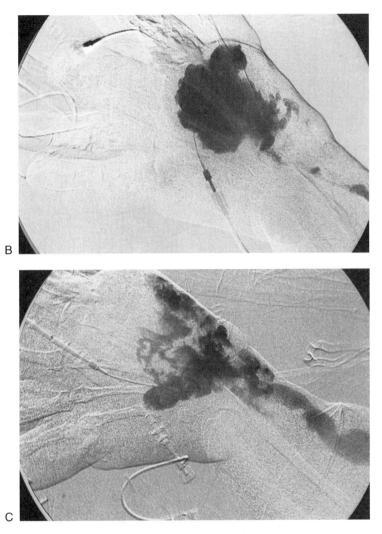

Figure 4. *(continued)*

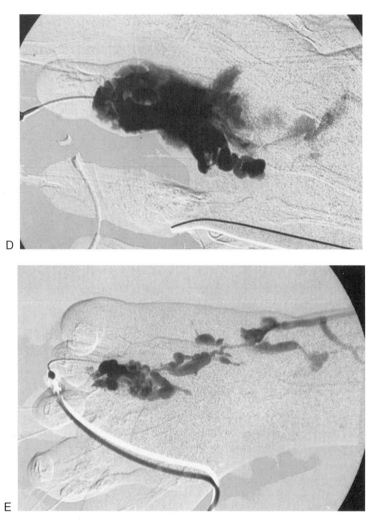

Figure 4. *(continued)*

other potential complication of treatment of intramuscular venous malformations, especially in the hand, is fibrosis.

Staged surgical resections or focal resection of intramuscular venous malformations is feasible, but is easier after sclerotherapy.[15,16]

Lymphatic Malformations

Lymphatic malformations represent abnormal collections of lymphatic channels or cysts that presumably result from obstruction of the developing fetal lymphatic system.[17] They are subdivided into microcystic forms, which tend to be seen peripherally, and macrocystic forms, the most extreme of which are seen centrally. Like venous malformations, these lesions can be focal or diffuse. The diffuse lesions involving the entire upper extremity often have massive macrocystic components in the axilla and upper thorax at birth. Lymphatic masses are often part of combined malformations, associated with capillary malformations of the skin (CLM), anomalous or malformed venous channels (LVM), or even focal high-flow lesions (LAVM).

Diagnosis

Lymphatic malformations appear as focal or diffuse enlargement of part or all of the upper extremity. The swelling is typically soft but nonpitting and not compressible. Overlying skin temperature and pulses are normal. The skin surface may appear normal, may be involved with a capillary malformation (port wine stain), and may demonstrate characteristic clear or black vesicles, which are part of the lymphatic malformation. These vesicles represent superficial extensions of the deeper lymphatic malformation and are often drain clear or blood-tinged fluid.

In general, lymphatic malformations grow proportionately with the child, although they characteristically demonstrate episodes of acute swelling, related to hemorrhage, obstruction or infection. Episodes of swelling are frequently associated with systemic illness such as viral infections. Infection, especially within diffuse lymphatic malformations, can result in septicemia. Hemorrhage into the macrocystic lymphatic malformations frequently results in a bluish discoloration of the skin.

Imaging

Imaging findings correlate with the size of the cystic or channel components of lymphatic malformations.[4] Ultrasound clearly shows the cystic components, with absence of vascular flow except for normal arterial flow in the septations (Figure 5). Microcystic forms may appear as amorphous echogenic areas of soft tissue thickening. No significant contrast enhancement is seen with CT and MRI (Figure 5). Due to their fluid content, they are generally diffusely of high-signal intensity on T2-weighted sequences;

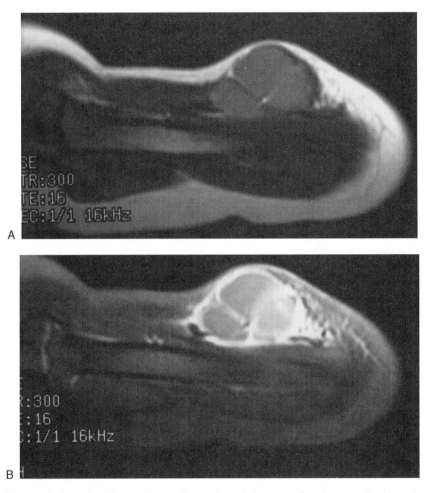

Figure 5. Localized lymphatic malformation of the arm. Sudden swelling in a 5-year-old girl. Bluish-color to the skin. **A:** Longitudinal T1-weighted MRI demonstates slightly hyperintense (due to the presence of blood) soft tissue mass. **B:** After gadolinium, the rim but not the contents of the mass are enhanced. **C:** Axial T2-weighted MRI demonstrates bright signal in the lower cyst. Upper cysts are darker because of blood. **D:** Gradient recalled echo image demonstrates no arterial flow in the lesion, and shows the proximity to the neurovascular structures. **E:** Direct contrast injection into the cystic lesion, digital subtraction technique, prior to sclerosis and injection.

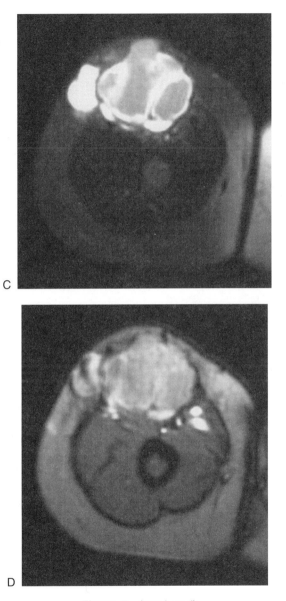

Figure 5. *(continued)*

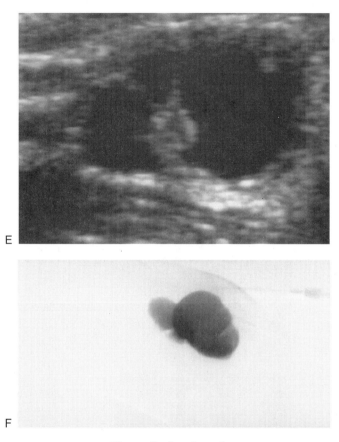

Figure 5. *(continued)*

macrocystic forms have clearly defined cysts or septations. Fluid-fluid levels and evidence of recent or old hemorrhage are frequent. Mixed lymphatic-venous malformations may demonstrate focal areas of enhancement or even phleboliths. Gradient recalled echo sequences typically demonstrate normal arterial channels. Adjacent veins are often dilated (Figure 5).

Treatment

Macrocystic lymphatic malformations, which typically involve the proximal upper extremity, axilla and chest wall, are generally treated by surgical resection.[15,16] Healing of the incisions may be slow due to fluid leakage. Likewise, localized lymphatic malformations of the fingers and hand are often managed by surgical resection. Diffuse lymphatic malformations are difficult to treat and are usually managed by tailored compression garments, pneumatic pumps, and in selected cases, surgical debulking.

Sclerosant injection is effective in treating focal macrocystic forms of lymphatic malformations. Sclerosants that have been used include doxycycline, bleomycin, sodium morrhuate, ethanol, Ethibloc, and OK432.[23,24] OK432 is a bacterial product, used predominantly in Japan, which produces a local inflammatory reaction followed by fibrosis. Ethibloc is a mixture of ethanol and amino acids derived from corn protein, which induces fibrosis through a foreign body reaction. Sodium morrhuate, ethanol, and doxycycline are sclerosants which damage the endothelial surface (and part of the wall in the case of ethanol). Ethibloc and OK432 are not approved for use in the United States.

Arteriovenous Malformations

An AVM is considered to be a developmental lesion consisting of an abnormal network of channels bypassing the capillary bed, and interposed between feeding arteries and draining veins.[9,13,15,16,25–28] Unlike the brain or lung, where AVM usually exhibits a discrete nidus, feeding arteries and draining veins, extremity lesions are generally diffuse, often including focal macroscopic AVF, in combination with much smaller communications between small arteries or arterioles and veins (Figures 6 and 7). AVM is assumed to be a congenital lesion; many are evident at birth with evidence of high flow, tissue overgrowth and overlying capillary malformation of the skin, while others are inapparent at birth and become symptomatic after injury, surgery or hormonal alteration, such as puberty or pregnancy. Patients with hereditary hemorrhagic telangiectasia characteristically develop telangiectasias and symptomatic AVMs over time. Two defects involving the endoglin gene have been identified in this condition; these defects result in defective endothelial cell function with resulting abnormal vascular structure.[9] Histologically, the telangiectasias and arteriovenous malformations lack capillaries; the venules are dilated with an excess of smooth muscle without elastic fibers. The exact factors that result in development or progression of symptoms in patients with AVM have not yet been identified. Unlike hemangiomas, histological examination of previously untreated AVM does not demonstrate evidence of endothelial cell proliferation. It is generally assumed that increase in size or extent of these lesions is related to dilatation of existing or potential arteriovenous shunts and the feeding and draining channels.

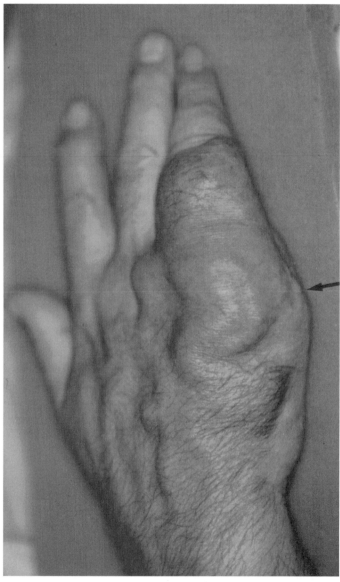

A

Figure 6. Fifty-year-old man with AVM of the right hand, who was relatively asymptomatic for many years after amputation of the fifth digit. He had progressive enlargement of the soft tissue mass and had recently developed a cutaneous ulcer (arrow) that did not heal. **A:** Clinical photograph demonstrated the amputation of the fifth digit, the soft tissue fullness of the fourth ray and prominent superficial veins.

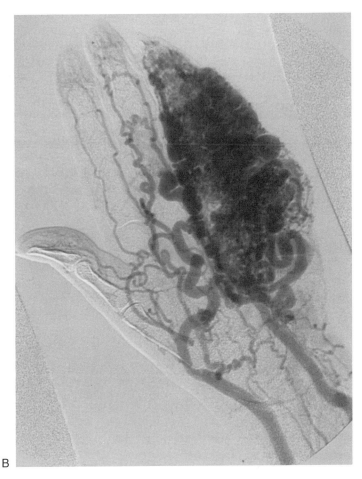

B

Figure 6. *(continued)* **B:** Brachial arteriogram prior to embolization, arterial phase demonstrates a diffuse AVM of the fourth and fifth rays with marked tortuosity of the third and fourth metacarpal and digital arteries.

Diagnosis

Like the other vascular malformations, AVM can be localized or diffuse. The overlying skin may be normal or have a capillary stain or blush and is generally hot to touch. Pulsations or thrill may be palpable in the highest flow lesions. The high-flow nature of an AVM can be easily confirmed by the application of a Doppler probe that demonstrates increased volume of the feeding arterial signal and, over the shunt itself, a continuous or to and fro sound. Arterial pulses above the malformation are in-

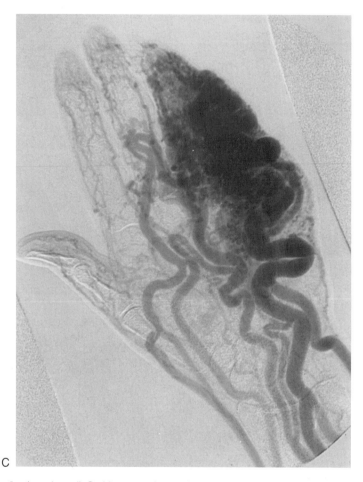

C

Figure 6. *(continued)* **C:** Venous phase demonstrating the AVM nidus and the dilated draining veins.

creased in comparison with the normal side and the superficial veins may be prominent. A positive Nicoladoni sign (slowing of the heart rate with application of a tourniquet) may be seen with extremely high-flow diffuse lesions. Hyperhydrosis and focal or diffuse enlargement of the extremity may occur.

Imaging

Helpful imaging studies include ultrasound with Doppler interrogation and MRI. Ultrasound confirms the high-flow character of the lesion; in particular, spectral analysis demonstrates high-velocity, low-resistance

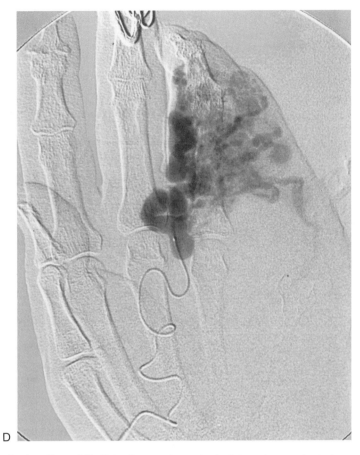

Figure 6. *(continued)* **D:** Selective angiography in the metacarpal arteries supplying the middle and ring fingers with a microcatheter demonstrates the marked tortuosity of the digital arteries. These vessels were embolized using polyvinyl alcohol foam particles and then sodium tetradecyl was injected interstitially in the soft tissue mass. Brachial arteriogram, arterial phase, following particle embolization demonstrates occlusion of arterial branches feeding the AVM.

feeding arteries, and often shows arterialization or turbulence of the venous waveform. MRI findings are variable, but typically include dilated feeding and draining vessels and thickening of the affected soft tissue planes (Figure 7).[2,4,5] Gradient recalled echo sequences that demonstrate high-flow vessels are excellent for assessment of the tissue extent. Magnetic resonance angiography is also useful for confirming the high-flow nature of the lesion and indicating which arteries are enlarged and therefore most likely supply the lesion.[7] Although AVM typically consists only of masses of enlarged vascular channels, associated edema or enhancement of tiny vessels may produce the appearance of a focal mass, includ-

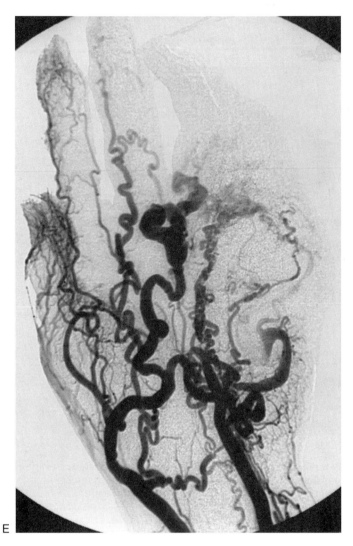

E

Figure 6. *(continued)* **E:** Venous phase demonstrating AVM nidus and the dilated draining veins.

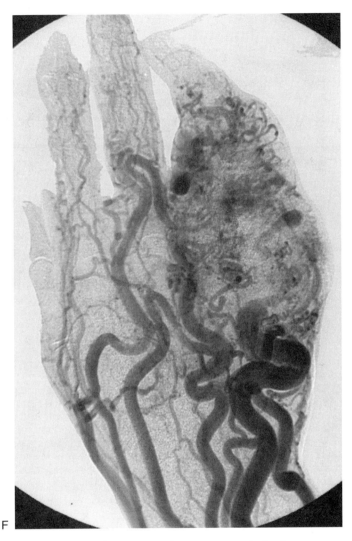

Figure 6. *(continued)* **F:** Brachial arteriogram postembolization, venous phase demonstrates perfusion of the distal ring finger, and markedly reduced flow in the AVM.

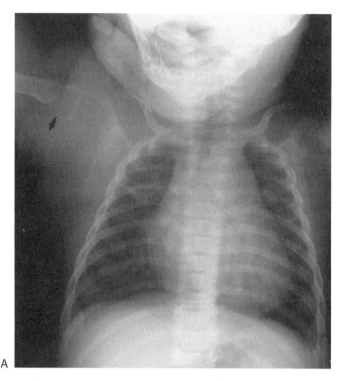

A

Figure 7. Diffuse AVM of the upper extremity (Parkes-Weber syndrome) in an infant with mild congestive heart failure and poor function of the arm. **A:** Chest radiograph demonstrates cardiomegaly, soft tissue enlargement, and defects in the right humerus. **B:** T1-weighted MRI shows extensive large flow voids, but no soft tissue mass. **C:** Magnetic resonance angiography showing the massively dilated vessels. **D:** Right brachial arteriogram shows discrete arteriovenous shunts into varicosities at the proximal arm and wrist, with diffuse vascular blush throughout the extremity. **E:** Venous phase, showing soft tissue blush and dilated draining veins.

ing increased signal on T2-weighted sequences and contrast enhancement, making differentiation from a hemangioma or sarcoma difficult. The clinical history and physical findings are usually sufficient to rule out av-neoplasm, but in some instances, diagnostic angiography or biopsy is necessary.

The characteristic angiographic finding in an AVM is the presence of arteriovenous shunting that results in early opacification of the draining veins.[29] The "nidus" may be discrete or diffuse and may consist of macroscopic AVF or multiple small channels. Feeding arteries frequently become tortuous and may develop aneurysms, especially in the hand.

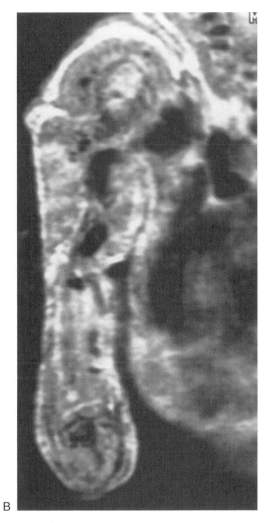

Figure 7. *(continued)*

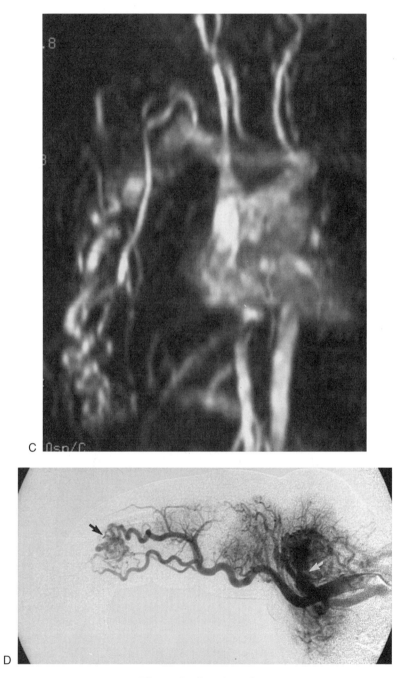

Figure 7. *(continued)*

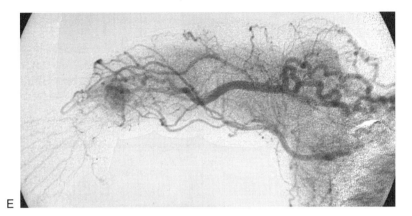

E

Figure 7. *(continued)*

Prognosis

In the series reported by Coombs et al,[8] 40% of AVMs were noted at birth and 34% presented after 10 years of age. Fifty percent of affected females had progression with puberty and 81% demonstrated worsening in response to hormonal change including puberty, birth control pill, and pregnancy. None of the male patients with upper extremity AVMs demonstrated progression of symptoms at the time of puberty. The prognosis of upper extremity AVM is variable, depending on the extent and number of feeding vessels. Those with a limited number of shunts and supply by only one vessel tend to remain relatively localized while diffuse lesions slowly enlarge, typically recruiting vessels in adjacent areas with gradually increasing thrill, worsening pain, and eventual vascular steal with distal ischemic pain and ulceration.[16,25,26] Diffuse extremity AVM frequently requires amputation to control pain.

Treatment

Treatment of AVMs of the upper extremity remains difficult. Surgical excision has a high reported incidence of recurrence or tissue loss, with the poorest results in diffuse lesions and those involving bone.[26] Asymptomatic AVMs are best managed conservatively with the use of tailored compression garments, especially during the periods of activity. Diffuse AVMs may present in the neonatal period with congestive cardiac failure (Figure 7). Superselective embolization of the macrofistulous components of the malformation, using permanent embolic material, may alleviate the cardiac overload.[14] Likewise, superselective embolization may be useful in treating surgically inaccessible symptomatic lesions.[14,25,27,28,30] Proximal embolization or ligation of feeding arteries is to be avoided at all costs. These procedures initially appear to reduce the arterial flow, but ultimately lead to increased distal tissue ischemia due to recruitment of collateral vessels by the AVM, and make subsequent treatment by embolization technically more difficult or impossible. Likewise, nonselective embolization of proximal feeding vessels such as the radial or ulnar artery is to condemned, as it will predictably result in distal tissue ischemia and loss. Unfortunately, diffuse AVMs of the hand and fingers are typically supplied by many tiny branches of the digital arteries, making cure by embolization extremely difficult or impossible. Recently, superselective embolization of arterial feeders, and direct injection of the nidus or draining vein using absolute ethanol, has been reported to result in cure of extensive AVM.[28] Ethanol is an extremely aggressive embolic agent and results in a significant rate of skin ulceration and neuropathy. Also, while it is very effective in macrofistulous AVM and in those with drainage into one or a small number of veins, it cannot be used in the "small vessel" AVM, due to the risk of tissue damage.

Congenital Arteriovenous Fistulae

Congenital AVF consists of a single communication between an artery and a vein. These most commonly occur in the head and neck area. Unlike AVM, the single hole AVF can be cured by ligation or by placement of an appropriate permanent embolic device across the fistula site (Figure 8).[20]

Acquired AVF, consisting of a single communication between artery and vein, may result from iatrogenic trauma, usually in the form of needle puncture (eg, venipuncture or arterial blood gas sampling).[31] The clinical findings may be similar to those in AVM. However, the localization over the antecubital fossa (Figure 8) or wrist, and the history of previous hospitalization may help in the diagnosis. Like congenital AVF, these lesions can be cured by embolization techniques or surgical ligation.

Acquired AVF may also result from penetrating trauma or surgical procedures. Chronic AVF may similate a diffuse AVM.[32] These lesions are much more difficult to manage than simple AVF and may require repeated embolization procedures.

Mixed Vascular Malformation Syndromes

The following are some of the combined vascular malformations that affect the upper extremities.[17]

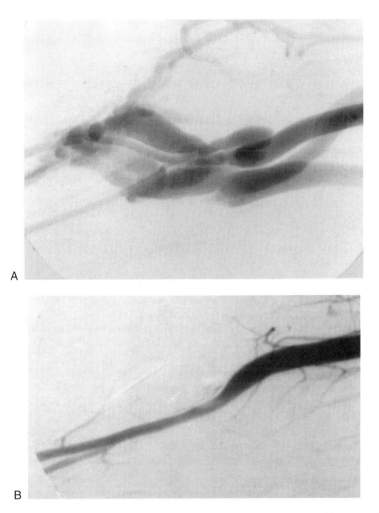

Figure 8. Antecubital arteriovenous fistula in a 7-year-old boy, possibly secondary to venipunctures during infancy. The child presented with a pulsatile mass, thrill, and bruit. **A:** Brachial arteriogram demonstrates dilatation of the brachial artery, and opacification of multiple dilated antecubital veins. **B:** Brachial arteriogram post-embolization of the vein immediately distal to the fistula with a small amount of tissue adhesive demonstrates occlusion of the fistula. Clinical follow-up demonstrated no evidence of recurrence of the shunt.

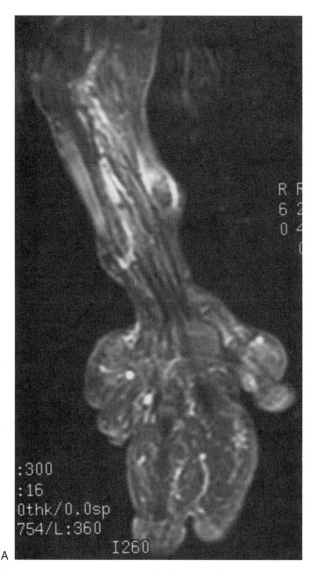

A

Figure 9. Klippel Trenaunay syndrome. This unfortunate youngster had involvement of both lower extremities and the right upper extremity with combined capillary lymphaticovenous malformation. **A:** T1–weighted MRI without contrast medium demonstrates soft tissue swelling, predominantly isointense to muscle. The high-signal areas represent fat.

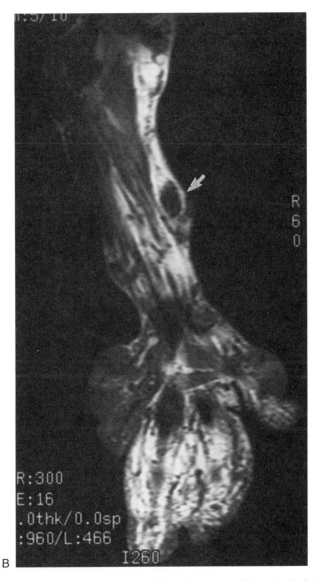

Figure 9. *(continued)* **B:** T1-weighted MRI of the arm and hand with fat suppression, after intravenous gadolinium administration demonstrates enhancement of the areas of soft tissue fullness of the second and third digits and some of the subcutaneous tissues of the forearm. The large area of absent enhancement (arrow) represents a thrombus, while the enhancing tissue is venous malformation.

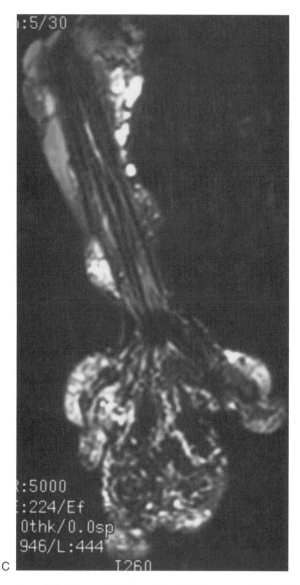

Figure 9. *(continued)* **C:** A heavily T2-weighted MRI demonstrates the lymphatic component of the malformation, which corresponds with the areas that did not enhance with contrast administration in Figure 7C. Note the discrete lymphatic cysts in the forearm (arrows).

Klippel Trenaunay Syndrome (CLVM)

Klippel Trenaunay syndrome (KTS) is a low-flow diffuse vascular and mesodermal malformation of the extremity. KTS usually affects the lower extremity, but the upper extremity is involved in 5% of patients. Components include capillary malformation (port wine stain) of the skin, lymphatic malformation, and venous malformation, usually consisting of anomalies and varicosities of the major conducting veins (Figures 9 and 10).[6,22,23,33]

Parkes Weber Syndrome

Parkes Weber Syndrome (CAVM) is a high-flow vascular malformation involving the entire extremity with overlying capillary malformation of the skin (Figure 7). Problems include congestive heart failure, tissue ischemia, and overgrowth.

Maffucci's Syndrome

Maffucci's syndrome (CVM plus dyschondroplasia) is a familial condition with capillary malformation of the skin, multiple venous malformations, and dyschondroplasia similar to Ollier's syndrome.

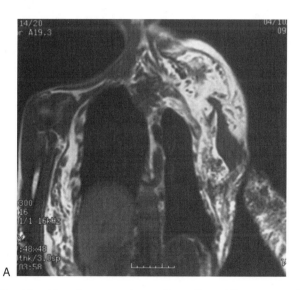

Figure 10. Combined low-flow vascular malformation of the upper extremity and thorax with predominant fatty content (CVVM). **A**: T1-weighted coronal MRI of the thorax demonstrates extensive soft tissue abnormalities, consisting of a combination of fat (increased T1 signal) and nodular areas of low signal. Note the deformity of the left hemithorax.

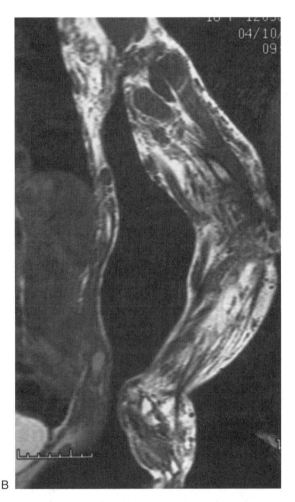

B

Figure 10. *(continued)* **B**. T1-weighted MRI of the upper extremity demonstrates an increase in fat and low-signal nodular abnormality. Contrast administration demonstrated minimal contrast enhancement.

Blue Rubber Bleb Nevus Syndrome

Blue Rubber Bleb Nevus syndrome (VM) is familial multiple progressive venous malformations, often involving the bowel. The most serious symptom is gastrointestinal bleeding and anemia, but upper extremity lesions can be symptomatic.

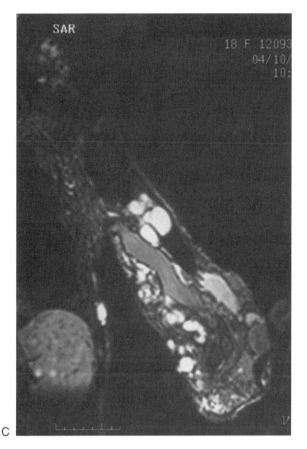

C

Figure 10. *(continued)* **C**. Heavily T2-weighted MRI of the left arm demonstrates macrocystic and microcystic lymphatic components, and a markedly dilated venous channel (V). Note, abnormal signal within the spleen.

Proteus Syndrome

Proteus syndrome (CVM plus) includes partial gigantism of the hands and/or feet, hemihypertrophy, macrocephaly, and/or other skull anomalies and nodular subcutaneous vascular (usually venous) malformations.

Bannayan Syndrome

Bannayan syndrome (LVM plus) includes macrocephaly plus multiple subcutaneous lipomas, venous malformations, and lymphedema.

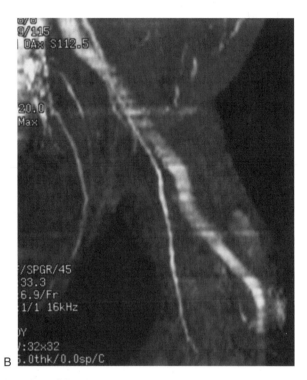

Figure 10. *(continued)* **D**. Magnetic resonance venogram of the left arm demonstrates the marked dilatation of the basilic and brachial veins.

References

1. Mulliken JB, Glowacki J: Hemangiomas and vascular malformations in infants and children: A classification based on endothelial characteristics. *Plast Reconstr Surg* 69:412–420, 1982.
2. Cohen JM, Weinreb JC, Redman HC: Arteriovenous malformations of the extremities: MR imaging. *Radiology* 158:475–479, 1996.
3. Burrows P, Robertson R, Barnes P: Angiography and the evaluation of cerebrovascular diseases of childhood. *Neuroimaging Clin North Am* 6:561–588, 1996.
4. Meyer JS, Hoffer FA, Barnes PD, Mulliken JB: Biological classification of soft-tissue vascular anomalies: MR correlation. *AJR* 157:559–564, 1991.
5. Rak KM, Yakes WF, Ray RL, et al: MR imaging of symptomatic peripheral vascular malformations. *AJR* 159:107–112, 1992.
6. Laor T, Burrows PE, Hoffer FA: Magnetic resonance venography of congenital vascular malformations of the extremities. *Pediatr Radiol* 26:371–380, 1996.
7. Disa JJ, Chung KC, Gellad FE, et al: Efficacy of magnetic resonance angiography in the evaluation of vascular malformations of the hand. *Plast Reconstr Surg* 99:136–147, 1997.

8. Coombs C, Upton J, Mulliken J: Vascular malformations of the upper limb: A review of 209 patients. *J Hand Surg*

9. Guttmacher AE, Marchuk DA, White JRI; Hereditary hemorrhagic telangiectasia. *N Engl J Med* 333:918–924, 1995.

10. Boon LM, Mulliken JM, Vikkula M, et al: Assignment of a locus for dominantly inherited venous malformations to chromosome 9p. *Hum Mol Genet* 3: 1583–1587, 1994.

11. Vikkula M, Boon LM, Carraway KL III, et al: Vascular dysmorphogenesis caused by an activating mutation in the receptor tyrosine kinase TIE2. *Cell* 87: 1181–1190, 1996.

12. De Takat G: Vascular anomalies of the extremities. *Surg Gynecol Obstet* 55: 227–237, 1932.

13. Malan E, Puglionisi A: Congenital angiodysplasias of the extremities. *J Cardiovasc Surg* 6:255–345, 1965.

14. Zuker RM, Burrows PE: Vascular problems in the hand. In: Marsh JL, ed. *Current Therapy in Plastic and Reconstructive Surgery.* Toronto: B.C. Decker; 1989, pp. 154–163.

15. Upton J, Coombs C: Vascular tumors in children. *Hand Clin* 11:307–335, 1995.

16. Upton J. Vascular malformations of the upper limb. In: Mulliken JB, Young AE, eds. *Vascular Birthmarks: Hemangiomas and Malformations.* Philadelphia: WB Saunders; 1988, pp. 343–380.

17. Mulliken J, Young A: *Vascular Birthmarks. Hemangiomas and Vascular Malformations.* Philadelphia: W.B. Saunders; 1988.

18. Burrows PE, Mulliken JB, Fellows KE, Strand RD: Childhood hemangiomas and vascular malformations: Angiographic differentiation. *AJR* 141:483–488, 1983.

19. Yakes WF: Extremity venous malformations: Diagnosis and management. *Semin Intervent Radiol* 11:332–339, 1994.

20. Burrows PE, Fellows KE: Techniques for management of pediatric vascular anomalies. In: Cope C, ed. *Current Techniques in Interventional Radiology.* Philadelphia: Current Medicine; 1995, pp. 12–27.

21. Dubois JM, Sebag GH, De Prost Y, et al: Soft-tissue venous malformations in children: Percutaneous sclerotherapy with Ethibloc. *Radiology* 180:195–198, 1991.

22. deLorimier AA: Sclerotherapy for venous malformations. *J Pediatr Surg* 30: 188–194, 1995.

23. Molitch HI, Unger EC, Witte CL, vanSonnenberg E: Percutaneous sclerotherapy of lymphangiomas. *Radiology* 194:343–347, 1995.

24. Ogita S, Tsuto T, Tokiwa K, Takahashi T: Intracystic injection of OK432: A new sclerosing therapy for cystic hygroma in children. *Br J Surg* 74:690–691, 1987.

25. Dickey KW, Pollak JS, Meier GH III, et al: Management of large high-flow arteriovenous malformations of the shoulder and upper extremity with transcatheter embolotherapy. *J Vasc Intervent Radiol* 6:765–773, 1995.

26. Gelberman RH, Goldner JL: Congenital arteriovenous fistulas of the hand. *J Hand Surg* 3:451–454, 1978.

27. Widlus DM, Murray RR, White RI Jr, et al: Congenital arteriovenous malformations: Tailored embolotherapy. *Radiology* 169:511–516, 1988.

28. Yakes WF, Rossi P, Odink H: Arteriovenous malformation management. *Cardiovasc Intervent Radiol* 19:65–71, 1996.
29. Bliznak J, Staple TW: Radiology of angiodysplasias of the limb. *Radiology* 110: 35–44, 1974.
30. Gomes AS: Embolization therapy of congenital arteriovenous malformations: Use of alternate approaches. *Radiology* 190:191–198, 1994.
31. Upton J, Sampson C, Havlik R, et al: Acquired arteriovenous fistulas in children. *J Hand Surg* 19:656–658, 1994.
32. Yakes WF, Luethke JM, Merland JJ, et al: Ethanol embolization of arteriovenous fistulas: A primary mode of therapy. *J Vasc Intervent Radiol* 1:89–96, 1990.
33. Gloviczki P, Stanson AW, Stockler GB, et al: Klippel-Trenaunay syndrome: The risks and benefits of vascular interventions. *Surgery* 110:469–479, 1991.

16

Complications of Vascular Access in the Upper Extremity

Ledford L. Powell, MD and Samuel E. Wilson, MD

General and vascular surgeons play a significant role in establishing vascular access for long-term hemodialysis patients, chemotherapy and parenteral nutrition patients. The most common indication for permanent vascular access is hemodialysis and the number of end-stage renal disease patients that require access for hemodialysis continues to grow. As a result, operations for the placement of grafts and other access devices have become the most commonly performed operation of the upper extremity. Surgeons must be able to not only perform these operations but recognize and treat their complications. Accordingly we have outlined the standard vascular access procedures and provided the treatment strategies for their complications.

Securing a site for repeated vascular access first became important in 1943 when Kolff and Berk[1] introduced extracorporeal hemodialysis. In early clinical trials, cutdowns on an artery and a vein with subsequent ligation were necessary for each hemodialysis. Reliable vascular access was only achieved when Quinton et al[2] Schribner and Dillard introduced the external teflon silastic catheter in 1960. Infection, thrombosis, and hemorrhage were not uncommon with usage of these percutaneous catheters. In 1966, Brescia and associates[3] published their results with the new radial artery to cephalic vein fistula constructed in the forearm. The later development of grafts using saphenous vein, human umbilical vein, bovine carotid artery, Dacron grafts, and polytetrafluoroethylene (PTFE) grafts have made high-flow long-term vascular access available to patients who do not have suitable vessels for autogenous fistulas.

From Machleder HI, (ed): *Vascular Disorders of the Upper Extremity*. Third Revised Edition. Futura Publishing Company, Inc., Armonk, NY, © 1998.

The importance of maintaining long-term vascular access becomes evident when we consider that more than 30% of hospital admissions for chronic hemodialysis patients are for vascular access complications.[4] Recognition, prevention, and management of these complications will improve the overall survival rate of hemodialysis patients.

Upper Extremity Access Sites

Vascular access sites in the upper extremity can be constructed in various ways depending on the location, size, and patency of the patient's vessels. Primary autogenous fistulas, having a superior patency rate and lower complication rate should be given initial consideration. The objective in long-term hemodialysis patients is to achieve vascular access that allows high-flow (approximately 300 mL/min) hemodialysis rates. The sites for potential placement are listed in Table 1. When selecting sites for hemodialysis, generally the most distal vessels are used initially, saving the more proximal vessels for future use. In practice, the arteriovenous fistula is established in the nondominant hand. The side of the artery-to-side vein configuration was described first; however, some surgeons advocate an end vein-side artery anastomosis because of the potential for distal venous hypertension or high-flow complications.[3] The end artery-to-end vein anastomosis has also been used (Figure 1).

If the distal vein has been used for previous shunts or is unavailable because of sclerosis of the cephalic vein from intravenous infusion, severe peripheral vascular disease, or if the veins are of inadequate diameter, one must proceed to more proximal vessels. The next choice is either an antecubital fistula from the brachial artery to the cephalic or basilic vein, or to use synthetic graft material, primarily PTFE. Options for grafts include a distal straight graft from the radial artery to the antecubital vein (Figure 2), a loop graft from the brachial artery to the antecubital vein

---

Table 1
Upper Extremity Sites for Permanent Vascular Access

1. Radiocephalic (Brescia-Cimino) autogenous fistula
2. Brachiocephalic or brachiobasilic autogenous fistula
3. Radial artery to antecubital vein straight graft
4. Brachial artery to antecubital vein loop graft
5. Brachial artery to axillary vein curved graft
6. Axillary artery to vein loop graft
7. Brachial artery to subclavian vein curved graft
8. Subclavian artery to subclavian vein loop or curved graft

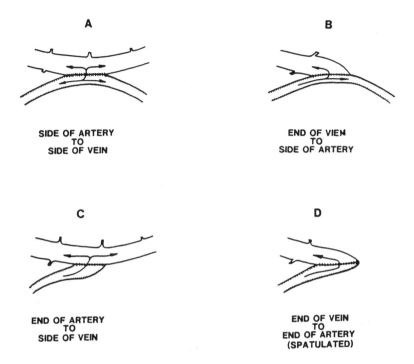

Figure 1: The various configurations of an autologous radiocephalic fistula.

(Figure 3), or an upper arm straight graft from the brachial artery to the more proximal axillary or basilic vein (Figure 4).

The natural history of vascular access is that of eventual failure; each construction has a variable but limited life span. The challenge is to provide access with the highest long-term patency and the least complications. Despite significant technical advances complications remain to be a persistent problem. Thrombosis and infection are the two most common complications leading to graft failure. Hemodynamic complications (steal syndrome, increased cardiac output and venous hypertension) and neurological complications occur less frequently. Although not a cause of graft failure, disabling neurovascular problems may develop making revision or excision of the conduit unavoidable. Prompt recognition and treatment of vascular access complications is an essential component in decreasing overall morbidity of chronic renal failure patients.

Thrombosis

Thrombosis is the most common complication of arteriovenous fistulas and grafts. In a retrospective study by Nakagawa et al[5] thrombosis accounted for approximately 78% of all complications of arteriovenous fistulas and grafts. The patency rate of the autogenous fistula is noted to be superior to that of the prosthetic graft.[5] Decreased fistula flow leading to thrombosis is the most frequent reason for graft failure, and is caused by inadequate arterial inflow or venous outflow obstruction. The etiologies of graft thrombosis may be considered as those causing early (0 to 3 months) or late (> 3 months) thrombosis. Early thrombosis is most commonly due to a technical error such as a choice of a poor vein or narrowing of the lumen of the artery or vein during the anastomosis. Occasionally failure to properly anticoagulate intraoperatively may cause clotting inside of

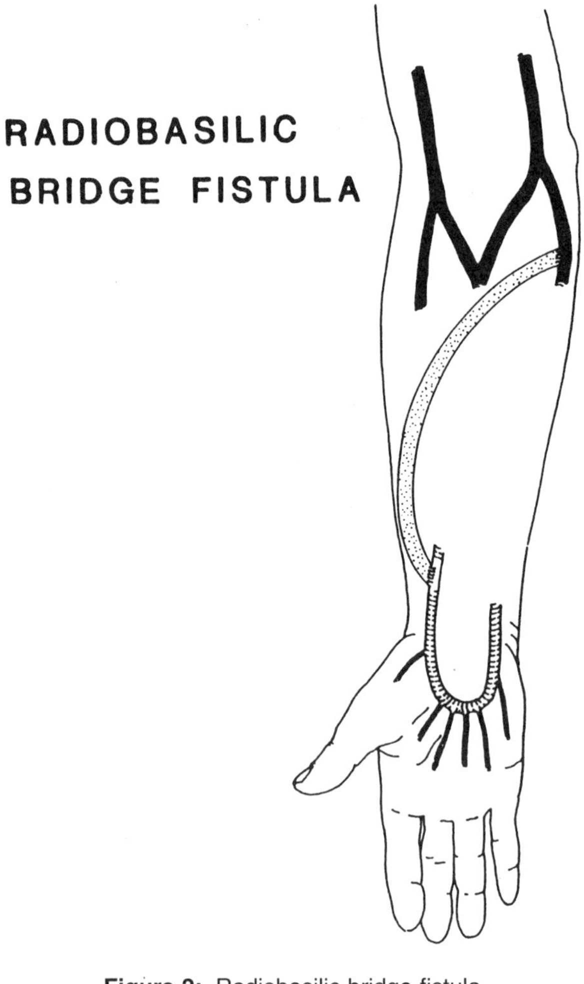

RADIOBASILIC BRIDGE FISTULA

Figure 2: Radiobasilic bridge fistula.

BRACHIOBASILIC LOOP FISTULA

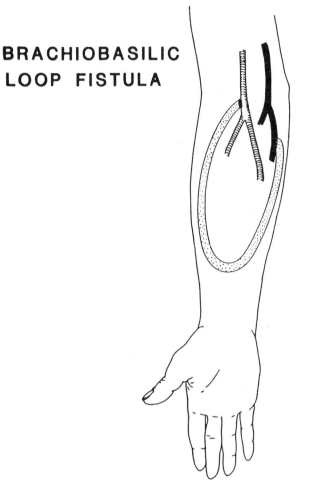

Figure 3: Brachiobasilic loop fistula.

the shunt. Thrombosis can also result from external compression for hemostasis, hypotension, dehydration, or early puncture of an inmature vein. It has been conceived that spasm of the artery after the operative manipulation leads to early thrombosis. Two prospective randomized trials using vasodilators such as PGE1 and nicardipine infusions have shown that without the use of these vasodilators there is a decrease in the anastomotic blood flow for as long as 20 minutes after the anastomosis is completed. This conceivably increases the early thrombosis rate. These studies have noted increased arterial inflow using these vasodilators but

BRACHIOAXILLARY FISTULA

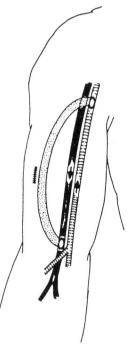

Figure 4: Brachioaxillary fistula.

have not changed the patency rate when compared to grafts constructed without the vasodilators.[6,7]

Late thrombosis can be due to hypotension, dehydration, compression, or trauma. However, it is more commonly due to an acquired stenosis of the runoff vein, attributed to mechanical endothelial damage from the shearing effect of the high pressure or the pulsatile arterial blood flow in the venous system.[4] In autogenous fistulas, the usual site of fibrosis is several centimeters proximal to the anastomosis on the venous side and is secondary to repeated trauma of needle puncture.[8] With grafts, the stenosis and subsequent thrombosis is usually at the site of the graft to vein anastomosis. A long stenosis inside of the graft may be due to chronic fibrin and cellular deposits.[9]

Thrombosis has an incidence of approximately 14% to 36%[10]; stenosis has an incidence of 34% to 63%[11]; subsequently, it has multiple modalities for diagnosis and treatment. Angiography confirms that most late occlusions are due to outflow abnormalities of the vein. Glanz et al.[9] reviewed 800 grafts and fistulas needing revision over a 2-year period. Of interest, 70% of the failures were due to outflow obstructions, 10% to inflow and 15% had combined lesions. Of the 70% with outflow obstruction, 21% of the lesions were proximal to the venous anastomosis, either at sites of compression or hypertrophied valves. Possible compression sites include the cephalic vein at the elbow, the axillary vein near the chest wall muscles with the arm adducted, or the subclavian vein as it crosses the ribs. Obstructing valves were found at the lower border of the subscapularis and in the subclavian vein, 2 to 3 cm proximal to the internal jugular junction.

The incidence of thrombosis may be estimated in terms of patency rates at different time intervals; immediate, 1, 2, and 3 years. Patency rates vary considerably from institution to institution and depends on the type and site of the fistula. The cumulative 3-year patency data collected from published results for the various access devices is shown in Figure 5. In general, autogenous fistulas have a higher early failure rate, ranging from 10% to 25%, while PTFE grafts average an initial 5% failure rate.[12–15] The superiority of the autogenous fistula to that of the prosthetic graft lies in the long-term patency rate with divergence in the outcome becoming statistically significant at 30 months.[13] Long-term data show the longest life expectancy for a PTFE graft at about 7 years while over 50% of autogenous fistulas are still patent at this time interval. Forearm grafts are generally preferred before establishing upper arm access. Most upper arm access grafts are placed after failure of forearm grafts. Dagher[16] quotes a

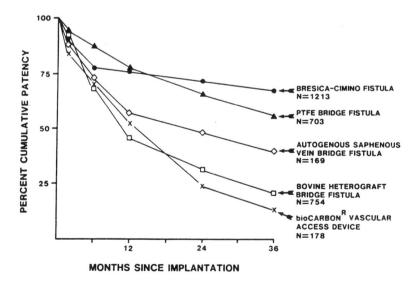

Figure 5: Patency rates for various types of vascular access.

surprising 70%, 8-year patency rate for the brachial artery-basilic vein PTFE fistula; however, the 50%, 3-year patency rate quoted by Dunlop et al[17] is more the norm. The patency rate for the radial to cephalic vein fistulas is quoted at 70% to 90%.[6,7]

Management options for the thrombosed graft include revising the graft via thrombectomy and/or patch angioplasty or thrombectomy and graft extension to an acceptable runoff vein. Alternatively, one can replace the entire graft. Given the limited number of access sites, local revision should be attempted whenever possible. Success rates for the various procedures vary greatly. In general, thrombectomy alone can be very successful for spontaneous thrombosis with no underlying anatomic abnormality as in hypotension or accidental compression. Palder and Kirkman[15] have an 87% success rate with revision of PTFE grafts. Patch angioplasty or a jump graft would be needed for outflow obstructions. Proximal lesions will require replacement of the graft. Approximately 40% of thrombosed grafts are not salvageable and must be reconstructed.[4] Thrombectomy and angioplasty is a commonly used procedure, the argument being that it works well for discrete lesions and saves proximal vessels for later revision. Thrombectomy and extension graft to a more proximal vein has the highest success rate by bypassing the outflow obstruction.[9,15] Interventional radiologists have introduced angioplasty with and without thrombolytics as a low-morbidity outpatient treatment for graft thrombosis. The 2-year patency rate of 24% does not compare with that of a revised graft. However, in recent studies, tissue plasminogen activator (TPA) has been shown to be successful in clot lysis in as high as 71% of thrombosed grafts.[10]

Prevention of both early and late thrombosis can be quite challenging. The judgment and technical error that contributes to early failure should be avoided with good preoperative and intraoperative evaluation of the patient. The superficial vein should be assessed preoperatively with and without a tourniquet for adequate flow. Inflow should be tested by palpating a strong pulse or measuring pressures in the brachial, radial, and ulnar arteries with the Doppler flow detector. Intraoperatively, it is imperative to use a precise, gentle technique to avoid vessel trauma and to check for high flow and an associated venous thrill before closure. Presence of low flow or a pulsatile vein flow indicates proximal stenosis and a poor prognosis.

Postoperatively, one must avoid hypotension, compressive dressings, blood pressure cuffs, intravenous cannulas, and phlebotomy in the graft arm. Caution is needed in patients with a maturing fistula undergoing unrelated operative procedures because the thrombosis rate has been reported to be as high as 22%.[18] The majority of late thrombosis are preceded by several weeks of difficulty with dialysis, such as high venous resistance, poor arterial inflow, or decreased thrill. When this occurs, a fistulogram needs to be obtained immediately.

Infection

Graft infection, the second most common graft complication after thrombosis, complicates 5% to 10% of vascular access procedures.[15] The decreased incidence of infection in upper extremity compared to lower extremity grafts is the major reason for preferring construction of upper extremity fistulas. Infection in general is second only to cardiovascular disease as a cause of serious morbidity and mortality in chronic renal failure patients.[19] Vascular access predominates as a source of infection.[20] The etiology of graft infections may be an extension of a superficial wound infection, or secondary infection of the graft or fistula with exogenous contamination during puncture, or bacteremic seeding.

Patients with chronic renal failure are thought to be at a higher risk for infection than the general population. Decreased immune response caused by granulocyte dysfunction and lymphopenia, altered skin and mucosal barriers, and increased colonization of patients and hemodialysis personnel with *Staphylococcus aureus* have all been implicated. Secondary infections can result from a break in sterile technique during needle insertion for hemodialysis or occasionally because of intravenous drug abuse. Brescia-Cimino fistulas have the lowest rate of infection, ranging from less than 1% to 3.5%, and forearm PTFE grafts have a 10% to 15% incidence.[12,13,21,22] Upper arm grafts tend to have a slightly higher infection rate than the autogenous fistula (2.5% to 6%).[16,17,23] Unless related to a postoperative complication, infections are discovered an average of 7 to 10 months after implantation.[13,15]

Taylor et al[24] described a 5% puncture infection rate of the arteriovenous fistula with no difference between home versus center directed dialysis. It was noted that the rate on puncture infections more than doubled after one puncture wound infection. The infection rate increased to 12% per year. Puncture infection rates were reported at 42% at 10 years for first infections while second puncture infection escalated to 40% at 4 years. Autogenous puncture infections were noted to be 0.02% over 10 years. The autogenous fistula group was much smaller and thus limits the application of these data, but the important fact is that the overall infection rate in the autogenous fistula group is much lower than that in the graft group. Taylor et al[24] also studied wound infections of grafts, unrelated to puncture wounds, as having an incidence of 3% per year. The incidence of these types of wound infections increased significantly in the population of patients that developed post-graft placement bleeds. The wound infection rate with autogenous grafts was low at 0.4%.

Prevention of infection requires strict adherence to sterile technique, both at the time of implantation and with each episode of hemodialysis whenever possible. The use of autogenous fistulas instead of grafts reduce the incidence of infection. Waiting for an adequate neointimal lining and subcutaneous incorporation prior to using a PTFE graft may help to decrease the local infection rate.[25] An antistaphylococcal agent is generally given in the preoperative period. Wound infections have been found to culture *Staphylococcal aureus* in greater than 70% of cases and *S. epidermidis* in 10% of cases.[24]

The management of the infected autogenous fistula requires ligation and excision of the involved segment. The infected wound should be left open and packed. It is occasionally possible to reconstruct the fistula proximally, utilizing the same vessel, through a clean incision. A graft that is infected in its entirety must be excised, as must any graft causing local hemorrhage, false aneurysm formation, or systemic sepsis. Localized cannulation site infections may be partially excised with flow restored by a bridge graft placed through a clean incision and routed through a new subcutaneous tunnel. Local debridement and other salvage risks run a higher risk for recurrent infection. The rate of total graft excision varies from 33% to 90%.[12,13,15] The overall graft salvage rate for wound infections has been reported at 60%. The highest success rate is with graft erosion and puncture wound infections (77% to 90%). Much lower rates of successful salvage procedures have been reported with grafts associated with an abscess. Graft salvage procedures should not be attempted when the entire tunnel is involved with one or many abscesses.

Steal Syndrome

Peripheral ischemia, secondary to the steal syndrome, is the most common symptom of local hemodynamic change produced by an upper extremity arteriovenous fistula. Vascular steal syndromes have been reported to have occurred in 8% of patients with autogenous antecubital fistulas compared to 1% of radiocephalic fistulas and 1.8% of PTFE bridge fistulas.[26] Amputations of the forearm have been reported in severe case of gangrene. Clinically steal syndrome is manifested by coldness, pain paresthesias, and weakness. The symptoms may be initially present only with exercise of the extremity or during dialysis, but may progress to rest pain in more severe cases. The diagnosis is not always clear because the symptoms may mimic the neuropathy of uremia and diabetes mellitus or the symptoms of obliterative arterial disease sometimes seen in patients with chronic renal failure.

Physiologically, the ischemia is due to retrograde flow from the ulnar artery through the palmar arches into the distal radial artery and into the venous system via the low resistance fistula or graft. The diagnosis can be made by the typical symptomatology and by directed flow studies, documenting retrograde flow and decreased blood pressures in the digits that increase with occlusion of the distal artery or fistula. A vascular steal occurs when an arteriovenous anastomosis is constructed with a side artery configuration. It is more pronounced with the high flow and large anastomosis of the brachial artery fistulas and grafts. Retrograde flow has been shown to occur quite commonly without symptoms. Haimov[26] measured fistula flow and convincingly demonstrated the presence and quantity of retrograde flow in patients at the time of operation. Brescia-Cimino fistulas had an average flow of 283 mL/min; two-thirds of them had retrograde flow in the distal artery and an average rate of 90 mL/min. The brachial artery to axillary vein grafts (8 mm) had an average flow of 1323 mL/min; 90% had retrograde flow with an average rate of 254 mL/min. Despite the documentation of retrograde flow few patients are symptomatic because of the collateral blood flow to the arm allows perfusion around the fistula and filling of the distal artery. Brescia-Cimino fistulas have an incidence of less than 2% while PTFE grafts of the forearm have an incidence of symptoms as high as 3%.[12] As many as 6% to 8% of larger brachioaxillary fistulas produce ischemic symptoms.[16,17,27]

It has been suggested that steal syndrome can be avoided if were constructed all of the arteriovenous anastomosis with an end artery configuration. This configuration can cause limb threat if this is the sole blood supply to the hand. Decreased flow seen with end artery configurations tend to make dialysis less efficient and increases the risk of thrombosis. Steal is much more common in the proximal fistulas and the larger grafts. Six-millimeter grafts or taper grafts have been used successfully to limit flow.

Moderate to severe ischemic symptoms should be treated because persistent ischemia can lead to permanent neuromuscular damage, particularly in diabetics. The choices for managing the ischemia include ligating the distal artery, which prevents retrograde flow by functionally converting the anastomosis to an end artery configuration, or restricting flow into the fistula by any one of a number of banding techniques. Ligating the distal artery compromises the dual blood supply to the hand should it be needed for future access and also decreases graft flow. The decrease in graft flow hampers the efficiency of dialysis and increases the risk of thrombosis. The goal of banding is to decrease the flow to 300 to 400 mL/min, which generally prevents ischemic symptoms, is adequate for dialysis, and is not prone to thrombosis. It was once thought that in order to have resolution of ischemic symptoms one would have to have return of the distal pulse. Studies have noted that symptoms of ischemia have resolved after outflow narrowing procedures despite the lack of return of a radial pulse. Rivers et al[28] showed that if the pulse volume recordings

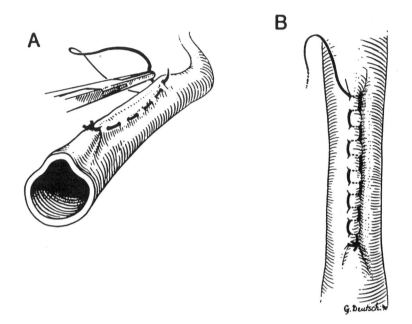

Figure 6: Technique for narrowing graft lumen.

(PVR) of the graft could be increased by 5 mm that most symptoms would resolve requiring less banding and thus a lower risk of thrombosis (PVR is a measurement taken at the base of the finger, correlating the volume of blood in a pulse with the height of the waveform created on a graph produced by the Life Sciences PVR IV machine). Narrowing of the graft outlet can be accomplished by placing interrupted sutures in the outlet to narrow the lumen (Figure 6), by insertion of an end-to-end PTFE interposition graft or conduit of smaller diameter,[29,30] or by encircling the conduit with simple PTFE band. In some patients with severe cases the fistula should be disconnected and the arteriotomy closed, attempting to restore normal flow to the hand.

Venous Hypertension

Venous stenosis proximal to the site of an arteriovenous fistula can cause increased venous resistance with eventual retrograde flow and valvular incompetence. Thrombosis of the axillary subclavian venous (ASV) system in patients with chronic renal failure undergoing hemodialysis is a consequence of central venous catheterization, unlike extrinsic causes for thrombosis such as the thoracic outlet syndrome or effort thrombosis, sometimes called Paget-Schroetter's syndrome, the incidence of the latter is unknown and requires, as part of the therapy for symptomatic patients, decompression of the thoracic outlet. With intrinsic axillary vein thrombosis secondary to catheterization, future complications are usually caused by arteriovenous fistulas constructed in the same extremity. The patient with asymptomatic axillary vein thrombosis who has an ipsilateral fistula can develop early and massive swelling of the entire forearm and brachium, such that even superficial venous distention is obscured and skin breakdown is a threat (Figure 7).

The incidence of ASV thrombosis after the placement of central venous access devices has been studied over the course of the last few years. For example, Deppe et al[31] found an incidence of 3.2% of symptomatic ASV thrombosis in 154 patients who had peripherally placed port devices between 1991 and 1994. The incidence of asymptomatic ASV thrombosis is at least twice that. For example, of 57 oncology patients who had routine venograms performed after central venous catheterization for chemotherapy, 10.5% had a silent complete thrombosis of the ASV and 46% had incomplete thrombosis. In fact, when counting the 78% who also had a fibrin sleeve, only 4 patients had a normal study.[32] From these data it is reasonable to predict an incidence of approximately 10% of ASV thrombosis in patients who have had central venous catheterization. The incidence of symptomatic ASV thrombosis in dialysis patients studied by Criado et al[33] was 14 of 158 (11.5%). All patients had significant arm swelling or dialysis graft thrombosis secondary to previous subclavian vein catheters.

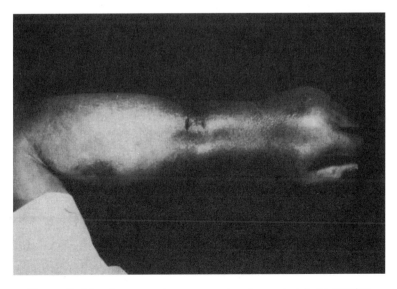

Figure 7: Massive arm edema secondary to venous hypertension.

ASV thrombosis was studied by Horne et al[34] who found that in 50 oncology patients with a silicone venous catheter device, routine venograms detected partial thrombosis in 30% as early as 6 weeks and complete thrombosis in 6% at 6 weeks. By 12 weeks, 10% of patients had already had ASV thrombosis. It was noted in another 30 patients who had previous catheterization, complete occlusion was noted in 30%, although only 6% had symptoms.[34] The reason that axillosubclavian thrombosis secondary to intrinsic causes is asymptomatic can be found in the development of rich collateral beds in the venous system of the neck and chest wall.[35] The risk of developing ASV thrombosis is 2.3% for internal jugular vein catheters versus 10% for subclavian vein catheters.

Color duplex ultrasound is an excellent technique for the diagnosis of ASV thrombosis. The key findings are visualization of the thrombus and absence of spontaneous flow with lack of respiratory phasicity. One may also find an incompressible vein and increased collaterals. The sensitivity of color duplex is 94%, and the specificity is 96%.[35] If the patient has an ASV thrombosis that is recognized preoperatively and another access site is available, it is better to relocate the graft to an extremity with patent venous outflow. In some cases this is not available and then surgical treatment of the ASV thrombosis needs to be addressed. The bypass operations available for symptomatic ASV thrombosis include transposition of the internal jugular to the axillary vein with end-to-side anastomosis, axillary to jugular vein PTFE bypass, and crossover PTFE bypass to the opposite axillary vein. In a comparison of percutaneous transluminal angioplasty versus bypass operation for ASV thrombosis, 13 patients had bypass and 15 had dilatation.[36] Relief of symptoms was 88% at 1 year and 71% at 2 years for bypass patients and for PTA patients the symptoms were relieved at a rate of 36% at 1 year and 0% at 2 years. Wisselink et al[37] noted that repeat angioplasty gave an 86% and 66% success rate at 1 and 2 years, respectively. It was concluded that repeat angioplasty came close to the success rate of bypass procedures. Another option for relief of the arm swelling associated with venous hypertension is to ligate the distal vein making certain that a more proximal blockage has been investigated and managed.

Congestive Heart Failure

Congestive heart failure is an unusual complication secondary to the systemic hemodynamic effects of arteriovenous fistulas. Theoretically, any fistula that decreases total peripheral resistance and increases venous return to the heart can lead to congestive heart failure. This is usually prevented by a compensatory increase in cardiac output by increasing the stroke volume, and contractility with minimal increase in the pulse. When

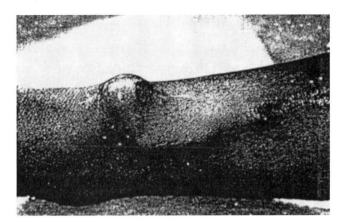

Figure 8: Venous aneurysm.

all compensatory mechanisms are effective, there is no decrease in systemic flow or pressure, venous pressures remain low, and the increase in cardiac output equals the flow through the fistula. If compensatory mechanisms fail, fistula flow exceeds the cardiac output and systemic flow and blood pressure decreases. This is compensated for by fluid retention, increased venous pressure and subsequent congestive heart failure. It is estimated that fistula flow equal to 20% to 40% of the preoperative cardiac output causes decreased systemic flow and that fistula flow greater than or equal to 60% causes congestive heart failure.[38-40] Patients with a decreased hematocrit, cardiomyopathy, coronary artery disease, and diabetes mellitus are at a greater risk.

The occurrence of fistula-induced cardiac failure is a rare but well documented event with an incidence of less than 1% in upper extremity fistulas.[22] It is more common with brachial artery fistulas with average flows of 600 mL/min than with radial artery fistulas, which average 200 to 400 mL/min. Flow rates vary considerably depending on the diameter of the fistula, inflow and outflow. In 1972 Ahearn and Maher[41] reported two patients with Brescia-Cimino fistulas and congestive heart failure in whom flow rates were measured at 2700 and 3800 mL/min.[42] Occluding the fistula caused the cardiac output to fall from 11.2 to 8.4 L/min. Anderson and colleagues[42] summarized six cases of anastomosis-induced congestive heart failure and reviewed another nine from the literature. All fistulas were radial or brachial artery fistulas and all of them had a documented decrease in cardiac output with fistula occlusion.

When a patient develops cardiac failure, the goal of treatment is to decrease flow through the fistula. If the patient has received a renal transplant then the treatment of choice is to close the fistula and repair the artery. For the majority of patients still requiring hemodialysis, revision with narrowing of the anastomosis, or construction of a new fistula will be required. Reduction of flow can be accomplished by placing a 1-cm PTFE cuff around the graft. Alternatively, the origin may be narrowed by several interrupted sutures. Intraoperative flowmeters are useful to document flow within the desired range of 300 to 400 mL/min. Flow less than 300 mL/min often results in thrombosis.

To prevent cardiac failure, it is necessary to keep fistula flow around 400 to 600 mL/min. To avoid excessive flow, a 6-mm tapered graft can be used. Special attention should be paid to high-risk patients, such as those with severe anemia, cardiomyopathy, known coronary artery disease, and diabetes mellitus. Preoperative evaluation of these high-risk patients may include an echocardiogram to evaluate contractility and septal and left ventricular function. Patients with such abnormalities should receive smaller grafts. Intraoperative flow studies can be used to calibrate the graft for desired flow.

Peripheral Neuropathy

Patient with chronic renal failure are at increased risk for peripheral neuropathies, either as a complication of chronic uremia or as a complication of diabetes mellitus. The conditions may produce polyneuropathies, however, several mononeuropathic conditions have been described in chronic renal failure patients with upper extremity fistulas.

A carpal tunnel-like syndrome was the first neurological complication that was reported by Mancusi-Ungaro et al[43] in 1976. The symptoms were consistent with those associated with median nerve compression, including pain, paresthesias and thenar wasting. Warren and Otiano[44] further elucidated the syndrome by documenting increased hand volumes in 23 dialysis patients with carpal tunnel syndrome among a study group of 36. In light of no identifiable anatomic abnormality, it was felt that the median nerve compression was secondary to the edema and the venous hypertension. In 1977, Harding[45] in two cases postulated that it was not secondary to median nerve compression but instead to neural ischemia, which was caused by vascular steal. Some credence was given to this theory by the partial resolution of symptoms by the ligation of the distal radial artery in one patient; however, complete relief in both patients was not obtained until the flexor retinaculum was released. Other neurological complications involving radial, ulnar, and median neuropathies were described in three cases by Reinstein.[46] All three cases were attributable to direct nerve compression: a basilic vein hematoma compressing the radial nerve, a basilic vein aneurysm compressing the median nerve, and a graft abscess compressing the median nerve.

The exact etiology of upper extremity fistula-induced peripheral neuropathy is not always clear. Fortunately, it is a rare complication occurring in less than 1% of all upper extremity fistulas. When direct nerve compression by a foreign body is apparent, treatment consists of removing the foreign body. When carpal tunnel syndrome exists, releasing the flexor retinaculum often relieves the symptoms. If these measures do not relieve the symptoms then the fistula may need to be closed and reconstructed in the other arm.

Prevention of neurological complications and their permanent sequelae depends on early diagnosis and surgical correction, if possible. Diabetics with severe peripheral vascular disease may be particularly at risk and should be watched closely, especially when high-flow shunts are placed.[47]

Aneurysms

Aneurysms and pseudoaneurysms are relatively uncommon complications of autogenous arteriovenous fistulas and prosthetic grafts. True aneurysmal dilatation is more common in autogenous fistulas, resulting from dilatation of the arterialized vein for hemodialysis. Pseudoaneurysms in both fistulas and grafts are secondary to a needle tear of the graft wall with resultant hematoma formation. In addition, false aneurysms can occur at both venous and arterial anastamotic ends of the graft. Infection is often implicated in the etiology of aneurysms. The frequency of aneurysm formation at the site of needle punctures and at the site of the venous anastomosis is approximately the same.[47]

The incidence of aneurysm formation varies from 1% to 10%, depending on the type of access (Figure 8).[12,14,26] Biological grafts have a higher rate of true aneurysm formation than prosthetic materials which tend to develop pseudoaneurysms. The time from graft construction to the appearance of this complication ranges from 18 to 35 months.[13,14] True aneurysms in autogenous fistulas can be treated by local revision if the overlying skin is not ulcerated. Pseudoaneurysms tend to enlarge, therefore, to avoid skin ulceration and potential hemorrhage, direct repair with suture or excision and replacement with a small interposition segment is recommended.

References

1. Kolff WJ, Berk WTJ: The artificial kidney: A dialyser with a great area. *Acta Med Scand* 117:121–134, 1944.
2. Quinton WE, Dillard D, Schribner BH: Cannulation of blood vessels for prolonged hemodialysis. *Trans Am Soc Artif Intern Organs* 6:104–109, 1960.

3. Brescia M, Cimino JE, Appel K, et al: Chronic hemodialysis using venopuncture and a surgically created arteriovenous fistula. *N Eng J Med* 275:1089–1092, 1966.

4. Nakagawa Y, Ota K, Sato Y, et al: Complications in blood access for hemodialysis. *Artif Organs* 18(4):283–288, 1994.

5. Owada A, Saito H, Mochizuki T, et al: Radial artery spasm in uremic patients undergoing construction of arteriovenous hemodialysis fistula: Diagnosis and prophylaxis with intravenous Nicardipine. *Nephron* 64:501–504, 1993.

6. Owada A, Saito H, Nagai T, et al: Prophylactic use of intravenous prostaglandin E for radial artery spasm in uremic patients undergoing construction of arteriovenous hemodialysis fistulas. *Int J Artif Organs* 17(10):511–514, 1994.

7. Wilson SE: Complications of vascular access procedures. In: Wilson SE, ed. *Vascular Access Surgery.* Chicago: Yearbook Medical Publishers; 1988, p. 285.

8. Hunter DW, SO, Samuel KS, et al: Failing or thrombosed Brescia-Cimino arteriovenous dialysis fistulas. *Radiology* 149:105–109, 1983.

9. Glanz S, Gordon DH, et al: The role of percutaneous angioplasty in the management of chronic hemodialysis fistulas. *Ann Surg* 206:777–781, 1987.

10. Andriana M, Drago G, Bernardi AM, et al: Recombinant tissue plasminogen activator (rt-PA) as first line therapy for declotting a hemodialysis access. *Nephrol Dial Transplant* 10:1714–1719, 1995.

11. Beathard GA, Welch BR, Maidment HJ: Mechanical thrombolysis for the treatment of thrombosed hemodialysis access grafts. *Radiology* 200:711–716, 1996.

12. Winsett OE, Wolma FJ: Complications of Vascular access for hemodialysis. *South Med J* 5:513–517, 1985.

13. Kherlakian GM, Roederscheimer LR, et al: Comparison of autogenous fistula versus expanded polytetrafluoroethylene graft fistula for angioaccess in hemodialysis. *Am J Surg* 152:238–243, 1986.

14. Reilly DT, Wood RFM, Bell PRF: Prospective study of dialysis fistulas: Problem patients and their treatment. *Br J Surg* 69:549–553, 1982.

15. Palder SB, Kirkman RL: Vascular access for hemodialysis: patency rates and results of revision. *Ann Surg* 202:235–239, 1985.

16. Dagher FJ: The upper arm AV hemoaccess: Long-term Follow-up. *J Cardiovasc Surg* 27:447–449, 1986.

17. Dunlop M, Mackinlay JY, Jenkins A: Vascular access: Experience with the Brachiocephali c fistula. *Ann R Coll Surg Engl* 68:203–206, 1986.

18. Berger A, Rosenberg N: Hypotension and closure of hemodialysis shunts. *Am Surg* 58:551–553, 1983.

19. Lundin AP, Alder A, Feinroth MV, et al: Maintenance hemodialysis: Survival beyond the first decade. *JAMA* 244:38, 1980.

20. Buckels JA: Management of infection in hemodialysis. In:*Vascular Access Surgery.* Wilson SE, ed. Chicago: Yearbook Publishers; 1988, p. 305.

21. Kim GE, Hovaguimian H, Matalou R: Vascular access for patients on long-term hemodialysis maintenance. *NY State J Med* 178–180, 1984.

22. Porter JA, Sharp WV, Walsh EJ: Complications of vascular access in a dialysis population. *Curr Surg* 42(4):298–300, 1985.

23. Hill SL, Seeger JM: The arm as an alternative site for vascular access for dialysis patients with recurrent vascular access failure. *South Med J* 78:37–40, 1985.

24. Taylor B, Sigley RD, May KJ: Fate of infected and eroded hemodialysis grafts and autogenous fistulas. *Am J Surg* 165:632–636, 1993.

25. Malone JM, Moore WS, Campagna G, et al: Bacteremic infectibility of vascular grafts: the influence of pseudointimal integrity and duration of graft function. *Surgery* 78:211–216, 1975.

26. Zibari GB, Landreneau MD, Rohr MS, Brown ST, McDonald JC: Complications from permanent vascular access. Abstracts of the Central Surgical Association. March 10, 1988, Columbus, Ohio.

27. West JC, Evan RD, et al: Arterial insufficiency in hemodialysis access procedures: Reconstruction by an interposition polytetrafluoroethylene graft conduit. *Am J Surg* 153:300–301, 1987.

28. Rivers SP, Scher LA, Veith FJ: Correlation of steal syndrome secondary to hemodialysis access fistulas: A simplified quantitative technique. *Surgery* 112:593–597, 1992.

29. Haimov M: Construction of vascular access using vascular substitutes. In: Haimov M, ed. *Vascular Access: A Practical Guide.* Mt. Kisco. NY: Futura Publishing Company, 1987, pp. 59–85.

30. Rubio PA, Farrell EM: *Atlas of Angioaccess Surgery.* Chicago: Yearbook Medical Publishers; 1983, pp. 238–245.

31. Deppe G, Kahn ML, Malviya VK, et al: Experience with the PAS port venous access device in patients with gynecologic malignancies. *Gynecol Oncol* 62(3):340–343, 1996.

32. Balestreri L, DeCicco M, Matovic M, et al: Central Venous catheter related thrombosis in clinically asymptomatic oncology patients: A phlebographic study. *Eur J Radiol* 20:108–111, 1995.

33. Criado E, Marston W, Jaque PF, et al: Proximal venous outflow obstruction in patients with upper extremity arteriovenous dialysis access. *Ann Vasc Surg* 8(6):530–535, 1994.

34. Horne MK 3rd, May DJ, Alexander HR, et al: Venographic surveillance of tunnelled venous access devices in adult oncology patients. *Ann Surg Oncol* 2:174–178, 1995.

35. Richard HM 3rd, Selby JB Jr, Gay SB, et al: Normal venous anatomy and collateral pathways in venous thrombosis. *Radiographics* 12:527–534, 1992.

36. Brothers TE, Morgan M, Robinson JG, et al: Failure of dialysis access: revise or replace? *J Surg Res* 60:312–316, 1996.

37. Wisselink W, Money SR, Becker MO, et al: Comparison of operative reconstruction and percutaneous balloon dilatation for central venous obstruction. *Am J Surg* 166:200–205, 1994.

38. Frank CW, Wang H, Lanerant J, et al: An experimental study of immediate hemodynamic adjustments to acute arteriovenous fistulae of various sites. *J Clin Invest* 34:722, 1955.

39. Leslie MB, Portin BA, Schenk WG: Cardiac output and posture studies in chronic experimental arteriovenous fistulas. *Arch Surg* 81:123, 1960.

40. George CRP, May J, Schieb M, et al: Heart failure due to an arteriovenous fistula for hemodialysis. *Med J Aust* 1:696, 1973.

41. Ahearn D, Maher J: Heart failure as a complication of hemodialysis arteriovenous fistula. *Ann Intern Med* 77:201, 1972.

42. Anderson CB, Codd JR, Graff RA, et al: Cardiac failure and upper extremity arteriovenous dialysis fistulas. *Arch Intern Med* 136:92, 1976.
43. Mancusi-Ungaro A, Cornes J, DiSpaltro F: Median carpal tunnel syndrome following a vascular shunt procedure in the forearm. *Plast Reconstr Surg* 57: 96, 1976.
44. Warren DJ, Otieno LS: Carpal tunnel syndrome in patients on chronic hemodialysis. *Postgrad Med J* 51:450, 1975.
45. Harding AE, LeFanv J: Carpal tunnel syndrome related to antebrachial Cimino-Brescia fistula. *J Neurol Neurosurg Psychiatry* 40:511, 1977.
46. Reinstein L, Reed WP, et al: Peripheral nerve compression by brachial artery-basilic vein vascular access in long-term hemodialysis. *Arch Phys Med Rehab* 65:142–144, 1984.
47. Wytress L, Markley HG, et al: Brachial neuropathy after brachial artery-antecubital vein shunts for chronic hemodialysis. *Neurology* 37:1398–1400, 1987.

Part IV

Vascular Manifestations of Systemic Disorders

17

Upper Extremity Manifestations of Systemic Vascular Disorders

David J. Klashman, MD, Swee Cheng Ng, MD, Dwight H. Kono, MD, and Harold E. Paulus, MD

Symptoms of vasculitis may first be noted in the upper extremity and can mimic diseases often seen by vascular surgeons. The recognition of vasculitis is important because specific medical treatment is often successful and surgical treatment, without adequate medical control of the underlying inflammatory process, is almost always unsuccessful. The manifestations of vasculitis involving the upper extremity and a brief overview of the various types of vasculitis are presented in this chapter.

Blood vessels are intimately involved with all inflammatory processes because they serve as a conduit for the various cellular mediators and effectors of inflammation. Depending on the severity of the inflammation, changes may range from a pericapillary infiltrate of mononuclear cells to frank necrosis of the vessel wall. The vasculitides comprise a group of clinically distinct syndromes in which there is primary inflammation of blood vessels, usually believed to be immunologically mediated, with histological evidence of vessel wall necrosis, fragmentation, and inflammatory cell infiltrate, primarily of polymorphonuclear leukocytes. Clinical evidence of inflammation, such as fever, leukocytosis, and elevated erythrocyte sedimentation rate (ESR), is generally present and each syndrome appears to have a characteristic distribution of organ involvement.

From Machleder HI, (ed): *Vascular Disorders of the Upper Extremity*. Third Revised Edition. Futura Publishing Company, Inc., Armonk, NY, © 1998.

Table 1
Classification of Vasculitis*

A. Infectious vasculitis
B. Noninfectious vasculitis
C. Vasculitis look-alikes

* Adapted from Lie JT: *J Rheum* 15:728—732, 1988.

Classification

Classification of vasculitis is difficult as the etiology and pathogenesis are still not fully understood. Many different classifications have been proposed and modified.[1-5] The classification recently suggested by Lie[5] seems to be most useful. This is shown in Table 1.

Infectious angiitis needs to be correctly diagnosed,[5] as specific antimicrobial therapy is required. Organisms that have been identified as causes of vasculitis include: spirochetes,[6] mycobacteria,[7] pyogenic bacteria,[8]

Table 2
Major Vasculitis Syndromes

Vessel Size	Necrotizing Vasculitis	Granulomatous Vasculitis	Associated Rheumatic Disease
Postcapillary venule	Leukocytoclastic vasculitis		
Small arteries	Erythema nodosa	Wegener's granulomatosis	Rheumatoid arthritis, Systemic lupus erythematosus
		Granulomatous angiitis of the CNS	Dermatomyositis of childhood
Medium arteries	Polyarteritis nodosa		Scleroderma (rare)
	Mucocutaneous lymph node syndrome	Allergic granulomatosis and angiitis	Acute rheumatic fever
Large arteries		Temporal arteritis. Takayasu's arteritis	Seronegative spondyloarthropathies Relapsing polychondritis Bechcet's disease* Cogan's syndrome

* May be secondary to vasa vasorum vasculitis.

Table 3
Overlap Syndromes of Noninfectious Angiitis*

Takayasu's arteritis with giant cell arteritis and necrotizing vasculitis
Takayasu's arteritis with polyarteritis nodosa
Takayasu's arteritis with Churg-Strauss/Wegener's
Giant cell arteritis with polyarteritis nodosa
Giant cell arteritis with Churg-Strauss
Polyarteritis nodosa with Churg-Strauss
Polyarteritis nodosa with Henoch-Schonlein
Polyarteritis nodosa with hypersensitivity angiitis

* Adapted from Hunder GG: ARA Biennial Review of Rheumatic Disease, Section VII, 1988.

fungi,[9] rickettsia,[10] viruses,[11-15] and human immunodeficiency virus (HIV).[16]

The noninfectious angiitis subgroup consists of various distinct clinical patterns of vasculitis. These are further classified according to the size of blood vessels predominantly involved, the histological finding of granulomatous changes and the presence or absence of a rheumatic disease (Table 2). Recognizing that this classification is not ideal, there are patients who have clinical features of two or more of the above clinical syndromes. These are called overlap vasculitis syndromes (Table 3).[17-19]

The final group of diseases are those that are noninflammatory, but clinically mimic vasculitis. These include coarctation-hypoplasia-dysplasia, atheroembolism, myxoma embolism, ergotism, neurofibromatosis, and idiopathic arterial calcification.[5]

Upper Extremity Manifestations

Nearly all vasculitides can affect the upper extremities. However, with the exception of Takayasu's arteritis (TA), thromboangiitis obliterans (Buerger's disease), and the digital vascular disease associated with scleroderma, severe RA and lupus erythematosus, such involvement is uncommon. Usually vasculitis tends to affect the lower extremities, and isolated upper extremity involvement is very rare.

The manifestations can be divided into the following areas: involvement of the skin, intermediate sized arteries (digital arteries and greater), peripheral nerves, and joints (Table 4). Small vessel vasculitis tends to have predominantly cutaneous and articular findings. In medium-sized vessel vasculitis, neuropathy and digital gangrene are more prominent. Large vessel vasculitis tends to spare the skin, joints and nerves, but has marked intermediate size vessel involvement causing bruits, diminished

Table 4
Upper Extremity Manifestations of Necrotizing Vasculitis

Vasculitides	Cutaneous*	Large Vessel†	Peripheral Neuropathy	Arthritis Arthalgias
Leukocytoclastic vasculitis	Palpable purpura, Petechiae to ecchymosis, Pustular eruption, Vesicles, Bullae, Small ulcers, Urticaria	0	Uncommon	Wrist and elbow most often
Polyarteritis nodosa	Subcutaneous nodules, Ecchymosis, Livedo reticularis, Ulcerative lesions	Gangrene of digits	Polyneuropathy mononeuritis multiplex	Common
Wegener's granulomatosis	Ulcerative nodules, Papular lesions, Vesicles, Petechiae, Churg-Strauss granuloma	Peripheral gangrene (rare)	Uncommon polyneuropathy mononeuritis multiplex	Common
Allergic angiitis granulomatis	Erythematous nodules, Ulcerative nodules, Ecchymosis, Plaques and pupuric papules, Churg-Strauss granuloma	Rare	Mononeuritis multiplex polyneuropathy	Uncommon
Temporal arteritis	0	Pulse, Bruit, Claudication	Rare	Rare unless polymyalgia rheumatica included
Takayasu's arteritis	0	Pulse, Bruit, Claudication	0	Transient during acute phase
Rheumatoid arthritis	Nailfold infarcts, Rheumatoid nodules, Cutaneous ulcers, Purpuric lesions	Digital Infarcts Peripheral gangrene	Uncommon unless vasculitis	All cases symmetric, small joints, usually erosive and deforming
Systemic lupus erythematosus	Petechiae, Cutaneous infarcts, Nailfold infarcts	Digital infarcts Peripheral gangrene	Mononeuritis multiplex polyneuropathy	Symmetric, nonerosive

* Digital artery and greater.   † Usually lower extremity.

pulses and intermittent claudication. Although the term claudication is generally accepted as ischemic pain of the extremities, it is defined in the dictionary as arterial spasm with subsequent painful cramping of the legs with lameness and has its origin from Emperor Claudius who "stumbled as he walked owing to the weakness of his knees."[20]

When upper extremity vasculitis is present, the particular type of vasculitis is generally identified by the patient's history as well as by physical and laboratory evaluations. The systemic necrotizing vasculitides generally have other areas of involvement, and manifestations of a rheumatic disease are almost always present if vasculitis is secondary to it. Upper extremity vasculitis only rarely occurs before other manifestations are present.

Rheumatic disorders can present with obstruction of the vessels of the upper extremity without an associated vasculitis. When faced with thrombosis of the vessels of the upper extremity one should consider the antiphospholipid syndrome that includes either the *lupus anticoagulant* antibodies or anticardiolipin antibodies. Much work has been done recently to advance the knowledge of this syndrome. The first description of the lupus anticoagulant antibody was probably in 1906 by Wassermann[21] in sera of patients with syphilis using a complement fixation test to detect regin. Later it was found that sera from subjects who do not have syphilis may give a so called "biological false-positive" test for syphilis. These included other infections, Jamaican neuropathy and autoimmune disorders like systemic lupus erythematosus (SLE).

In 1952,[22] there was a report of two patients with SLE, hemorrhagic disorders, prolonged prothrombin and whole blood clotting times, and biological false-positive tests for syphilis. Speculation about a relationship between this circulating anticoagulant and a false-positive test for syphilis ensued within a few years.

Although originally associated with bleeding, it soon became evident that hemorrhagic abnormalities were rare in patients with this so-called lupus anticoagulant. Paradoxically it was found to be associated with thrombosis.[23] The sites of thrombosis are leg veins in 66%, cerebral vessels in 25%, and peripheral arteries in 10%.[24] Antiphospholipid antibodies (including either lupus anticoagulant antibodies and/or anticardiolipin antibodies) have also been found to be associated with recurrent fetal loss, thrombocytopenia, hemolytic anemia, Evan's syndrome, livedo reticularis, transient cerebral ischemia, migraine, and chorea.[25]

The many tests available to look for the antiphospholipid antibodies using different sources of phospholipid, eg, cardiolipin.[21] When a patient presents with unexplained thrombosis of arteries or veins it is prudent to look for the antiphospholipid antibodies using one or more of these tests. The patient may or may not have features of SLE or other connective tissue disease.

Treatment of the initial thrombotic event is anticoagulation. Two retrospective studies have suggested that maintaining an international normalized ratio (INR) in the 3.0 to 4.0 range with warfarin greatly reduces the risk of a recurrent thrombotic event in patients with the antiphospholipid syndrome.[26,27] Associated connective tissue disease is treated on its own merit. There had been some enthusiasm to treat the presence of the antiphospholipid antibody with corticosteroids to prevent recurrent thrombosis or recurrent abortions. However, this has been disputed as the level of the antiphospholipid antibody fluctuates spontaneously and a rising antibody titer does not predict thrombotic events[28] (and therefore does not justify therapy).[29]

Etiology and Pathogenesis

Environmental agents are known to trigger the development of some types of vasculitis in susceptible individuals. Infections are an important cause and can include multiple types of infections involving viruses, bacteria, fungi and parasites.[30] HIV-associated vasculitis in a variety of forms has been increasingly recognized.[16,31] Hepatitis C virus has been implicated as the etiology of essential mixed cryoglobulinemia.[32]

Drugs can also cause vasculitis, usually small vessel vasculitis (Table 5).[33-48] As many of these drugs are commonly used, it is important to remember that removal of the offending agent can result in cure of the

---

Table 5
Some Drugs That May Induce Vasculitis

1. Illicit drugs	Methamphetamine
	Cocaine
2. Thrombolytic agents	streptokinase
	anisoylated plasminogen streptokinase activator complex
3. Antithyroid drugs	propylthiouracil
4. Hypoglycemic drugs	Metformin
5. Nasal decongestants	Phenylpropanolamine
6. Acne drug	Isotretinoin
7. Antibiotics	Vancomycin
8. Anticonvulsants	Phenytoin
9. Antiarrhythmic	Quinidine
10. NSAID	Phenylbutazone
11. Asthma drugs	Cromolyn sodium
12. Antihypertensive	Hydralazine
13. H_2 Blockers	Cimetidine

vasculitis. More recently antiretroviral agents used to treat HIV including zidovudine and didanosine have been associated with drug-induced vasculitis.[49] Biological agents including hematopoietic growth factors, interferon, and monoclonal antibodies representing a clinically significant new area of medical therapeutics are gaining approval for treatment of a variety of disorders. As experience with these new medications increases, associations with drug-induced vasculitis are being observed. In particular granulocyte colony-stimulating factor (G-CSF) has been particularly noted to have potential vasculitis inducing toxicity.[50,51]

Although infrequent, vasculitides can be associated with malignancy either as a true paraneoplastic syndrome, malignancies masquerading as vasculitides, and vasculitides masquerading as malignancies.[52]

It is known that a single agent can cause a diversity of clinical manifestations in different individuals, again indicating that host responses are important. For example, hepatitis B virus infection can cause: hepatitis ranging in severity from mild transient hepatitis, to chronic persistent hepatitis, to chronic active hepatitis, to acute fulminant hepatic necrosis[15]; hepatocellular carcinoma[53]; asymptomatic carrier state; a prodromal transient serum sickness-like illness with arthritis, urticaria, and mild glomerulonephritis; polymyositis/dermatomyositis[54]; glomerulonephritis[55]; and necrotizing vasculitis.[56]

It is not known why exposure to an antigen predisposes some persons to develop vasculitis but not others who are exposed to the same antigen. The genetic predisposition of patients to develop vasculitis has been studied and some relation between vasculitis and human leukocyte antigen (HLA) subtypes has been found. Specifically, giant cell (temporal) arteritis (GCA) has been linked with HLA-DRB1*04 alleles.[57] In contrast, an association between Wegener's granulomatosis and any defined HLA allele has been excluded by molecular investigation.[58]

Immune complexes appear to play a role in the development of some forms of necrotizing vasculitis. The sequence of events leading to small and medium sized vessel necrotizing vasculitis appears to start with immune complex deposition in the vessel wall, followed by activation of complement, migration of polymorphonuclear leukocytes with liberation of lysosomal enzymes and destruction of the vessel wall. Evidence supporting this hypothesis includes:

(1) The classic Arthus reaction.[59] After immunization of an animal by systemic injection of an antigen, subsequent subcutaneous injection of the antigen leads to deposition of antigen-antibody complexes in and around blood vessels, activation of complement, polymorphonuclear leukocyte migration with release of lysosomal enzymes, and edema and hemorrhage 4 to 10 hours later. Similar findings occur after systemic injection of antibody fol-

lowed by subcutaneous injection of antigen (passive Arthus reaction) or systemic injection of antigen followed by subcutaneous injection of antibody (reverse passive Arthus reaction).

(2) Serum sickness model.[60,61] Eight to 14 days after intravenous injection of heterologous serum protein or preformed immune complexes, animals develop arthritis, glomerulonephritis, and vasculitis.

(3) Animal models.[61] Vasculitis can be seen in association with immune complex deposition in animal models such as NZB/NZW mice, Aleutian mink disease and mice with lymphocytic choriomeningitis virus infection.

(4) Findings in patients with vasculitis, which may include elevated levels of immune complexes and depressed complement levels in serum,[62,63] histological similarity between above animal models and necrotizing vasculitis of postcapillary venules,[61,63] the finding of immunoglobulins and complement in vessel walls by immunofluorescent technique,[63,64] and serum sickness in humans.[65]

Certain features appear to be important for the development of immune complex vasculitis:

(1) Mechanical factors. Lesions tend to occur in areas of high turbulent flow such as branching points, bifurcations, coarctation,[66] and with hypertension.[67] These lesions may be inhibited by depletion of platelets. Dependent areas are often affected by cutaneous vasculitis,[68] again suggesting a role for hemodynamic forces. The pattern of cutaneous vasculitis has been shown to depend on the anatomic sites of involvement and flow patterns.[64]

(2) Platelets. The role of platelets is not entirely clear, but they probably release vasoactive amines leading to increased vascular permeability.[61]

(3) Vascular permeability.[69] Increased vascular permeability appears important for the deposition of immune complexes in vessel walls. It is mediated in part by mast cell degranulation,[70] platelets, and histamine and serotonin.[61] With increased permeability, deposition of immune complexes[71] can be seen in vessel walls.

(4) Characteristics of the immune complexes. In early studies looking at immune complex deposition in vessels, it was found that large immune complexes greater than 19S formed in slight antigen excess were best able to be deposited in vessel walls with increased permeability.[62] Net charge, properties of the antigen, and degree of ability to fix complement did not appear to be significant variables.[69]

(5) Complement. Depletion of C3 by cobra venom prevents the development of vasculitis despite immune complex deposition.[72]
(6) Inflammatory cells. Polymorphonuclear leukocytes appear responsible for the phagocytosis of immune complexes,[73] as well as the release of lysosomal enzymes causing vessel wall destruction. Depletion of polymorphonuclear leukocytes by treatment with nitrogen mustard abolishes the development of vasculitis despite the deposition of immune complexes. Coincident with the appearance of polymorphonuclear leukocytes in lesions, there is rapid disappearance of immunoglobulin and complement within 18 to 48 hours after initiation of the Arthus reaction.[73] Decreasing chemotaxis and enzyme secretion by treatment with prostaglandin E_1 markedly suppresses the reverse passive Arthus reaction in rats[74] again supporting the role of polymorphonuclear leukocytes.

Factors that lead to the development of immune complexes are less well understood. A slower rate of clearance of immune complexes from the circulation by the reticuloendothelial system may play a role by allowing immune complexes time to localize in blood vessels. Clearance of carbon particles or large immune complexes has been shown to decrease once saturation of the reticuloendothelial system occurs, and in animal models correlates with the finding of immune complexes or particles in blood vessels.[75] In several rheumatic diseases that are associated with immune complexes, an increase in the rate of clearance of a lipid emulsion by the reticuloendothelial system has been found.[76] However, using another system, a decrease in the rate of clearance of radiolabeled IgG-sensitized red blood cells by the reticuloendothelial system was noted in SLE,[77] Sjøgren's syndrome (SS),[78] and certain vasculitides.[79] A decrease in this prolonged rate of clearance has been reported after plasmapheresis.[79] Another possibility for the persistence of antigen could be decreased antibody response resulting in an inability to completely clear the antigen.[80]
The pathophysiology of the granulomatous vasculitides is not known. It may be the result of cell-mediated immune injury.[81] Circulating immune complexes themselves may trigger a granulomatous response.[82] In several of these syndromes the inflammatory infiltrate consists of activated T lymphocytes and macrophages. Class II major histocompatibility complex (MHC) expressing dendritic cells with a putative antigen-presenting function have been identified within lymphocyte infiltrates in temporal arteritis and in polyarteritis nodosa (PAN).[83–85] Molecular studies have demonstrated clonal expansion of selected T cell populations in inflammatory foci, possibly recognizing a disease-relevant antigen.[85] The expansion of T lymphocytes bearing particular T-cell receptor V-beta families observed in Kawasaki disease is suggestive of a mechanism involving

superantigens in the pathogenesis of the condition.[86] T lymphocyte activation and mechanisms that mediate vascular injury appears to be heterogeneous among the different vasculitic syndromes.[85]

The identification of the antineutrophil cytoplasm antibody (ANCA) may be a step toward better understanding of the pathogenesis of Wegener's granulomatosis. It was first reported in 1985[87] that 25 of 27 sera from patients with Wegener's granulomatosis had this antibody (initially called anticytoplasmic antibody) while none of 500 sera from normal subjects nor 175 sera from patients with related diseases had this antibody. This work was substantiated by another group[88] who reported the presence of this antibody in 18 of 32 sera of patients with Wegener's granulomatosis, but not in 730 other sera. Correlation between titers of these antibodies and disease activity further suggested that their occurrence was not simply an epiphenomenon. However it was the also shown that this antibody is not specific for Wegener's granulomatosis.[89] It was detected in the sera of patients with microscopic polyarteritis, Churg-Strauss, and Kawasaki disease.

Immunofluorescence is the current ANCA screening technique. Three different fluorescence patterns can be distinguished including fine granular cytoplasmic (C-ANCA), perinuclear (P-ANCA) and diffuse atypical (A-ANCA) patterns. C-ANCA is a seromarker for Wegener's granulomatosis and is mostly induced by antibodies to proteinase 3. P-ANCA is mostly induced by antibodies to myeloperoxidase and is a seromarker for microscopic polyangiitis (MPA). P-ANCA and A-ANCA have been detected in a variety of other vasculitides, collagen vascular, inflammatory bowel and liver diseases. Currently this antibody can be considered a useful test for the diagnosis of systemic vasculitis, particularly Wegener's granulomatosis.[90,91]

Some evidence suggests a possible role of ANCAs in the pathogenesis of associated vasculitides.[85] *In vitro* studies show that ANCA promote neutrophil activation and endothelial injury.[92,93] Animal models of ANCA-induced vasculitis and glomerulonephritis have been developed.[94,95]

The role of adhesion molecules in the development of vascular inflammation is a topic of increasing research interest.[85,96] Vascular endothelial cells exhibit a wide range of regulatory functions, mediated in large part by adhesion molecules in addition to growth factors and cytokines. Increased expression of adhesion molecules in various vasculitides has been demonstrated.[85,96,97] Soluble adhesion molecules are being investigated as possible markers of vasculitic disease activity.[98]

Although some advances have been made in the understanding of the pathogenesis of vasculitis and the identification of newer antibodies can aid in the management of vasculitis, further investigations still need to be done.

Small and Medium Vessel Vasculitis

Leukocytoclastic Vasculitis

The descriptive terms leukocytoclastic vasculitis (LCV), hypersensitivity vasculitis, and allergic vasculitis have been applied to the findings associated with necrotizing vasculitis of the postcapillary venule. LCV is the most common type of vasculitis and generally has the best prognosis. A causative factor or an associated disease (Table 6) is often found, so that the finding of LCV generally warrants a search for one.

The clinical features of LCV are influenced by the associated conditions, but certain generalities can be made.[99,100] Persons of all ages are affected. In some, a preceding flu-like illness can be identified. Constitutional symptoms such as fever, malaise, and myalgia may develop, but are less common than in PAN. The skin is affected in all patients. A wide variety of cutaneous lesions can occur, the most characteristic being multiple nonblanching palpable purpura (Figure 1). Other manifestations include petechiae, ecchymoses (confluent purpura), urticaria, vesicles, bullae, ulcers, and pustular eruptions. Lesions are symmetric, occur in crops on dependent surfaces, and generally evolve from petechiae to palpable purpura and then may progress to a plaque-like lesion or a bulla, which may become ulcerated. Only a small number of patients develop ulcerations. Dependent edema can occur. Pain and a burning or tingling sensation often accompany the vasculitic skin lesions, but about 30% have no symptoms. Arthritis or arthralgia occurs in about 40% of cases, usually involves the knees, ankles, wrists, or elbows, is not destructive, and usually lasts only a few days. Renal involvement occurs in about half of the cases, with hematuria due to glomerulonephritis the most common finding. A small number of patients progress to kidney failure. Gastrointestinal symptoms of abdominal pain, anorexia, nausea, and emesis are common, but transient and of minor consequence. In a few patients, catastrophic gastrointestinal manifestations such as perforation, intussusception, gastrointestinal bleeding, and infarction of bowels may occur.[101] Involvement of the lungs, peripheral nerves, central nervous system (CNS), and the heart may occur, but is not common.

In the upper extremity the manifestations of LCV are limited to the cutaneous lesions, which involve the arms in about 40% of the cases,[100] arthritis or arthralgias (wrist 28%, elbow 23%, hands 14%, shoulders 7%),[100] and rarely peripheral neuropathy. Gangrene does not occur without involvement of larger muscular arteries.

Diagnosis is confirmed by biopsy of involved skin. The histological picture can vary depending on the severity and stage of the lesion, but there is always involvement of the postcapillary venules and sometimes

---

Table 6
Conditions Associated with Leukocytoclastic
Vasculitis (LCV)

Subsets of LCV
　Benign leukocytoclastic vasculitis
　Chronic urticaria
　Serum sickness
　Henoch-Schonlein purpura
　Essential mixed cryoglobulinemia
Rheumatic Diseases
　Polyarteritis nodosa
　Rheumatoid arthritis
　Systemic lupus erythematosus
　Mixed connective tissue disease
　Sjogren's syndrome
　Dermatomyositis
　Goodpasture's syndrome
　Scleroderma
　Rheumatic fever
　Relapsing polychrondritis
Drugs (See Table 5)
Neoplasms
　Lymphomas and lymphosarcomas
　Chronic lymphocytic leukemia
　Waldenstrom's macroglobulinemia
　Multiple myeloma
　Cancers
Infections
　Viral
　Subacute bacterial endocarditis
　Acute bacterial infections especially gonococcemia
Physical Agents
　Cold
　Mechanical trauma
　Environmental allergens–pollen, contactants, food
Miscellaneous
　Benign hypergammaglobulinemic purpura
　Chronic hepatitis
　Primary biliary cirrhosis
　Retroperitoneal fibrosis
　Ulcerative colitis
　Intestinal bypass
　α-1-antitrypsin deficiency
　Influenza vaccination
　Congenital deficiency of C1q, C2, or C3
　Erythema elevatum diutinum
　Livedoid vasculitis (atrophic blanche)

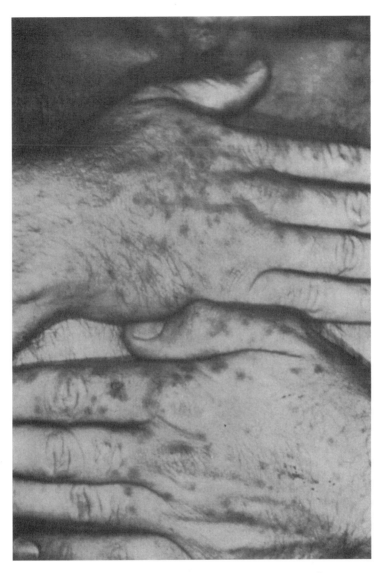

Figure 1. Petechiae and purpura of the hands in Henoch-Schönlein purpura.

of arterioles and capillaries, with polymorphonuclear leukocyte infiltration and nuclear fragmentation (leukocytoclasis), necrosis of the vessel wall, fibrinoid deposits, and sometimes hemorrhage and thrombosis.[1,99,102,103] Laboratory tests are utilized to search for an associated condition. No specific tests for LCV exist other than the biopsy. The ESR is often elevated.[99] Depressed complement components and an elevated rheumatoid factor may be found.

The prognosis of LCV is in part dependent on the associated condition if one exists. However, LCV is generally self-limited and the outlook is good, especially if only the skin is involved.[104] Treatment involves identifying and eliminating any underlying precipitating factors. Antihistamines, nonsteroidal anti-inflammatory drugs, sulfone and antimalarials are sometimes effective for the cutaneous manifestations.[105] Elevation of the legs and elastic stockings may help dependent edema. For severe cutaneous lesions a brief course of prednisone 40 to 60 mg a day may be beneficial. In chronic or recurrent LCV, besides systemic steroids, azathioprine and colchicine appeared to be effective.[105] Steroids have also been used for joint and gastrointestinal[101] manifestations, but appear to be of less value for renal impairment.[103] The use of chronic steroid or cytotoxic agents should be avoided in patients with disease limited to the skin.[104]

Subgroups of Leukocytoclastic Vasculitis

Chronic urticaria.[106–108] A hypocomplementemic vasculitis was described in 1973 by McDuffie et al[106] in four patients with recurrent urticarial, erythematosus, and hemorrhagic skin lesions which on biopsy showed LCV. Constitutional symptoms, arthritis, abdominal pain, and rarely glomerulonephritis were present. LCV has since been found to occur in 20% to 25% of patients with chronic urticaria (duration longer than 6 weeks) both with and without hypocomplementemia. Hypersensitivity to potassium iodide and congenital deficiency of Clq, C2, and C3 have also been associated with hypocomplementemic vasculitis. Urticaria tends to be recurrent and troublesome, but systemic manifestations are generally not serious.

Serum sickness[61,65] is a prototype for immune complex-mediated diseases and the syndrome closely resembles animal models. Exposure to heterologous serum or certain drugs leads to fever, arthralgia, urticaria, lymphadenopathy and occasionally mild glomerulonephritis and polyneuropathy. The time course is characteristic, with onset 7 to 10 days after initial injection (or after 1 to 4 days if there has been previous exposure to the antigen). Resolution of symptoms takes place within 2 weeks of discontinuing the antigen. Because the manifestations are transient, symptomatic treatment with antihistamines and nonsteroidal anti-inflammatory agents may be sufficient. Rarely, corticosteroids are necessary to relieve severe symptoms.

Henoch-Schönlein purpura (anaphylactoid purpura) (HSP)[109–115] is an acute transient LCV with characteristic features. Most cases occur in children between 2 and 10 years of age although infants and adults are sometimes affected.[100] There is an increased incidence during spring and often a preceding viral illness. Fever, palpable purpura, arthritis, abdominal pain, and mild glomerulonephritis are classically seen. Kidney involvement is usually manifested by mild hematuria, but can rarely lead to progressive glomerulonephritis and renal failure. Persisting heavy proteinuria and severe glomerular changes most accurately predict renal failure.[111] Rarely, gastrointestinal involvement can be severe with intussusception in children, gastrointestinal hemorrhage, infarction, perforation, stricture and pancreatitis. While abdominal pain occurs in 42% to 58% of patients with HSP, significant surgical lesions occur in only 2% to 6%, and are unlikely to occur prior to the cutaneous rash.[112] Neurological complications are rarely seen. Headaches and mental status changes are most frequent, followed by seizures, focal neurological deficits, mononeuropathies and polyneuropathies.[113] As in LCV, the pathogenesis appears to involve immune complex deposition. Immunoglobulin A (IgA) is elevated in about half of cases, and IgA and complement can be identified in kidney and blood vessel walls. An abnormal IgA immune response to respiratory or gastrointestinal antigens has been postulated. It has been shown that there is a selective increase in the number of circulating IgA producing lymphocytes during disease activity suggesting a pathogenic role of this immunoglobulin.[114] Most cases spontaneously resolve and treatment is supportive. In a few cases, corticosteroids have been helpful for severe arthritis or for gastrointestinal involvement; however, progressive renal disease does not appear to respond well and other treatment such as cytotoxic agents may need to be considered.

Essential mixed cryoglobulinemia.[116–122] The finding of mixed cryoglobulinemia in patients without lymphoproliferative, collagen vascular, or chronic infectious disease has been called essential mixed cryoglobulinemia. However, in many cases hepatitis C virus has been implicated[32] and it may take up to 10 years before an underlying malignancy or autoimmune disease manifests itself. The average age of onset is about 50 years and there is a 2:3 female predominance. The disease is characterized by cutaneous LCV (palpable purpura), arthralgia-arthritis, variable renal manifestations (usually glomerulonephritis), a high incidence of asymptomatic hepatic involvement, and less commonly, vasculitis of the gastrointestinal tract, peripheral nerves, CNS, lungs, and heart. Along with the mixed cryoglobulins, elevations in immunoglobulin, rheumatoid factor, and ESR, as well as depression of complement components are often found. The disease tends to be chronic and recurrent. Treatment is symptomatic unless severe cutaneous, renal, neurologicAL, or vascular insufficiency to a major organ occurs. The most effective therapy is that which is directed toward the underlying etiology; treatment of hepatitis C with interferon-α may induce remissions of associated cryoglobulinemia.[123]

Plasmapheresis or cryoglobulin-apheresis have been successful. Steroids and cytotoxic agents have sometimes been of benefit.

Polyarteritis Nodosa

PAN is a necrotizing vasculitis of small and medium size muscular arteries. It can present in a multitude of ways depending on the number and extent of organ systems involved, and diagnosis can be difficult and delayed.[124] Cytotoxic agents have markedly improved the outlook of this disease,[125,126] but it is essential to diagnose PAN before major irreversible organ dysfunction occurs.

In autopsy series there is generally a higher incidence of renal, cardiac, and gastrointestinal involvement than in clinical studies (Table 7), reflecting the poorer prognosis when these organs are affected. As opposed to allergic granulomatosis, the lungs are generally spared except for bronchial artery involvement.

Small- and medium-sized muscular arteries are segmentally involved, primarily at bifurcations and branching points, especially where a smaller vessel takes off.[124] Aneurysms are often seen and granulomas may occur (6%). Veins and arterioles are spared.

Four histological stages in the evolution of PAN lesions have been described[124]: (1) degenerative stage with degeneration of the media; (2) acute inflammatory stage with primarily polymorphonuclear infiltration of the vessel wall, destruction of the media and elastica, and sometimes aneurysm formation; (3) granulation stage with proliferation of fibroblasts and replacement of the vessel wall by granulation tissue associated with

Table 7
Organ Involvement in PAN*

Organ	Autopsy	Clinical
	% Involvement in PAN*	
Kidney	85	71
Heart	76	19
GI tract	51	27
Skeletal muscle	39	53
Peripheral nerves	27	10
CNS	19	37
Skin	20	53
Testes	19	
Liver	66	

* Polyarteritis nodosa.

marked intimal proliferation; and (4) healed scar tissue stage. Lesions in all stages of evolution can be seen. Clinically, the first stage is generally latent and without symptoms, the second stage is associated with organ ischemia and rarely with rupture of aneurysms, the third stage has further vascular occlusion with anemia and marked constitutional symptoms, and the fourth stage generally has organ dysfunction remaining from previous vascular occlusion.

Subclinical vasculitis involving cerebral and coronary vessels, as well as corticosteroid usage, is believed to predispose to subsequent atherosclerosis with late cerebrovascular accidents and myocardial infarctions.[127] The incidence is not known, but PAN is an uncommon disorder with the number of reported cases at large referral centers being 2.9 to 8.8 cases per year.[125,127,128] Males (1.7 to 1, male to female ratio) between 40 and 60 years of age are most often affected,[125–128] but it can be found in females and in any age group.

Constitutional symptoms, abdominal pain, musculoskeletal discomfort, and peripheral neuropathy are common initial symptoms.[129,130] The distribution and severity of the vasculitis are highly variable, resulting in a multitude of clinical presentations.

Kidney involvement is frequent and often asymptomatic. Vasculitis of the arcuate and interlobular arteries, infarcts, and glomerulonephritis are commonly found. Abnormal urine findings such as proteinuria, hematuria, and casts are nearly always found when renal vasculitis occurs.[131] Hypertension is common. Refractory secondary hyper-reninemic, hyper-aldosteronemic hypertension has been described.[132] Hemorrhage from a ruptured aneurysm leading to a perinephric hematoma can rarely occur.[133]

Involvement of the nervous system is common, clinically easy to detect, and plays a major role in the diagnosis of PAN. Peripheral neuropathy tends to occur early and may be the presenting symptom. It can present as single or extensive mononeuritis (multiplex), small patches of hypesthesia in the distribution of small cutaneous nerves, or as a distal polyneuropathy.[134] Up to 40% in one series had no sural nerve conduction and were found to have vasculitis on biopsy, despite the absence of neuropathy on examination.[135] The CNS Tends to be affected late or as part of a widely disseminated vasculitis.[136] Findings range from headaches, blurred vision, seizure (only during acute disease), cranial nerve palsy, hemiparesis, cerebellar ataxia, toxic psychosis, and meningoencephalitis.[134,136] Spinal fluid sometimes contains a mild increase in protein. Electroencephalogram (EEG), computed axial tomography (CAT) scan, and brain scan are not diagnostic. Magnetic resonance imaging (MRI) was shown to be a sensitive method for detecting brain lesions but is not specific for PAN.[137] CNS findings in many instances may represent late vascular changes exacerbated by hypertension and corticosteroid therapy rather than active inflammation.[134]

Musculoskeletal involvement tends to be mild with myalgias, arthralgias, and a nonerosive, oligoarticular arthritis, but a destructive arthritis has been reported.[138] Vasculitis has been found in biopsies of skeletal muscles.[128]

A wide array of cutaneous findings have been described, most commonly a nonspecific maculopapular, purpuric, urticarial, or petechial rash.[139] The presence of either a characteristic painful nodular lesion, ulceration, or livedo reticularis suggest medium size vessel involvement. Pruritus, Raynaud's phenomenon, nail fold, and digital pulp lesions, splinter hemorrhages, gangrene, and ecchymosis are uncommon findings.[128,139–141] A benign form of PAN that involves primarily the skin has been described.[128,141]

Any portion of the gastrointestinal tract can be involved. Nonspecific abdominal pain, weight loss, anorexia, vomiting, and abdominal distention are common.[142] Hepatomegaly, elevated liver enzymes, gastrointestinal and intra-abdominal hemorrhage, ulcers, infarction, perforation of bowel, peritonitis, pancreatitis, and localized involvement of the appendix or gallbladder are seen,[125–128,130,140–143] An acute abdominal catastrophe requiring surgical intervention may rarely occur[125,130,140,142,143] and carries a high mortality rate. Spontaneous splenic rupture in PAN Has been reported.[144]

Cardiac involvement is associated with a poorer prognosis. Congestive heart failure, atrial arrhythmias, conduction defects, pericarditis, and myocardial infarctions can be seen.[129,132,133]

Respiratory involvement may present clinically with asthma, nonspecific dyspnea, hemoptysis or be asymptomatic. In a report of 17 patients, alveolar shadowings were seen in 6, and pulmonary function tests performed on 7 patients showed airway obstruction in 5 and diffusion abnormalities in 3. No consistent relation between asthma, pulmonary infiltrates, ear, nose, and throat symptoms, and eosinophilia was observed.[140] Other areas of involvement include the eye, ear, breast, epididymis, and testis. Several disease conditions are associated with PAN (Table 8).

Results of laboratory tests reflect systemic inflammation or immune complex disorder, and end organ involvement. There is leukocytosis, anemia and, in around 90%, an elevated ESR.[125,127,128,135] Immune complexes, cryoglobulin, rheumatoid factor, low-titer ANA, and depressed complement levels are sometimes found.[127,135,140]

Involvement of the upper extremities is nearly always associated with disease elsewhere. Cutaneous findings as described above are more common on the lower extremities. Peripheral neuropathy often affects the upper extremities. Patients may suddenly develop a wrist drop. Vascular occlusion with gangrene and ulcers can occur (Figure 2). PAN involving

---

Table 8
Conditions Associated with Polyarteritis Nodosa*

Infections
　　Hepatitis B virus
　　Streptococcal infection (including rheumatic fever)
　　Endocarditis
　　Acute serous otitis media
　　Cytomegolovirus
　　Trichinosis
Collagen Vascular Diseases
　　Systemic lupus erythematosus
　　Rheumatoid arthritis
　　Relapsing polychondritis
　　Scleroderma (progressive systemic sclerosis)
　　Dermatomyositis
　　Giant cell arteritis
　　Sjogren's syndrome
　　Leukocytoclastic vasculitis
Drugs
　　Sulfonamides
　　Amphetamine drug abuse
　　Allergic hyposensitization therapy
Miscellaneous
　　Essential mixed cryoglobulinemia
　　Cogan's syndrome
　　Enteritis
　　Hairy cell leukemia
　　Mesenteric arteritis following surgical repair of aortic coarctation

---

* Adapted from Cupps TR, Fauci AS: Necrotizing vasculitis of the polyarteritis nodosa group: The Vasculitides. In: *Major Problems in Internal Medicine*, Vol. 21, p 37, Smith LH Jr (ed), W. G. Saunders Co. Philadelphia, 1981.

the lower extremities with periosteal new bone formation has been described.[145]

Diagnosis of PAN is made by the finding of vasculitis of small to medium sized vessels on biopsy or angiographic demonstration of microaneurysms. Biopsy of involved skin, sural nerve (with abnormal nerve conduction), muscle, testes, and viscera will usually show vasculitis. Blind biopsies of uninvolved areas are generally unrewarding,[128,140] although it has been suggested that early renal biopsy may lead to early diagnosis of PAN.[146] Angiograms of renal, hepatic, and mesenteric arteries may show characteristic microaneurysms. However, angiographically similar lesions have rarely been described in Wegener's granulomatosis, SLE, mucocutaneous lymph node syndrome, atrial myxoma, bacterial endocarditis (mycotic aneurysms) and although not quite similar, fibromuscular

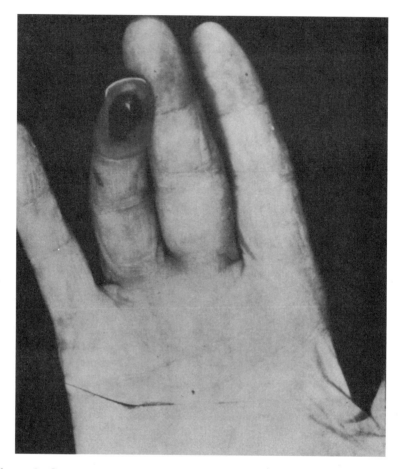

Figure 2. Gangrene and cyanosis of finger tips seen with polyarteritis nodosa. Similar-appearing lesions can be seen with any digital artery occlusive disese.

dysplasia and pseudoxanthoma elasticum.[140] In PAN, microaneurysms can be found in the absence of clinical involvement of the kidneys.[140]

It cannot be overemphasized that treatment must be started before significant organ damage has occurred. Treatment, although markedly improving the overall prognosis, cannot vitalize infarcted tissue. The 5-year survival without treatment is about 13%,[125,128] with corticosteroids about 50%,[125,127,128] and with cytotoxic agents 80%.[125] Kidney and gastro-intestinal vasculitis are associated with a poorer prognosis.[127] Cutaneous PAN does not require intense treatment to bring about remission. Topical steroids, colchicine, dapsone or moderate oral corticosteroids therapy for 3 to 6 months may induce a remission.[141]

Cyclophosphamide[147] and azathioprine[125] are the primary cytotoxic agents utilized. Remission in advanced PAN[147] and improvement of renal and neurological deficits[134] have occurred with the use of these agents.

Microscopic Polyangiitis

Recent studies[148] favor the recognition of a distinct form of systemic vasculitis called MPA. MPA is characterized histologically by necrotizing involvement of small sized vessels including capillaries, venules and arterioles and the absence of granulomata. Controversy exists as to whether MPA is a subset of PAN[149] versus a distinct entity.[150] Clinically MPA is distinctively characterized by rapidly progressive glomerulonephritis, pulmonary alveolar hemorrhage and a relapsing and remitting course.[148] The perinuclear pattern of the antineutrophil cytoplasmic antibody (P-ANCA) has been associated with MPA up to 80% of cases.

Allergic Granulomatosis and Angiitis

The triad of eosinophilia, asthma, and systemic necrotizing vasculitis was identified as a separate entity by Churg and Strauss in 1951.[151,152] Allergic granulomatosis and angiitis (AGA) is considered to be of the PAN group of vasculitides and occupies one end of the spectrum of PAN to overlap syndromes with AGA.[3]

The pathological findings can be divided into vasculitis and lesions of extravascular tissue.[151] The vasculitis involves medium and small arteries in a manner similar to PAN but, in addition, there is an intense eosinophilic infiltrate, multinucleated giant cells, and involvement of small and medium sized veins.[151,153] The characteristic extravascular lesion is the granulomatous nodule. It is generally less than 1 mm in size and consists of a central eosinophilic core of necrotic cells and degenerating collagen fibers surrounded by radially arranged macrophages and giant cells.[151] Nodules have been found in the heart, lung, kidney, gastrointestinal tract, liver, spleen, genitourinary tract, and skin.[151,153] This fibrinoid eosinophilic granulomatous nodule differs from the more coagulative or liquefactive epithelioid granuloma of Wegener's granulomatosis.[153] Immunochemical studies on tissue obtained from a patient who died of Churg-Strauss syndrome showed large amounts of eosinophilic cationic protein and eosinophil protein "X" in the granulomata. Eosinophil cationic proteins are thought to be involved in the development of lesions in AGA.[154,155]

AGA affects patients of any age, with the average age being in the 40s.[151,153] Males predominated in one study[153] and females in another.[151]

Fever, weight loss, and fatigue commonly occur. The organ involvement is similar to PAN except for less frequent and less severe kidney, and increased upper and lower respiratory tract involvement.[151,153] Asthma occurs in nearly all cases. A short duration of asthma prior to the onset of vasculitis is considered a poor prognostic sign.[153] Asthma usually abates when the vasculitis appears. The chest x-ray is often normal. When infiltrates occur, they range from a transient patchy pneumonitis to, less commonly, bilateral noncavitating nodules or diffuse interstitial disease.[153] The absence of asthma does not exclude the diagnosis of AGA.[156]

Nasal manifestations are common and include a history of allergy with nasal obstruction and rhinorrhea, nasal polyps, nasal crusting, sinusitis, and rarely perforation.[157] Differentiation from Wegener's granulomatosis, polymorphic reticulosis (midline granuloma), and infectious rhinitis may be difficult.

Ocular manifestations are rare. They include conjunctival nodules, episcleritis, marginal corneal ulceration, panuveitis, and ischemic retinopathy with amaurosis fugax.[158,159]

Cutaneous features are the most common manifestations in the upper extremity. Three kinds of lesions can be found: (1) an erythematous maculopapular lesion resembling erythema multiforme; (2) hemorrhagic lesions from petechiae to ecchymoses, sometimes with necrosis or urticarial wheals; and (3) subcutaneous and cutaneous tender nodules which are usually multiple and of symmetric distribution.[160] Only the nodules are characteristic of AGA, but they also have been described in Wegener's granulomatosis, bacterial endocarditis, SLE, and RA. In these cases, however, there was no eosinophilic infiltrate.[160] This AGA nodule can be confused with granuloma annulare, rheumatoid nodules, erythema elevatum, diutinum, xanthoma, abscess, pyoderma gangrenosum, and chronic infectious granulomas.[160] Cutaneous infarcts, ulcers, peripheral neuropathy, and arthritis can also be found.[151,153,160] Other organ involvement includes the thymus,[156] prostate,[161] kidney, CNS, and heart.[162]

Leukocytosis with eosinophilia (up to 29,000), anemia, and an elevated ESR occur in nearly all patients. The eosinophil count and ESR appear to correlate with disease activity.[151,157] Elevated IgE, rheumatoid factor, and circulating immune complexes have been found in a few cases.[153,163]

Characterization of cellular immunity in Churg-Strauss syndrome has been done in one patient and a low proportion of suppressor/cytotoxic lymphocytes and a high helper/suppressor ratio were seen throughout the course of the disease. Hyperimmunoglobulinemia and immune complexes were present. With therapy immunoglobulin levels and circulating immune complex levels decreased.[164]

AGA must be differentiated from: (1) granulomatous diseases: Wegener's granulomatosis, midline granuloma (polymorphic reticulosis), infection (fungal, tuberculosis, syphilis, leprosy), eosinophilic granuloma, bronchocentric granuloma, necrotizing sarcoid-like granuloma; (2) vasculitides: PAN, HSP, drug-induced vasculitis; and (3) eosinophilic disorders: hypereosinophilic syndromes, chronic eosinophilic pneumonia, allergic bronchopulmonary aspergillosis, and hypersensitivity pneumonitis.

Similar to PAN, the use of corticosteroids has increased the 5-year survival from less than 10%[151] to 62%.[153] When administered, a prompt improvement generally results. Pulse methylprednisolone has been tried in a patient who had not responded to high doses of prednisone. After four doses of methylprednisolone 1 gm daily, there was dramatic clearing of the pulmonary infiltrate.[165] Immunosuppressive agents, such as cyclophosphamide or azathioprine, are probably as effective in AGA as they are in PAN, but experience is limited.[126,163,166,167] Local treatment of nasal manifestations is useful.[157]

Wegener's Granulomatosis

Wegener's granulomatosis is a necrotizing granulomatosis vasculitis of small arteries and veins, classically with involvement of the lungs, upper respiratory tract, and kidneys.[168–170] A limited form sparing the kidneys has also been recognized.[171] Wegener's granulomatosis can affect any age group, with the mean age about 40 years. Presenting symptoms are usually referable to the upper respiratory tract, and include rhinorrhea, sinusitis, otitis media, nasal and oral ulcerations, and hearing loss. A few patients present with cough, chest pain, and hemoptysis. Constitutional symptoms such as fever, malaise, fatigue, anorexia, and weight loss are common.

The lungs[168,172] are involved in over 95% of cases, but only about one-third have symptoms. The chest roentgenogram is abnormal with a nodular infiltrate being most common. Nodules are usually 1 to 9 cm in size, may cavitate, may be unilateral or bilateral, single or multiple, may be fleeting, and may wax and wane without relevance to the overall disease course. Hilar adenopathy is rare. Pleural involvement can occur. Respiratory involvement may occur late. The patient may present with severe glomerulonephritis and the proper diagnosis may be missed for several years.[173]

The upper respiratory tract[168] is involved in 90% of cases, and includes findings of sinusitis, mucosal ulceration, nasal perforation, and saddle nose deformity. Secondary bacterial infections, especially with *Staphylococcus aureus*, can occur. Kidney involvement[168,169,172] can be found in 85%, with an abnormal urine sediment the most common finding. Hypertension is unusual. Renal biopsy may demonstrate focal segmental glomerulonephritis or other glomerular lesions, including diffuse proliferative glomerulonephritis with crescents. Renal vasculitis, renal artery aneurysm, granuloma, and interstitial nephritis are uncommonly found. Inapparent renal disease is common and 50% of biopsies may show glomerulonephritis in the absence of clinically detectable renal disease. Urologic manifestations can include ureteral infiltration with obstruction, prostatic involvement, penile involvement with necrosis, and involvement of the testes.[174,175]

Joint pain[168,169] tends to be polyarticular and is common. The skin[176,177] is involved in 40% to 50% of cases; the manifestations are highly variable and include necrotizing vasculitis, palisading granuloma (Churg-Strauss granuloma), granulomatous vasculitis, vesicles, pustules, petechiae, ecchymoses, and pyoderma gangrenosum. Ulcerative and papular lesions are the most common type of skin involvement after changes associated with terminal uremia are excluded. Skin involvement may precede other evidence of disease by months.

In about half of cases the eyes[168,169] are affected with a necrotizing vasculitis that may manifest as keratoconjunctivitis, scleritis, episcleritis, proptosis, vasculitis of the optic nerve, uveitis, corneal degeneration, lacrimal duct occlusion, retinal artery occlusion, or scleromalacia perforans. Serous otitis media from blockage of the eustachian tube occurs in about a third of cases. Purulent otitis media may develop secondarily. Granulomatous otitis may also occasionally occur.

Cardiac[168,169] involvement occurs less often; pericarditis, coronary vasculitis, endocardial and valvular lesions, and pancarditis have been described. Peripheral neuropathy and granulomatous vasculitis involving the brain and cranial nerves as well as a diffuse cerebritis can be seen.[178]

Upper extremity involvement is uncommon and limited to cutaneous, joint, and peripheral nerve manifestations.

Laboratory tests, although not diagnostic, are helpful. The cytoplasmic pattern of C-ANCA has been detected in sera of these patients and the antibody titer seems to correlate with disease activity. The ESR rate is elevated, often greater than 100 mm/h, and generally correlates with the activity of the disease. Often there is an increase in leukocyte and platelet counts, immunoglobulins, and rheumatoid factor (60%). Proteinuria or hematuria is present in 80% of cases. The chest x-ray is almost invariably abnormal.[168,170,172] Sinus films often show pansinusitis, and sinus tomograms may help delineate erosions. CT scans may be helpful in evaluating ocular, orbital, or cerebral involvement.[179] Renal angiogram may show aneurysms.[179]

Diagnosis is based on finding the characteristic histological picture on biopsy. Open lung biopsy has the greatest chance of making the diagnosis. Kidney biopsy generally demonstrates glomerulonephritis, but in the absence of vasculitis can only be suggestive of Wegener's granulomatosis, although, the presence of glomerulonephritis helps rule out other entities such as lymphomatoid granulomatosis and midline granuloma (polymorphic reticulosis). Biopsy of the upper respiratory tract may be helpful if granulomatous vasculitis is found. The differential diagnosis is long and includes other vasculitides, infections, neoplasms, granulomatosis diseases, and Goodpasture's syndrome (Table 9).

Before cytotoxic agents the prognosis was uniformly dismal with a mean survival of 5 months from diagnosis. Only 10% of patients were alive after 2 years.[180] With cytotoxic therapy up to 93% of patients have been reported to achieve complete remission.[169,170,180,181] Cyclophosphamide in a dose of 1 to 4 mg/kg per day, depending on the severity of the manifestations, along with prednisone 1 mg/kg per day, is the usual initial

Table 9
Differential Diagnosis of Wegener's Granulomatosis

Vasculitis—Necrotizing
  Polyarteritis nodosa
  Systemic lupus erythematosus
  Scleroderma
  Dermatomyositis
  Sjogren's syndrome
  Leucocytoclastic vasculitis
Infections
  Tuberculosis
  Histoplasmosis
  Blastomycosis
  Coccidiomycosis
  Syphilis
  Leprosy
  Streptococcus pneumonia
  Parasitic
Neoplastic
  Nasopharyngeal carcinoma
  Primary and metastatic lung cancer
  Lymphoma
  Sarcoma
Granulomatous Diseases
  Sarcoidosis
  Berylliosis
Vasculitis—Granulomatous
  Churg-Strauss
  Lymphomatoid granulomatosis
  Midline granuloma
  Granulomatous angiitis of the CNS
Miscellaneous
  Goodpasture's syndrome

treatment.[169] Some patients are responsive to a less toxic regimen of monthly pulse cyclophosphamide. Corticosteroids are tapered after the disease is under control and cyclophosphamide is generally continued in tapering doses until the patient has been in complete remission for at least 1 year. Local care and prevention of infection are important in the management of sinusitis and otitis. Renal involvement usually responds to medical therapy, but if necessary has been treated with dialysis[182] and kidney transplant has been successful.[183] Unfortunately despite the initial success with cyclophosphamide, approximately 50% of Wegener's granulomatosis patients will relapse within 5 years, thus much attention has been focused on devising relatively nontoxic therapies to prevent relapse. Data has been reported supporting the use of either trimethoprim-sulfamethoxazole[184] or methotrexate[185] in preventing Wegener's granulomatosis disease relapse.

Large Vessel Vasculitis

Large vessel vasculitis is seen primarily in TA, temporal arteritis and in association with certain rheumatic diseases, notably, the seronegative spondyloarthropathies (ankylosing spondylitis, Reiter's disease, ulcerative colitis, psoriasis), relapsing polychondritis, Behcet's disease, and Cogan's syndrome. Isolated cases have also been described in association with RA,[186] SLE,[187] and scleroderma.[188] These vasculitides must be distinguished from the aortitis seen with syphilis, mycotic aneurysms, or rheumatic fever.[189] Upper extremity involvement is seen more frequently in the primary vasculitides than in the aortitis associated with the rheumatic diseases.

Takayasu's Arteritis

TA is an inflammatory and stenosing vasculitis of large and intermediate sized arteries. It and temporal arteritis are sometimes classified together as GCA because of similar histological findings, but each has distinct clinical features (Table 10).

TA affects females in more than 9 of 10 cases. The majority have onset of symptoms between the ages of 10 and 30 years. It has a worldwide distribution[190] and is the likely cause of acquired coarctation of the aorta.[191] The etiology is not known. Anti-aorta antibodies have been described.[192] TA appears to be associated with an immune response gene in the D locus.[193]

The clinical manifestations have been divided into an early systemic (prepulseless) stage and a late occlusive (pulseless) stage.[194–197] The sys-

Table 10
Giant Cell Vasculitides*

	Takayasu's Arteritis	Temporal Arteritis
Age of onset	10–30 years	50–70 years
Sex	90% females	54%–79% females
Clinical features	Early systemic phase,	Constitutional manifestations,
	Late occusive phase	Localized areas of ischemia, Association with polymyalgia rheumatica
Vessel involvement	Aorta and its major branches, Pulmonary arteries, stenosis and/or dilatation, Dissections rare	Medium to large sized vessels especially temporal artery, A systemic arteritis, Aortitis similar to Takayasu's arteritis may rarely occur
Histology	Panarteritis with mononuclear cell infiltrate, Some giant cells, Intimal proliferation, Fibrosis, Calcification	Panarteritis with mononuclear cell infiltrate, Frequent giant cells, Intimal proliferation, Fragmentation of the internal elastic lamina
Major complications	Cerebrovascular accident, Myocardial infarction	Ocular involvement (blindness)
Diagnosis	Arteriography, Biopsy	Biopsy of any involved vessel, usually temporal artery
Treatment	Corticosteroids may help the acute stage	Excellent response to corticosteroids

* Adapted from Fauci AS, Haynes BF, Katz P: The spectrum of vasculitis: Clinical, pathologic, immunologic, and therapeutic considerations. *Ann Intern Med* 89:660—676, 1978.

temic phase can be identified in one-half to two-thirds of cases and consists of (1) constitutional symptoms (fever, anorexia, weight loss, night sweats); (2) a variety of nonspecific symptoms (arthralgias, myalgias, skin rash, pleuritis, pericarditis, cough); and (3) sometimes transient evidence for local circulatory deficits (dizziness, syncope, claudication, angina, and hypertension). Local pain over an artery has been noted in up to a third of cases. This stage lasts several weeks, then resolves. It may be followed immediately or after a latent, silent period lasting as long as several decades, by the chronic occlusive arteritis of the pulseless phase. The differentiation of the early and late phases of TA is not always clear-cut. Patients with symptoms of the early phase of TA coexisting with complications of the late phase have been described.[198]

The occlusive arteritis characteristically involves the aorta, the branches of the aortic arch, and the pulmonary arteries. The distribution of involvement has been classified into four types.[199] Type I: localized to the aortic arch and its branches; type II: localized to the descending thoracic and abdominal aorta; type III: combined features of type I and II; and type IV: involvement of the pulmonary artery. In a retrospective analysis of 50 Japanese patients who underwent total aortography, 86% had panaortitis. Twenty-one pulmonary arteriograms were done; 86% showed abnormalities.[200] Clinical features are related to the specific artery involved and include: absent pulses (especially radial, ulnar, and carotid), tenderness over arteries, bruits, claudication, systemic hypertension from decreased renal perfusion, ocular involvement (retinal arteriovenous anastomosis), CNS ischemia (syncope, cerebrovascular accident), cardiac (palpitations, angina, congestive heart failure, myocardial infarction, aortic insufficiency, pericarditis), and pulmonary hypertension.

Upper extremity involvement is characterized by diminished or absent pulses, claudication, and rarely Raynaud's phenomenon. Gangrene is very rare because the gradual onset of occlusion permits the formation of adequate collateral circulation.[201]

TA has also been described to be associated with interstitial lung disease,[202] glomerulonephritis,[202,203] and erosive arthritis.[204]

Laboratory tests[195] often show moderate leukocytosis and slight normochromic normocytic anemia. The ESR is usually elevated during the acute phase and tends to return to normal during the chronic phase. In some studies it has been useful as an index of disease activity and as a guide for adjusting steroid dosage.[205] Immunoglobulins are often elevated. Plain x-rays may show changes suggestive of aneurysmal dilatation. Aortography[206] reveals the coarctation, occlusion, and aneurysmal dilatation of the chronic phase (Figure 3). Stenosing aortitis is considered unique to TA. Doppler studies and ophthalmodynamometry to assess flow, and echocardiogram to record dilatation of the aortic root are sometimes helpful. Intravenous digital subtraction angiography has been shown to have certain advantages over conventional angiography as it gives an overview of the entire cardiovascular system using 120 to 150 mL of contrast media, is safer, less invasive, requires less skill, is rapidly performed and more cost effective. However it has drawbacks, ie, coronary ostial stenosis and aortic regurgitation may not be adequately visualized, bowel gas may obscure renal lesions, patient breathing or motion causes artifacts, and it is difficult to assess thickening versus calcification in the aortic wall. It may show reduced density of opacification and less fine detail of arteries and caution must be exercised when giving this

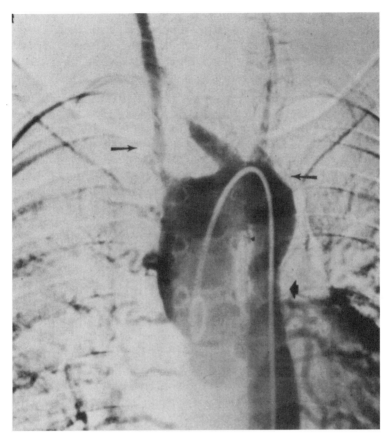

Figure 3. Aortography in Takayasu's aortitis. Characteristic stenoses involving the aorta and major aortic branches can be seen.

amount of dye to patients with impaired cardiac or renal failure.[207] MRI is thought to be inadequate as a screening examination at this time although magnetic resonance angiography (MRA) techniques are being developed.

Pathologically there is periarteritis with mononuclear and GCA (less abundant than temporal arteritis) infiltrate, intimal proliferation, fibrosis, and calcification which may be both dystrophic and secondary to atherosclerotic changes. Aneurysmal dilatation or constriction of arteries is common. Dissection is rare.

The survival rate 5 years after an established diagnosis of TA is about 83%.[196] Treatment with steroids during the active stage is usually helpful.[195] Prevention of stenosis or aneurysms with prolonged steroid therapy has been found in a few studies.[196,205] Cyclophosphamide has been used together with steroids with good effect.[208] Vascular surgery should not be performed during periods of active inflammation, but is of benefit in selected cases, especially those with hypertension secondary to aortic and renal lesions.[209] Success with renal artery reconstruction is limited,[194] but good results have been reported with aortic valve replacement,[210] coronary artery bypass,[211] and aortic arch bypass.[212] For cases with severe ischemia of the upper extremity, modified bypass procedures have been done. These include subclavian-subclavian, axilla-axillary, and femora-axillary bypass using autogenous vein or Dacron graft. Excision and graft replacement is always indicated for aneurysm, for fear of rupture.[213] Percutaneous transluminal balloon angioplasty of the aorta and renal arteries has been done successfully.[214, 215] Medical management of hypertension, congestive heart failure, and renal insufficiency is important. Captopril, a converting enzyme inhibitor has been shown to be very useful for hypertension and congestive cardiac failure.[216] Use of aspirin or other methods of anticoagulation has not been helpful.

Temporal Arteritis

Temporal arteritis or GCA is a systemic segmental granulomatous panarteritis involving large to medium size arteries with a propensity for extracranial and aortic arch involvement.[217–219] It has a tendency to affect arteries with abundant elastica.[220,221] Characteristic clinical features combined with biopsy findings distinguish temporal arteritis from other vasculitides (Table 10).

The etiology and pathogenesis are not known and although immunologic mechanisms appear to be important,[222–225] findings have not been consistent.[226] Excessive solar or other actinic radiation have been proposed to be risk factors for vascular accidents in temporal arteritis.[227] HLA-DRB1 genes may represent an important risk factor in the development of GCA.[193]

The incidence of temporal arteritis is between 11.7 to 16.8 cases per 100,000 persons 50 years or older[228, 229] with a prevalence of 133 cases per 100,000 persons in the same age category.[228] One study of patients over age 65 years showed a prevalence of 33 of 1000 and incidence of 4 of 1000.[230] Nearly all cases occur in patients over 50 years old with an average age of 69 or 70.[228, 229, 231–234] Temporal arteritis has been uncommonly found in 40 to 50 year olds and rarely in pediatric patients.[217, 235] In the younger age group, TA is more likely. Females are affected in 54% to 79% of cases[217,219,228,231–233] and Caucasians are nearly exclusively afflicted.[236] Familial associations have been described, but are rare.[237]

The clinical manifestations can be divided into constitutional (systemic) and specific (localized) findings. Specific symptoms are related to the area of arterial involvement and are more likely to lead to a correct early diagnosis. Constitutional findings include: headache (in up to 97% of cases; usually of recent onset or with a change in character), fever (21% to 80%; up to 103°F reported), polymyalgia rheumatica (30% to 50%), weight loss, anorexia, malaise, depression, myalgias, and arthralgias.[217,228,231,237–239]

A multitude of specific or localized findings have been reported in temporal arteritis. The most striking is ophthalmic involvement which has been reported in 5% to 57% of cases[217,228,232,240] with blurring of vision, diplopia, or transient to permanent loss of vision. Arteritis of the posterior ciliary artery with ischemic optic neuritis is the most common cause of blindness.[217] Once ocular damage (blindness) has occurred, it is usually permanent.[239,240] Claudication commonly involves the jaw (20% to 67%) or a lower extremity (5% to 8%).[217,228,241,242] Facial neuralgia and vertigo can be seen.[217] Other areas of involvement are less common, but should be considered as possibly temporal arteritis in an elderly Caucasian patient with an elevated ESR. Liver involvement with elevated alkaline phosphatase and transaminase is common, but reported cases of hepatic necrosis,[243] hepatic artery vasculitis,[244] or granulomatosis hepatitis[245] are rare. CNS involvement with seizures, hemiparesis, brain stem ischemia, and subarachnoid hemorrhage can be found and usually are due to carotid or vertebral artery involvement.[217,246] Gangrene of the scalp[247–249] and tongue claudication, Raynaud's phenomenon or infarction[241,247,249,250] have been reported. Other areas of involvement include the aorta,[217,231] peripheral nerves,[251] gallbladder,[238] mesentery often with PAN,[239,252] and heart.[252,253]

Temporal arteritis is closely related to polymyalgia rheumatica (PMR) although the exact nature of this relation is not known.[254] PMR can be found in 30% to 50% of patients with temporal arteritis and temporal arteritis can occur in 15% to 80% of patients with PMR.[217,228,233] PMR is characterized by often symmetric proximal muscle pain, joint pain, morning stiffness, constitutional symptoms such as fever, malaise, anorexia and weight loss, elevated ESR, the absence of another rheumatic condition, and a prompt and dramatic response to corticosteroids.[212, 231] Symptoms of PMR are probably related to a low-grade synovitis[255] and not to muscle involvement.[256] Biopsy of the temporal artery has shown arteritis in the absence of symptoms of temporal arteritis in up to 40% to 50%.[228,231,256] Serious ophthalmic artery involvement has occurred in patients on low-dose corticosteroid treatment for PMR.[238,257,258] The PMR-temporal arteritis complex can often mimic other diseases, and present as a malignancy,[232,259] fever of unknown cause,[217,228,232,259,260] anemia,[228,232,259] neuropathy,[232,239]psychiatric problems,[217] and claudication.[232, 261, 262]

Aortic arch involvement with temporal arteritis can be seen in 7% to 15% of cases.[218,228,262,263] In a large autopsy series, 0.4% of over 20,000 postmortem examinations revealed aortic involvement with GCA.[264] Involvement of the aortic arch by temporal and TA is similar, with biopsies in both[262] showing GCA. Differentiation is usually made by demographic features, temporal artery involvement which rarely occurs in TA, and the fact that TA usually leads to stenosis rather than aneurysms formation (Table 10).

Temporal arteritis can affect the upper extremity by isolated involvement of the axillary or brachial arteries,[234,261,263,265,266] or more commonly, as part of an aortic arch syndrome.[228,233,262,264,267–273] Findings include claudication, diminished or absent pulses, bruits, and Raynaud's phenomenon.

Claudication of the upper extremities can be unilateral or bilateral[262] and can involve the shoulders alone.[267] Symptoms are usually weakness and a tingling sensation with use of the arms, that is relieved by rest.[232,261,262,267,274] Diminished or absent pulses as well as asymmetric blood pressures can be found,[261,268,275] although normal pulses can be present despite significant proximal narrowing because of the formation of adequate collateral circulation. Bruits are common,[234,261] and have been noted in up to 57% of patients with temporal arteritis compared with 12% of controls.[234] Raynaud's phenomenon has been observed and is usually associated with aortic arch involvement.[267, 275] Gangrene of the upper extremity does not appear to occur. Even in the lower extremity where gangrene can rarely be found, it has been secondary to arteriosclerosis obliterans[262] or PAN.[248]

The most common laboratory abnormality is an elevated ESR,[217,228] although rare cases of a normal ESR with biopsy-proven temporal arteritis have been described at the time of diagnosis[276–278] or with relapse.[258] The finding of an elevated ESR without an obvious cause should make temporal arteritis a consideration. Other findings include a normochromic normocytic anemia[217, 219]; elevated immunoglobulins[217]; elevated acute phase reactants such as α_3 -globulin, fibrinogen, C-reactive protein, α_1-antitrypsin, orosomucoid, and haptoglobin[279]; and elevated liver enzymes especially the alkaline phosphatase.[219,225] The rheumatoid factor and ANA are normal.[219, 256] In general, the laboratory abnormalities correct with treatment,[228,243,275] and form the basis for monitoring therapy.

Angiograms of areas involved with temporal arteritis show long segments of smooth arterial stenosis in the absence of irregular plaques or ulcers,[262] however, these findings have been found to be diagnostically sensitive, but not specific in two studies[280,281] and not sensitive or specific in another.[282]

Biopsy of the temporal artery can provide definitive diagnosis of temporal arteritis. On pathological sections a panarteritis involving the whole thickness of the artery with inflammatory cells composed of histiocytes, lymphocytes, epithelioid cells mainly in the area of the internal elastic lamina, intimal proliferation, fragmented and duplicated internal elastic lamina, and occasionally fibrinoid necrosis can be seen.[217,220,221,283] The pathology is similar to TA.[283] Even with a normal temporal artery on physical examination, biopsy may be positive.[221,231,261,262,273,284–286] Other sites of involvement besides the temporal artery have included facial artery,[241,261] occipital artery,[261] prostate,[257] bone marrow,[287] and arteries supplying other areas noted in the clinical features section if localized symptoms are present. When biopsies of the temporal artery have been obtained, skip (segmental) lesions have been noted in 28% with foci as short as 333 μm, and in 4% biopsy was normal in one artery but abnormal in the contralateral artery.[288] Biopsy of the temporal artery should be several centimeters long with frequent sectioning and if negative on one side, the contralateral artery should be biopsied even if it is normal to physical examination. Corticosteroids can be started before biopsy is obtained. In a review of 76 patients with TA who developed tongue and scalp necrosis (after temporal artery biopsy) it was cautioned that this is a risk inherent in taking a biopsy under local anesthetic with a vasoconstrictor.[289]

Corticosteroids almost always produce improvement in symptoms within 4 to 72 hours[217,290] and correction of laboratory abnormalities in about 1 to 3 weeks.[231] Initial dosage is 40 to 60 mg daily followed by tapering after 1 to 4 weeks,[231] with maintenance dosage usually between 5 and 12.5 mg daily.[228,229,231] Alternate day administration of steroids does not adequately control disease, even after initial induction with daily corticosteroids, in 33% to 60% of cases.[291, 292] This may be tried, however, to prevent steroid side effects. Duration of therapy is usually at least 1 to 2 years.[217,228,231,265,293,294] A mean duration of 5.8 years (range 0 to 12.8 years) was reported in a series of 90 patients.[295] Therapy needs to be individualized.[273,293] In severe sight-threatening disease, pulse intravenous methylprednisolone 1 gm every 12 hours for 5 days has been used successfully.[296] Nonsteroidal anti-inflammatory agents may help the myalgias and arthralgias, but do not treat the arteritis and may mask the symptoms of active temporal arteritis, permitting the subsequent development of loss of vision.[297,298] Cyclophosphamide may be of benefit in cases refractory to steroids.[299] The use of methotrexate[300] has become popular in attempts to spare steroid dosage, although large controlled trials confirming its efficacy are lacking. In a controlled double-blind study involving 31 patients with GCA over 52 weeks, azathioprine was shown to have a steroid-sparing effect.[301] Dapsone has been reported to be useful.[302] Cyclosporin A was used effectively for a patient with GCA with reduction in dose of steroid required.[303] Surgical repair of aortic aneurysms[270,271] sometimes requiring aortic valve replacement,[271] and axillary artery reconstruction has been successful. In arm ischemia secondary to temporal arteritis, the response to steroids is usually adequate to eliminate the need for early surgical intervention.[304]

Vasculitis Associated with Rheumatic Diseases

A wide range of vessels from venules to medium size arteries to large arteries may develop vasculitis in rheumatic diseases. Involvement of venules to medium size arteries is most commonly seen in SLE and RA, but can be seen rarely in scleroderma, dermatomyositis, mixed connective tissue disease, and rheumatic fever. Large vessel involvement, primarily aortitis, most commonly occurs in the seronegative spondyloarthropathies, although it has also been described in relapsing polychondritis, Cogan's syndrome, and rarely in RA, scleroderma, and SLE. In general, upper extremity manifestations of vasculitis are more common in the rheumatic diseases with small to medium size vessel vasculitis and almost never present in the rheumatic diseases with predominantly aortitis.

Vasculitis Associated with Rheumatoid Arthritis

The finding of vasculitis in patients with RA is uncommon but can be serious.[305] Manifestations such as nail fold or nail edge lesions are seen in only 5.5% to 7.9% of outpatients[294,306]; ulcers were present in only 12 of about 2000 outpatients,[307] but 3.9% to 8.3% of inpatients with RA.[308,309] In general, the age and sex distribution is similar in patients with or without vasculitis. Patients with vasculitis usually have longstanding definite or classic RA with positive rheumatoid factor, nodules and erosions.[310,311] The average duration of RA before the onset of vasculitis is 9 to 13.6 years[310,311] with a wide range of 3 months to 30 years.[311–313] Thus, by the time vasculitis appears, the diagnosis of RA has been obvious. The manifestations of RA vasculitis can be highly variable depending on the vessel size and location. The severity and outcome generally are similar to that of the primary vasculitides, with postcapillary venule (LCV) involvement causing palpable purpura and having a more benign course than (PAN-like) vasculitis of medium sized arteries which often is associated with serious complications. The onset of vasculitis is usually abrupt and without prodromal symptoms. Active vasculitis may last several days to a few weeks, and is followed by slow healing over several months.[311] Vasculitis often occurs without exacerbation of the underlying arthritis.[311,314]

Cutaneous features are the most common, occurring in 88% of patients with RA vasculitis in one study. Findings include: (1) small areas of ischemia affecting the digital pulp and nail fold or nail edge (Figure 4); (2) cutaneous ulcers (Figure 4), that are shallow, well demarcated, painful, and with scant drainage, and very slow to heal; (3) purpuric lesions ranging in size from petechiae to large ecchymoses sometimes evolving into ulcers; (4) gangrene of the distal part of an extremity (Figure 5); and

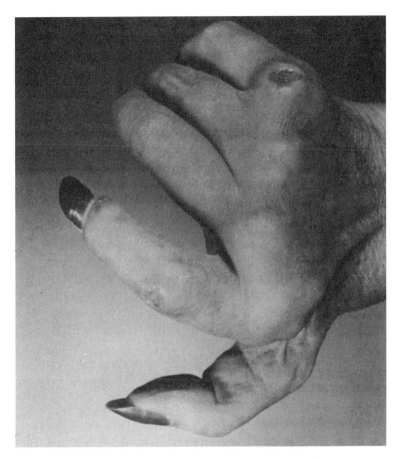

Figure 4. Digital ulcers in rheumatoid vasculitis.

(5) subcutaneous nodules. Rarely, biopsy of pyoderma gangrenosum demonstrates vasculitis however, vasculitis may not always be found with this lesion. Raynaud's phenomenon can sometimes occur.[306,308–310,315–319]

A peripheral neuropathy or a mononeuritis multiplex can be found in 42% to 60% of cases with cutaneous vasculitis associated with RA and the deficit (eg, wrist drop) often develops during a few hours to a few days, with characteristic numbness, paresthesia, and weakness. Other organs are involved less frequently and may be an isolated finding or part of a systemic PAN-like vasculitic picture. Vasculitis may involve muscle, often without symptoms, mesenteric arteries, coronary arteries, kidney, CNS, testes, and adrenals. A case of fibrosing alveolitis has been reported.[222,310–313,320–328]

Upper extremity findings are common in patients with RA vasculitis.

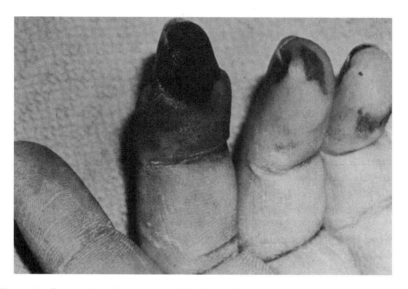

Figure 5. Cyanosis and gangrene of the finger tips with rheumatoid arthritis. (Courtesy of Yale B. Bickel, M.D.)

All the cutaneous manifestations can affect the upper extremity. Nail fold and digital pulp lesions are probably due to ischemia and thrombosis of capillary loops. Each lesion generally resolves over a few weeks however, they rarely may evolve into gangrene. Nail fold infarcts may be related to the use of the hand since they were absent in a paralyzed hand. Their location may correlate with areas of blanching on hand gripping. Brachial arteriograms of RA patients with vasculitic lesions of the hand show irregularity, narrowing, or obliteration of arterial lumens up to digital artery size. Biopsies of nail fold and digital infarcts initially show acute necrosis, followed by hyperkeratosis and hyperpigmentation. When vessels are present in the biopsy specimen, an obliterative endarteritis without inflammatory cells is usually found. In RA, vasculitis may cause neuropathy involving the upper extremity.[306,315,316,320,329]

RA patients with vasculitis usually have a higher incidence of other extra-articular manifestations including: subcutaneous nodules which may themselves be caused by vasculitis; pericarditis; and episcleritis.[310–312,320,330]

Laboratory findings suggest that immune complexes may play an important role in the pathogenesis of RA vasculitis. Nearly all patients have high titers of IgM-rheumatoid factor. However, IgG-rheumatoid factor and 7S-IgG-rheumatoid factor are also increased, and appear to correlate better with the presence of vasculitis. Circulating immune complex concentrations have been noted to be elevated by the Clq-binding assay,

Raji cell assay, and anticomplementary activity, but not in all cases. Other findings include: decreased complement in many cases a slight increase in frequency of positive ANA, a trypsin sensitive, RNase and DNase resistant ENA[323] and mixed cryoglobulinemia in some cases. The ESR is often elevated, but, unlike other vasculitides, it does not correlate with the activity of the vasculitis.[310–315,320,322,323,325,331–340]

Pathological sections of vessels have shown at least two patterns: (1) a necrotizing vasculitis involving venules similar to LCV[310,332] or small and medium sized arteries indistinguishable from PAN[141,311,320]; and (2) a bland intimal proliferation associated with fibroblasts and mucoid material, without inflammatory cells, sometimes with thrombotic occlusion, involving the digital arteries.[316,320] Sural nerve biopsies have shown immunoglobulin and complement deposits in vessel walls,[324,341] epineurium and endoneurium. Immunoglobulin and complement deposits in blood vessels of uninvolved forearm skin have been demonstrated with RA vasculitis, but are also associated with increased circulating immune complexes, subcutaneous nodules, and elevated rheumatoid factor.[342] Biopsy of uninvolved lower extremity skin showed only a slight increase in immunoglobulin deposits in patients with vasculitis, because of a high incidence of such deposits in seropositive RA patients without vasculitis.[343] Location and hydrostatic differences may account for the discrepancy. Rectal mucosal biopsy can sometimes be utilized to diagnose vasculitis.[310]

The natural history of RA vasculitis is highly variable. With postcapillary venule involvement[317] or isolated nail fold lesions,[306,315] the prognosis is good. However, with small artery vasculitis (PAN-like) the outlook is poor. Bywaters and Scott[315] noted mortality in 10 of 34 such patients over a 5-year observation period and Scott et al[310] in 13 of 50 patients after a 2-year follow-up. With neuropathy the prognosis tends to be worse.[310] Ferguson and Slocum[344] noted a 40% mortality if mononeuritis multiplex affected three to four extremities. The finding of a necrotizing vasculitis on rectal biopsy is also associated with a poorer prognosis.[310]

Treatment of RA vasculitis depends on the severity and type of vasculitic lesion. With nail fold lesions, close observation and treatment of the underlying RA suffices. Nonsteroidal anti-inflammatory drugs have not been of benefit.[310] A few anecdotal cases of benefit from penicillamine have been reported, but its onset of action is delayed.[345] Corticosteroids have clearly been of benefit in some cases, but in others have not controlled the vasculitis.[309,316,344] Cyclophosphamide alone has also been of benefit.[311,320] Chlorambucil was effective in five cases,[346] but azathioprine was not particularly beneficial in a small controlled study.[347] High-dose pulses of intravenous corticosteroids in conjunction with cyclophosphamide have resulted in healing of ulcers[314] and decreased mortality[310] in retrospective case studies. One open study showed that combined intravenous methylprednisolone with intravenous cyclophosphamide resulted in more frequent healing of vasculitis ulcers and neuropathy. In addition, there was a lower incidence of relapse, fewer serious complications and a lower mortality rate.[348] Plasmapheresis has been used successfully in a few patients however, many of these patients were also taking cyclophosphamide.[335,339,349] Low-dose methotrexate has been found to be useful for cutaneous vasculitis in RA.[350] Local wound care of ulcers and gangrene is important. Skin grafting of ulcers has been successful despite the high doses of steroids necessary to control the vasculitis.[309] Amputation of digits or extremities is sometimes necessary. A coronary artery saphenous vein bypass graft was successfully performed for RA-associated coronary vasculitis and angina.[327] Intravenous infusion of prostacyclin has resulted in healing of intractable vasculitic ulcers of the leg due to RA.[351]

Vasculitis Associated with Systemic Lupus Erythematosus

Vasculitis is a common finding in SLE. The most frequent site of involvement, the skin, develops vasculitis in 21% to 70% of cases.[240,352-356] The age and sex distribution of subjects with or without vasculitis is similar. The vasculitic lesions seen are not specific for SLE. Like RA, digital vasculitis and upper extremity involvement occur much more often than in the primary vasculitides.

Small and medium sized vessels are affected and the manifestations vary widely depending on the distribution and site of the vessel involved. Vasculitis may occur at any time during the course of SLE and may even precede other findings of SLE by many years.[357,358] Cutaneous findings range from common digital vasculitic lesions, nail fold infarcts, and periungual erythema, to less common LCV with palpable purpura and urticaria, nodules, livedo reticularis, ulcers, and gangrene.[240,352-364] Cerebral vasculitis can occur with sometimes devastating results.[352,353,365,366] Transverse myelopathy can rarely develop[367] and peripheral neuropathy is seen.[135,352] Vasculitis of the gastrointestinal tract can present as an acute abdomen with perforation, infarction of bowel, ruptured hepatic aneurysm, intussusception, or gastrointestinal bleeding, as well as pancreatitis, malabsorption, and protein-losing enteropathy.[353,368-371] Other areas of involvement include the eye with vasculitis of small arterioles and capillaries,[372] pulmonary artery,[373] renal artery with necrotizing vasculitis[374] and microaneurysms,[375] heart with coronary arteritis and myocardial infarction,[376] and placenta.[377] SLE is also associated with ascites, pleural effusion,[378] and thrombophlebitis.[379] A fulminant PAN-like vasculitis involving predominantly medium size arteries can occur.[352,380]

Upper extremity manifestations of vasculitis in SLE are frequently found, and comprise cutaneous findings, peripheral neuropathy, and rarely diminished pulses.[240,352-354,357,361,362] Digital and nail fold infarcts

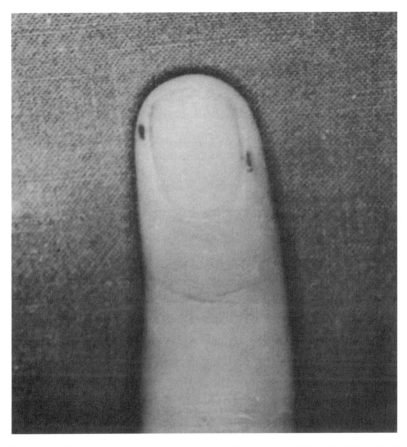

Figure 6. Characteristic nailfold infarction. (Courtesy of Yale B. Bickel, M.D.)

(Figure 6) are the most common upper extremity findings. Ulcers nearly always occur on the lower extremity and only very rarely appear on the forearm. Raynaud's phenomenon occurs in 10% to 40% of cases, but may or may not be associated with vasculitis. Ischemic changes and gangrene of extremities occur in about 1% of SLE patients[364] and often affect the upper extremity. Raynaud's phenomenon need not be present for this to occur. Pulses are nearly always intact.[357] Other less common upper extremity findings include: livedo reticularis,[357,358,360,381] thrombophlebitis, nodules, splinter hemorrhages, and Osler's nodes.[352,354,357,382,383]

Laboratory tests such as antinuclear antibody titer, complement levels, anti-DNA antibody titer, and circulating immune complexes, do not distinguish vasculitis from other manifestations of SLE.[384, 385] Active SLE can sometimes occur without abnormal serologies[353] and markedly abnormal serologies can occur in the absence of active SLE.[386] Cryoglobulins are usually not elevated.[387] SLE patients with vasculitis have been reported to have an IgG antibody that reacts with endothelial cells[388]; however, another study was unable to find this antibody by another method.[389] A precipitating antibody to DNA by electroimmunodiffusion is more common in SLE patients who have vasculitis.[390] Vasculitis and Raynaud's phenomenon have developed in a C6 deficiency SLE-like syndrome.[391] The presence of the antiphospholipid antibody is associated with an increased risk of thrombosis of vessels.[21-25,28,29,392] The lupus band test (granular immunofluorescent staining of immunoglobulins and complement at the dermal-epidermal junction on skin biopsy) does not correlate with SLE vasculitis.[393,394] When medium sized vessel involvement occurs angiographic findings are similar to those in PAN. Biopsy of involved areas shows necrotizing vasculitis with fibrinoid necrosis and a polymorphonuclear leukocyte infiltrate[364] ranging from LCV[359,371] to PAN-like medium size vessel vasculitis. In general, the arteries involved tend to be smaller than those seen with PAN.[395] Deposits of immunoglobulin and complement are often detected in the vessel walls.[359,375,389,395]

The course and prognosis of vasculitis with SLE is highly variable and difficult to separate from the other manifestations of SLE. Involvement of larger vessels or viscera is associated with a poorer outlook. The presence of cutaneous vasculitis should arouse suspicion of possible visceral vasculitis.[352,359,369] Livedoid vasculitis may serve as a cutaneous marker of CNS lupus.[396]

Corticosteroids are the mainstay of therapy, but high doses are required.[352,354,362,364,385,387,397] One gram intravenous pulses of methylprednisolone are sometimes effective when usual oral doses fail.[398,399] Cytotoxic agents such as azathioprine, 6-mercaptopurine, nitrogen mustard, cyclophosphamide, and chlorambucil have been of benefit in steroid unresponsive cases.[205,355,368,382] Stellate ganglion block for gangrene,[364] antimalarials,[400] and nonsteroidal anti-inflammatory agents have not been successful. Chronic urticarial vasculitis has been treated successfully with dapsone in a few cases.[401]

Vasculitis Associated with the Spondyloarthropathies

The vasculitis which develops in the spondyloarthropathies is limited to proximal aortitis. It is more likely to be seen in Reiter's syndrome and ankylosing spondylitis, but can sometimes be seen in psoriatic arthritis and rarely with arthritis associated with inflammatory bowel diseases or juvenile RA.[186,402-407]

Aortic insufficiency has been reported in 3.0% to 10.7%[403,408,409] of ankylosing spondylitis subjects and was found to be secondary to aortitis in 2.6% on postmortem examination.[406] Aortic insufficiency tends to be a late manifestation of spondylitis and develops an average of 11 to 15 years after the onset of arthritis.[402,405] However, the murmur has been detected before the onset of spondylitis[410] or may develop as late as 30 years after.[403] As with the demographics of the spondyloarthropathies, Caucasian males are almost exclusively affected.[402,408,411]

The usual manifestation of aortitis is aortic insufficiency, due to the loss of elastic tissue supporting the aortic ring, resulting in a dilated incompetent aortic valve orifice. The aortic insufficiency may lead to congestive heart failure, and angina. However, symptoms indicative of the severity of aortic regurgitation may be missed because of the limited mobility imposed by the arthritis. Intermittent or permanent atrioventricular conduction disorders range from first degree heart block to, less commonly, left bundle branch block, second degree block, and complete heart block and have been noted in 27% to 75% of patients with aortic regurgitation, probably from extension of the inflammation to involve the atrioventricular node and bundles.[186,402,403,406,408,411–415]

Aortitis is nearly always confined to the ascending aorta, although, rarely, large aneurysms of the descending thoracic aorta[415–417] and the proximal abdominal aorta have been found.[406]

A patient with a nonocclusive saccular aneurysm of the left coronary artery has been described.[405] However, unlike temporal arteritis and TA, the aortitis associated with the spondyloarthropathies does not cause narrowing or occlusion of the branches of the aorta.

The development of aortitis is usually associated with more severe spondyloarthropathy, with a higher incidence of peripheral joint involvement, iritis, or conjunctivitis.[402–404,412,414] Pericarditis is sometimes seen and a case has been described of hemodynamically significant mitral regurgitation because of inflammation extending to the base of the anterior mitral leaflet.[410] No specific arteritis lesion occurs in the upper extremity.

Laboratory tests do not help in identifying those patients who have aortitis. Two-dimensional echocardiogram is useful in detecting preclinical aortic root involvement.[418] The ESR is often elevated in the spondyloarthropathies and does not appear to correlate well with aortitis and aortic insufficiency. A subaortic septal bump, characteristic of aortitis from the spondyloarthropathies can be seen on left ventriculogram. On pathological examination there is widening of the aortic ring and arch with retraction of the aortic cusps, rolling of the free margins, and with chronic involvement, scarring of the aortic cusps with areas of calcification. Early, the aorta has focal areas of thickening, media and elastica destruction with inflammatory infiltrates, ingrowth of granulation tissue and obliterative endarteritis of the vasa vasorum. This is followed by focal replacement of the media with fibrous tissue leading to thin areas of scarred aorta.[402,403,406,408,412–414,416,419]

The aortic insufficiency tends to be mild and chronic; however, when heart failure occurs, it has developed as early as the first year of disease,[405,410] or as late as 20 years[408,410] after the detection of aortic regurgitation. The role of the nonsteroidal anti-inflammatory agents, corticosteroids, cytotoxic agents, or plasmapheresis in the treatment of aortitis has not been established because of the variability of the natural history and the rarity of the disease. Medical treatment of congestive heart failure and arrhythmias is important.[402] Aortic valve replacement,[403,411,420] mitral valve replacement, and resection of a descending thoracic aneurysm[409] have been successful.

Relapsing Polychondritis

Vasculitis is often found in relapsing polychondritis (RP). The disease itself is uncommon, immunologically mediated and characterized by three or more findings of: (1) chondritis of the ear; (2) a nonerosive, seronegative, oligo- or polyarticular inflammatory arthritis; (3) nasal chondritis; (4) ocular inflammation; (5) respiratory tract chondritis; and (6) audiovestibular damage.[421-425] Fever and constitutional symptoms are often present. The onset usually occurs in the third to sixth decades of life and there is a slight male predominance. In 25% to 35% of cases there is an associated autoimmune or rheumatic disease. Glomerulonephritis is unusual but has been reported[426] as well as recurrent oral ulcerations.[427] Vasculitis is a prominent feature and is present in 25% to 56% of patients.[428]

A wide spectrum of vasculitis can be seen with RP. Aortitis is the most characteristic and is similar to the aortitis of ankylosing spondylitis and Reiter's syndrome. Nearly all cases occur in males. Involvement of the ascending aorta and aortic valve ring leading to aortic insufficiency and/or dissection is most commonly seen. Involvement of the descending aorta and abdominal aorta with dissection or rupture can also occur. First-degree atrioventricular block, presumably from extension of the aortitis to involve the conduction system of the heart, is sometimes found.[421-424,428-431] Histologically there is extensive vascularization and lymphocytic cuffing around the vasa vasorum of the outer aortic media, loss and fragmentation of elastic tissue, an increase in collagen, and a decrease in mucopolysaccharide content.

Other types of vasculitis seen in association with RP include: cutaneous small vessel vasculitis, Wegener's granulomatosis, PAN, temporal arteritis, and TA.[421,428,432-437]

The upper extremity is generally not affected by the vasculitis associated with RP, although cutaneous small vessel vasculitis may affect the upper extremity and a left subclavian aneurysm[438] has been reported.

The only diagnostic laboratory test for RP is biopsy of involved cartilage. The ESR is often elevated, and circulating immune complexes and antibodies to type II collagen (more against native rather than to denatured collagen) have been detected.[439] Deposits of immunoglobulin and complement may be detected in affected cartilage by direct immunofluorescence.[440,441]

A wide variability in severity and course can be seen. There is a 22% to 30% mortality primarily from airway collapse or cardiovascular involvement.[421] In a review of 112 patients the most frequent causes of death were infection, systemic vasculitis and malignancy and only 10% of the deaths could be attributable to airway obstruction.[442] Treatment has included nonsteroidal anti-inflammatory agents,[421,443] dapsone,[444] colchicine for chondritis,[445] and corticosteroids.[421,422,428,430, 444] For severe manifestations immunosuppressive agents such as 6-mercaptopurine, azathioprine, cyclophosphamide and cyclosporin A have been used.[421,446] Surgery is often essential in the management of aortitis, with aneurysm resection, aortic valve replacement, and aortic valvuloplasty.[422,424,428–430]

Scleroderma

Vascular involvement is an almost invariable feature of scleroderma (progressive systemic sclerosis). Symptoms include digital infarcts, digital ulcers, Raynaud's phenomenon, and gangrene. However, the underlying disorder is not a necrotizing vasculitis, but a noninflammatory intimal proliferation with occlusion of the microvasculature and small arterioles. Necrotizing vasculitis similar to PAN and aortitis has been reported.[188,205,447–450]

The compromised blood flow to the digits make it difficult for digital ulcers to heal and may result in digital infarcts and gangrene. Digital calcinosis further compound the problem.

Many vasodilating drugs, eg, methyldopa, phenoxybenzamine and prazosin have been tried.[451] The use of nifedipine (a calcium channel blocker) has met with some success in the treatment of digital ulcers.[452] Prostaglandin E_1 infusion via central venous catheter has been reported to produce improvement of Raynaud's phenomenon and ischemic ulcers healed in 54% of cases.[453] Superimposed infection is treated with antibiotics.

Surgical treatment with preganglionic sympathectomy had been recommended for gangrene or digital pain not responding to medical treatment.[454] As a last resort, the gangrenous digit has to be amputated. Calcinosis cutis, which is disabling, can be excised, but the patient should be warned of possible delayed healing, residual numbness and recurrence of the calcium deposit.

Dermatomyositis

Childhood dermatomyositis is usually associated with an angiopathy. However, it is generally a non-necrotizing, lymphocytic to noninflammatory vasculopathy involving primarily capillaries and small arteries and veins.[453–458] Diffuse vasculitis (nail bed telangiectasia, digital ulceration, and infarction of the oral epithelium) is associated with more severe disease.[459] Uncommonly, a necrotizing vasculitis similar to PAN may be seen[460] and ischemic ulcerations of the upper extremity digits has been reported.

In adults, cutaneous vasculitis is reported to be associated with dermatomyositis rather than polymyositis. There is dissociation between cutaneous vasculitis and vasculitis in muscle biopsy and a suggestion that cutaneous vasculitis may be a marker for an occult malignancy.[461]

Mixed Connective Tissue Disease

Mixed connective tissue disease is a rheumatic disease with features in common with SLE, scleroderma, and polymyositis associated with high titers of antibody against a ribonucleoprotein.[462] Vasculitis is generally not a feature of mixed connective tissue disease. Ischemic changes with ulceration can be seen,[463,464] but are most likely secondary to intimal proliferation4[65,466] without necrotizing vasculitis.

Sjögren's Syndrome

Vasculitis is an extraglandular manifestation of primary SS that was seen in one series in 9 of 70 patients.[467] An acute necrotizing medium vessel vasculitis simulated PAN except that it did not form aneurysm. One patient developed finger gangrene requiring amputation. A small vessel vasculitis was of the hypersensitivity type, localized mainly in the skin. Dermal vasculitis in a group of patients with SS was studied[468,469] and two pathological types were identified: one LCV and the other mononuclear. The leukocytoclastic vasculitis was associated with hyperglobulinemia and high titers both of Ro and La (anti-SSA and anti-SSB) autoantibodies and of other autoantibodies. The mononuclear vasculitis generally was not associated with high antibody titers. Approximately 70% of patients with SS and cutaneous vasculitis developed peripheral and CNS disease.

Miscellaneous Vasculitides

Mucocutaneous Lymph Node Syndrome (Kawasaki Disease)

Mucocutaneous lymph node syndrome or Kawasaki disease is an acute illness of infants and small children in which vasculitis, mainly of the coronary arteries, often develops. The syndrome is characterized by: (1) spiking fevers lasting more than 7 days; (2) bilateral conjunctival injection; (3) oropharyngeal erythema that later leads to dry, cracked lips; (4) indurated edema and erythema of the hands and feet followed about 2 weeks later by desquamation of the skin from fingertips and toes; (5) an erythematosus polymorphous rash; and (6) nonsuppurative cervical lymphadenopathy.[470–472] To make a secure diagnosis, 5 of the 6 features should be present and other conditions excluded.[473] Rarely, adolescents and young adults are affected.[474]

The clinical course consists of three phases: (1) an acute febrile phase lasting up to 14 days with the previously listed findings; (2) a subacute phase lasting from 10 to 25 days associated with resolution of the acute phase and the development of dry, cracked lips, desquamation of skin, and arthralgia or arthritis; and (3) a convalescent phase with gradual resolution of symptoms. Children who develop arthritis before 10 days tend to have a polyarticular disease and those with later onset arthritis tend to have oligoarticular disease. Uncommon findings include diarrhea, urethritis with sterile pyuria, mild aseptic meningitis, focal encephalopathy, mild hepatitis with jaundice, otitis media, pleuritis, pneumonitis, and hydrops of the gallbladder.[475] The disease is usually self-limiting except for 1% to 2% who most often die suddenly from coronary arteritis.[471,476]

Coronary arteritis has been noted in nearly 100% of postmortem examinations,[476,477] and coronary aneurysms have been detected in nearly 20% of patients.[478] The pathology of the arteritis is an inflammatory necrotizing panarteritis similar to PAN.[476,478] In autopsy studies, vasculitis commonly involves the large arteries such as the aorta and its branches. Medium size to small arteries and veins are less often affected.[477] In spite of these findings, clinical manifestations are rare, with isolated reports of symptomatic distal aortic aneurysm,[479] ruptured hepatic aneurysm,[480] mesenteric infarction,[481] gallbladder necrosis,[481] ruptured aortic aneurysm with cardiac tamponade,[482] and ruptured iliac artery aneurysm.[476] Upper extremity involvement has been rarely reported with gangrene due to axillary artery aneurysm with obstruction.[481–484]

Laboratory tests although nondiagnostic are characterized by elevation of the ESR, neutrophilia, slight anemia, and increased hepatic function tests during the acute febrile phase; thrombocytosis during the subacute phase; and resolution of these abnormalities during the convalescent phase. An acute rise and convalescent fall of immunoglobulins, presence of circulating immune complexes peaking on day 30 of illness and a universally elevated C_3 from weeks 1 to 3 are some of the immunologic abnormalities seen in Kawasaki syndrome.[472] The electrocardiogram may be abnormal during the acute phase, probably from myocarditis. Coronary artery aneurysms have been detected by angiography and echocardiography. MRI is thought to be inadequate as a screening examination.[485]

Aspirin is symptomatically helpful for treatment during the acute phase. However it has been suggested that it is difficult to achieve therapeutic concentrations of salicylate in Kawasaki disease.[486] Antibiotics and steroids have not been of benefit.[472] Surgery may be indicated in selected cases. Coronary artery bypass grafting has been successful in few cases with symptomatic coronary artery aneurysms.[480,482] Obstruction, rupture, or aneurysmal dilatation of arteries may require surgical repair.[476,479-482] Prostaglandin E_1 infusion has been used for severe peripheral ischemia.[484]

Multicenter randomized trials have demonstrated that high-dose intravenous gammaglobulin given early in the disease reduces the frequency of coronary artery abnormalities.[487-489] Currently it is recommended that patients with Kawasaki disease seen in the first 10 days of illness receive intravenous gamma globulin at a dose of 400 mg/kg per day for 4 consecutive days.

Primary Angiitis of the Central Nervous System

Primary angiitis of the CNS[490] is a granulomatosis and/or necrotizing inflammatory vasculitis of arterioles, capillaries and venules predominantly limited to the brain and spinal cord. The leptomeninges are commonly affected. The etiology is not known, but the sparing of the media and intima suggests that the agent causing angiitis may reach the vessel from without rather than by a hematogenous route.[491] Adults 40 to 70 years of age are most commonly affected. Symptoms vary from headache and confusion to focal neurological deficits, cranial neuropathy or spinal cord involvement. Untreated, there is nearly always progression to multifocal neurological deficits leading to coma and death after a few days to several years. Treatment with steroids has been of some benefit, and cyclophosphamide and azathioprine may be of value.[490]

Cogan's Syndrome

Cogan's syndrome is a rare disorder that affects young adults with episodes of acute interstitial keratitis and vestibuloauditory dysfunction,[492] as well as some systemic manifestations.[493-495] In a few cases it has been associated with a necrotizing vasculitis similar to PAN[496,497] and aortitis.[498,499] In one study, 12 of 18 patients developed vasculitis and the median duration from onset of disease to development of vasculitis was 7 months.[500] Upper extremity involvement is rare with one report of chronic venous inflammation at the site of thrombosis in the right arm of the patient.[500]

Behcet's Disease

In 1937, a Turkish dermatologist described a syndrome of recurrent oral and genital ulcers associated with eye lesions, that now bears his name.[501] The multisystemic nature of Behcet's disease has since been described.

No specific diagnostic test exists and diagnosis relies on finding a characteristic constellation of manifestations (Table 11). Aphthosis is mandatory. The etiology and pathogenesis are not known.[502-505] Disease susceptibility genes, studied in large independent British and Japanese surveys, are HLA B51 and HLA DRW52.[502]

Behcet's disease is most common in the Eastern Mediterranean area and Japan. The onset is usually before age 45 and the prognosis is worse in the younger patient.[503,504]

Manifestations include oral ulcers that are painful, recurrent, multiple, and on biopsy resemble typical canker sores. They have regular borders and usually heal without scarring within 10 days. Genital ulcers occur on the scrotum, penis, vulva, and vagina. The latter may be painless and may not be brought to the physician's attention. Recurrences of genital ulcers are less frequent than those of oral lesions. Eye involvement with anterior and posterior uveitis is a serious manifestation. About 70% to 80% of patients with posterior uveitis progress to loss of visual acuity and about half ultimately progress to blindness.[503,504] The mean time from onset of eye involvement to blindness is about 5 years.[504] Cutaneous findings are varied and include erythema nodosum, superficial thrombophlebitis, acneform rash, and hypersensitivity of the skin; in 60% to 70% of patients a characteristic aseptic pustule develops at the site of a pin prick. The mechanism of this Bechcetin reaction is not known but is thought to be related to increased chemotaxis. The arthritis is nondestructive, usually asymmetric, recurrent, and usually involves the ankles, elbows, knees, wrists and sacroiliac joints. Nonspecific gastrointestinal symptoms are present in at least 50% of patients and of minor consequence.[506] However, intestinal ulcers, most often in the ileocecal area, can give rise to severe pain, perforation, melena, and abdominal mass.[503]

With neurological involvement, CNS manifestations predominate[505,507,508]; the peripheral nerves tend to be spared. Epididymitis occur

Table 11
Diagnostic Criteria of Behçet's Syndrome* Behçet's Syndrome
Research Committee of Japan, 1972

Major Criteria	Frequency %*
Recurrent aphthous ulceration in the mouth	99
Skin lesions	66
e. nodosum-like lesions	
subcutaneous thrombophlebitis	
hypersensitivity of the skin	
Eye lesions	66
recurrent hypopyon iritis or iridocyclitis	
chorioretinitis	
Genital ulcerations	80
Minor Criteria	
Arthritis symptoms and signs	55
Gastrointestinal lesions	50
Epididymitis	8
Vascular lesions	24
Central nervous system involvement	22
brain stem syndrome	
meningo-encephalomyelitic syndrome	
confusional type	
Diagnostic Categories of Behçet's Syndrome	
Complete type: all four major criteria during the clinical course of the patient	
Incomplete type: (a) three of four major criteria	
(b) recurrent hypopyon iritis or typical chorioretinitis and one other major criteria	

* Adapted from Rose GA, Spencer H: Polyarteritis nodosa. *Q J Med* 26:43—81, 1957, and Liebow AA: The J Burns Amberson lecture—pulmonary angitis and granulomatosis. *Am Rev Respir Dis* 108:1—18, 1973.

in 4.5% to 8% of male patients. The heart, lungs, kidneys, and liver are infrequently affected.

Vasculitis occurs in about one-fourth of cases[503,504] and four types have been recognized: (1) arterial occlusions; (2) aneurysms of the aorta or other large arteries; (3) occlusion of any vein including the superior and inferior vena cava; and (4) varices. A lymphocytic vasculitis of capillaries and venules can be seen in various organs[504,509,510] and may play a role in the development of large vessel arteritis. Large artery involvement occurred in 10 of 450 patients and usually occurs late in the disease. Occlusion of the subclavian, brachial or radial artery may present as pulseless disease.[511] Gangrene has been reported, but usually involves the lower extremity.[507,512,513]

Vascular involvement in the upper extremity is uncommon, but arterial occlusions or aneurysms of the subclavian, brachial, radial, and ulnar arteries, and occlusion of the subclavian vein, superior vena cava, and axillary vein have been observed.[504]

Laboratory tests may show a transient elevation of the ESR, leukocytosis, raised C-reactive protein and elevated immunoglobulins during a relapse.[503] The CSF IgM index was found to be higher in patients with active neuro-Behcet.[514] Vascular, neurological, or gastrointestinal involvement is associated with a poor prognosis. Death is usually the result of rupture of an aneurysm, perforation of intestines or severe CNS involvement. Treatment is largely unsatisfactory[503–505] and there are no large controlled trials. Steroids are used topically for aphthous ulcers and systemically for ocular and neurological disease.[505] A wide array of other therapeutic agents have been reported to be of benefit in some patients and include: immunosuppressive agents (especially chlorambucil or azathioprine for ocular involvement), levamisole, transfer factor, interferon-α colchicine, and fibrinolytic drugs. Cyclosporin A has been reported to be useful in severe Behcet uveitis not responding to other therapy, as well as for the mucocutaneous lesions.[515–518]

Thromboangiitis Obliterans

In 1908, Buerger described a segmental, thrombosing, and inflammatory vascular disease causing severe ischemia of the extremities in predominantly young male cigarette smokers.[519] The resemblance of atherosclerosis, systemic embolization and peripheral thrombosis led Fischer in 1957[520] and Wessler et al in 1960[521] to question the existence of thromboangiitis obliterans (TAO) or Buerger's disease. However, in spite of the fact that early studies of TAO included patients with arteriosclerosis, subsequent reports[522–528] clearly define TAO as a distinct entity on the basis of characteristic clinical presentation, radiographic and pathological findings, prognosis and therapeutic response.

TAO is not a necrotizing vasculitis, but an inflammatory vascular thrombosis with relative sparing of the vessel wall. It very often involves the upper extremity and its presentation can mimic a necrotizing vasculitis.

TAO, despite varying diagnostic criteria, is an uncommon disease. In the United States an incidence of 7 to 8 cases per 100,000 white males age 20 to 40 years, has been estimated.[528] Large centers may see anywhere from 0 to 20[521,529] new cases per year. As a cause of arterial occlusive disease, it usually accounts for less than 17% of cases in men less than 40 years of age.[521,525,529,530]

Men between 20 and 40 years of age are most often affected.[519,522–525,527–536] Women account for less than 2% of cases and do not appear to have any racial predisposition. In males, there is an increased incidence in Asian and in some studies in Jewish populations.[520,531.] However, this has not been confirmed by others.[523–525] Blacks have a low incidence. For unclear reasons, smoking is strongly associated with TAO.[521,526.] Nearly all patients who develop TAO are cigarette smokers and when compared with all other treatment modalities, abstinence from tobacco alone has given the best results. Often patients continue smoking despite continued symptoms of vascular ischemia and multiple amputations.[524,536] A case of TAO was reported in a 38-year-old man that was associated with smokeless (chewing) tobacco. Treatment with nifedipine, and antiplatelet therapy and total abstinence from tobacco resulted in resolution of symptoms.[537]

Findings reflect arterial insufficiency and thrombophlebitis of the extremities. Early in the disease, claudication, migratory thrombophlebitis or ischemic pain involving a single lower extremity is most commonly found. With progression, involvement of other extremities, ulceration, and gangrene occur. Claudication of the instep is found in 25% to 100% of patients.[523,524,530,531,533,538] due to popliteal artery involvement.[539] This may uncommonly progress to involve the calf. Burning and aching ischemic rest pain is common, up to 78% to 100% in some series, and is often increased out of proportion to visible signs of ischemia, The area involved may be discolored, hypohidrotic, cold, and markedly tender. Decreased or absent pulses are common distal to the popliteal and brachial arteries. More proximal involvement or bruits suggest arteriosclerosis obliterans.

Thrombophlebitis is usually migrating and occurs in 27% to 100% of cases.[523–525,529–533,538] Ulcerations and gangrene are present in about half of patients and begin distally. Malleolar and pretibial ulcers as seen in venous stasis and in vasculitis are not described. Raynaud's phenomenon has been described in up to 57% of cases.[524,531] Subungual-splinter hemorrhages have been detected as an early finding in a few cases.[540]

TAO primarily involves the extremities. Cases with cerebrovascular,[541]mesenteric,[519,542], celiac,[543] descending aorta,[538] heart,[531] and spermatic arteries[522] have been described, but are rare and in many instances secondary to atherosclerosis.[520,521] The absence of systemic involvement as well as the lack of constitutional symptoms help distinguish TAO from necrotizing vasculitis.

The same manifestations of TAO occur in both the upper and lower extremities. Although involved less often, because of the rarity of atherosclerosis in the arms, upper extremity manifestations are more specific for TAO.[522,525,531] Only a small percentage (5%) of patients start with symptoms in the upper limb.[531] However, as the disease progresses upper extremity involvement increases to 14% to 100%.[539] When angiography was performed on all cases of TAO, asymptomatic occlusive disease was found in several patients and the earliest lesions most commonly involved the digital arteries.[544] An aneurysm of the radial artery in a patient with TAO has been reported.[545] Routine laboratory tests have not been of value in the diagnosis of TAO.

Angiography of involved vessels provides important diagnostic information. Individual findings are not diagnostic, but in combination are characteristic of TAO.[523] In TAO there is nearly always involvement only of small and medium vessels, sparing large arteries proximal to the brachial and popliteal arteries. Upper extremity vessels are often involved. The distribution is in a segmental rather than a diffuse pattern, and smooth-lined even walls rather than an irregular surface are seen on angiography.[522] Findings such as spider-legs, or tree-root configuration of collateral vessels, cork screw tortuosity of vessels due to recanalization, and rippling, corrugated, segmental stenoses[522–524] are considered characteristic findings. However, they may be seen in atherosclerosis and other conditions.[525,526]

Arteriograms of the upper extremities show primarily digital involvement although any size vessel up to the radial and ulnar arteries may be involved.[522,544] Lesions can be segmental or involve the whole length of the artery. Tortuosity of collateral and digital arteries can be seen.[544]

The lesions in TAO are limited to small and medium sized vessels, are segmental in distribution, and can be seen in all stages of evolution.[523,524] Random sections may demonstrate focal lesions.[522] The pathological findings have been divided into three stages to correspond with the evolving thrombosis: (1) the acute stage; (2) the subacute stage; and (3) the chronic stage. On gross examination, the acute and subacute stages appear as a friable brown-red thrombus. In the chronic stage the artery is a fibrotic cord sometimes bound together with vein and nerve trunks.[546]

The histology[522–524,546] of the acute stage consists of dense aggregates of polymorphonuclear cells (micro-abcess), monocytes, and giant cells in a fresh or organizing thrombus. There is infiltration of the vessel wall with polymorphonuclear cells and chronic inflammatory cells, but the vessel wall is intact with preservation of the elastic lamina and media. In the subacute phase, mononuclear cells and giant cells predominate within the lumen. The vessel wall contains a mild inflammatory infiltrate. The chronic stage spans a wide spectrum of fibrotic occlusions, with a variable amount of chronic infiltrate, lymphoid aggregates and perivascular fibrosis. Recanalization is present. Throughout all stages there is a relative lack of necrotizing and degenerative changes in the vessel wall. Only the histology of the acute stage is diagnostic of TAO.[521]

The etiology and pathogenesis are not known. The strong association of TAO with smoking has suggested an etiologic role, but more information as to the mechanism involved is needed. Other conditions associated with TAO include: trauma, cold exposure, wet conditions, and fungal infections.[522,531]

The role of the immune system has not been studied sufficiently to draw any conclusions. One group of patients with TAO was found to have normal values for immunoglobulins, complement titers, B and T cells, and mitogen transformation of lymphocytes, but 35% had circulating antibodies to heat-denatured human collagen.[547] In contrast, another study found elevated immunoglobulins, decreased complement titers, normal reactions to dinitrochlorobenzene, and inhibition of leukocyte migration when exposed to arterial antigen.[548]

Abnormalities in the coagulation system have been sought in order to explain the vascular thromboses. Increased platelet aggregation in the acute occlusive stage of both TAO and arteriosclerosis obliterans has been found,[549,550] as well as an increased heparin precipitable fraction of fibrin.[551] Whether these findings represent the cause of, or the consequence of the thrombus formation is not known.

Genetic factors may be important in the pathogenesis. There is an increase in TAO in certain ethnic groups such as Japanese, Koreans, and Ashkenazi Jews.[520,531] In one study several cases within families were found.[531] An increased incidence of HLA A9 and B5 was found in one study,[552] whereas another found no increase in any specific HLA type, but a decreased frequency of HLA B12.[553] An increased frequency of ABO blood type B was found in a series of Indian patients with TAO.[554]

Patients with TAO have only a slight increase in mortality rate, with a 5-year survival of 93.1% compared with 97.7% in normals and 75.6% in those who have arteriosclerosis obliterans.[525] The rate of amputation varies from 15% at 10 years in an outpatient survey in the United States,[528] to 58% at 9 years in Java.[534] The major goals of treatment are to prevent amputation and to decrease ischemic pain.

Complete abstinence from smoking is the best and only successful therapy that is well documented.[519,522–526,528–531,533,534] However, TAO occurring 15 years after cessation of smoking has been described.[555] Sympathectomy has been tried with good results when performed in the early phase,[523,556] but generally with only transient improvement.[522,530,533] Vascular reconstruction has generally not resulted in long-term patency except when the distal anastomosis has been proximal to the popliteal bifurcation and even then long-term patency occurred only in patients who had stopped smoking.[557,558] Endarterectomy has not given good long-term results.[557] Long-term results of omental transplantation show it to be effective in TAO but no in atherosclerotic disease.[559] Prednisone,[523] adrenalectomy,[530] and azathioprine 100 to 200 mg per day for 4 to 5 months[531] are of questionable value. Intravenous prostacyclin,[560] prostaglandin E,[561] and hypervolemic treatment with dextran[562] have been tried with some success. Meticulous care of the ischemic area to prevent further injury or infection is important.

References

1. Zeek PM: Periarteritis nodosa and other forms of necrotizing angiitis. *N Engl J Med* 248:764–772, 1953.
2. Fauci AS, Haynes BF, Katz P: The spectrum of vasculitis: Clinical, pathologic, immunologic, and therapeutic considerations. *Ann Intern Med* 89:660–676, 1978.
3. Cupps TR, Fauci AC: The vasculitides. In: Smith LH, Jr, ed. *Major Problems in Internal Medicine*. Volume 21. Philadelphia: WB Saunders Co.; 1981.
4. Fan PT: A clinical approach to systemic vasculitis. *Semin Arthritis Rheum* 9: 248–304, 1980.
5. Lie JT: Classification and immunodiagnosis of vasculitis: A new solution or promises unfulfilled? *J Rheumatol* 15:728–732, 1988.
6. Jordaan HF: Widespread superficial thrombophlebitis as a manifestation of secondary syphilis: A new sign. *S Afr Med J* 70:493–494, 1986.
7. Fountain JA, Werner RB: Tuberculous retinal vasculitis. *Retina* 4:48–50, 1984.
8. Bodaghi E, Kheradpir KM: Vasculitis in acute streptococcal glomerulonephritis. *J Pediatr Nephrol* 8:69–74, 1987.
9. Anevato PA, Eisses JF, Mezger E, et al: Nocardia asteroides aortitis with perforation of the aorta. *Hum Pathol* 16:743–746, 1985.
10. DeMicco C, Raoult D, Benderitter T, et al: Immune complex vasculitis associated with Mediterranean spotted fever. *J Infect* 14:163–165, 1987.
11. O'Donohue JM, Enzmann DR: Mycotic aneurysm in angiitis associated with Herpes zoster ophthalmicus. *AJNR* 8:615–619, 1987.
12. Sandler A, Snedeker JD: Cytomegalovirus infection in an infant presenting with cutaneous vasculitis. *Pediatr Infect Dis J* 6:422–423, 1987.
13. Li-Loong RC, Coyle PV, Anderson MJ, et al: Human serum parvovirus associated vasculitis. *Postgrad Med J* 62:493–494, 1986.
14. Inman RD, Hodge M, Johnston ME, et al: Arthritis, vasculitis and cryoglobulinemia associated with relapsing hepatitis A virus infection. *Ann Intern Med* 105:700–703, 1986.
15. Inman RD: Rheumatic manifestations of hepatitis B virus infection. *Semin Arthritis Rheum* 11:406–420, 1982.
16. Libman AS, Quismorio FP, Stimmler MM: Polyarteritis nodosa-like vasculitis in human immunodeficiency virus infection. *J Rheumatol* 22:351–355, 1995.
17. Hunder GG: Clinical and therapeutic issues in vasculitis. *ARA Bienniel Review of Rheumatic Disease*, Section II. 1988.
18. Leavitt RY, Fauci AS: Polyangiitis overlap syndrome: Classification and prospective clinical experience. *Am J Med* 81:79–85, 1986.
19. DeShazo RD, Levinson AI, Lawless OJ, et al: Systemic vasculitis with coexistence of large and small vessel involvement: A classification dilemma. *JAMA* 238:1940–1942, 1977.
20. Crowley JG: Axillary arteritis (letter). *N Engl J Med* 306:1297, 1982.
21. Harris EN, Gharani AE, Hughes GRV: Anti-phospholipid antibodies. *Clin Rheum Dis* 11:591–609, 1985.
22. Conley CL, Hartmann RC: A hemorrhagic disorder caused by circulating anti-

coagulant in patients with disseminated lupus erythematosus. *J Clin Invest* 31: 261–262, 1952.

23. Boey ML, Colaco CB, Gharavi AE, et al: Thrombosis in SLE: Striking association with the presence of circulating lupus anticoagulant. *Br Med J* 287: 1021–1023, 1983.
24. Pabinger-Fasching I: Lupus anticoagulants and thrombosis: A study of 25 cases and review of the literature. *Haemostasis* 15:254–262, 1982.
25. Alarcon-Segovia D: Pathogenetic potential of antiphospholipid antibodies (editorial). *J Rheumatol* 15:890–893, 1988.
26. Rosove MH, Brewer PM: Antiphospholipid thrombosis: Clinical course after the first thrombotic event in 70 patients. *Ann Intern Med* 117:303–308, 1992.
27. Khamashta MA, Cuadrado MJ, Mujic F, et al: The management of thrombosis in the anti-phospholipid syndrome. *N Eng J Med* 332:933–937, 1995.
28. Sturfelt G, Nived O, Norberg R, et al: Anticardiolipin antibodies in patients with systemic lupus erythematosus. *Arthritis Rheum* 30:382–388, 1987.
29. Lockshin MD: Anticardiolipin antibody (editorial). *Arthritis Rheum* 30: 471–472, 1988.
30. Lie JT: Vasculitis associated with infectious agents. *Curr Opin Rheum* 8:26–29, 1996.
31. Gherardi R, Belec L, Mhiri C, et al: The spectrum of vasculitis in human immunodeficiency virus-infected patients. *Arthritis Rheum* 36:1164–1179, 1993.
32. Pascual M, Perrin L, Giestra E, et al: Hepatitis C virus in patients with cryoglobulinemia type II. *J Infect Dis* 169:569–570, 1990.
33. Matick H, Anderson D, Brumlik J: Cerebral vasculitis associated with oral amphetamine overdose. *Arch Neurol* 40:253–254, 1983.
34. Kaye BR, Fainstate M: Cerebral vasculitis associated with cocaine abuse. *JAMA* 258:2104–2106, 1987.
35. Noel J, Rosenbaum LH, Gangadharan V, et al: Serum sickness like illness and leucocytoclastic vasculitis following intracoronary arterial streptokinase. *Am Heart J* 113:395–397, 1987.
36. Bucknall C, Darley C, Flax J, et al: Vasculitis complicating treatment with intravenous anisoylated plasminogen streptokinase activator complex in acute myocardial infarction. *Br Heart J* 59:9–11, 1988.
37. Carrasco MD, Riera C, Clotet B, et al: Cutaneous vasculitis associated with propylithiouracil therapy. *Arch Intern Med* 147:1677, 1987.
38. Reidy TJ, Upshaw JD Jr, Chesney TM: Prophylthiouracil-induced vasculitis: A fatal case. *South Med J* 75:1297–1298, 1982.
39. Klapholz L, Leitersdorf E, Weinrauch L: Leucocytoclastic vasculitis and pneumonitis-induced by metformin. *Br Med J (Clin Res)* 293:483, 1986.
40. Maertens P, Lum G, Williams JP, et al: Intracranial hemorrhage and cerebral angiopathic changes in a suicide phenylpropanolamine poisoning. *South Med J* 80:1584–1586, 1987.
41. Epstein EH Jr, McNutt NS, Beallo R, et al: Severe vasculitis during isotretinoin therapy. *Arch Dermatol* 123:1123–1125, 1987.
42. Markman M, Lim HW, Bluestein HG: Vancomycin-induced systemic granulomatous vasculitis. *South Med J* 79:382–383, 1986.
43. Gaffey CM, Chun B, Harvey JC, et al: Phenytoin-induced systemic granulomatous vasculitis. *Arch Pathol Lab Med* 145:2051–2052, 1986.

44. Shalit M, Flugelman MY, Harats N, et al: Quinidine-induced vasculitis. *Arch Intern Med* 145:2051–2052, 1985.
45. Leung AC, McLay A, Dobbie JW, et al: Phenylbutazone-induced systemic vasculitis with crescentic glomerulonephritis. *Arch Intern Med* 145:685–687, 1985.
46. Grisold W, Jellinger K: Multifocal neuropathy with vasculitis in hypereosinophilic syndrome: An entity or drug-induce effect? *J Neurol* 231:301–306, 1985.
47. Doherty M, Maddison PJ, Grey RH: Hydralazine-induce lupus syndrome with eye disease. *Br Med J (Clin Res)* 290:675, 1985.
48. Mitchell GG, Magnusson AR, Weiler JM: Cimetidine-induced cutaneous vasculitis. *Am J Med* 75:875–876, 1983.
49. Calabrese LH, Duna GF: Drug-induced vasculitis. *Curr Opin Rheum* 8:34–40, 1996.
50. Jain KK, Basel MD: Cutaneous vasculitis associated with granulocyte colony-stimulating factor. *J Am Acad Dermatol* 31:213–215, 1994.
51. Johnson ML, Grimwood RE: Leukocyte colony stimulating factors. *Arch Dermatol* 130:77–81, 1994.
52. Fortin PR: Vasculitides associated with malignancy. *Curr Opin Rheum* 8:30–33, 1996.
53. Shafritz DA, Shouval D, Sherman HI, et al: Integration of hepatitis B virus DNA into the genome of liver cells in chronic liver disease and hepatocellular carcinoma: Studies in percutaneous liver biopsies and post-mortem tissue specimens. *N Engl J Med* 305:1067–1073, 1981.
54. Mihas AA, Kirby D, Kent SP: Hepatitis B antigen and polymyositis. *JAMA* 239:221–222, 1977.
55. Combes B, Shorey J, Barrera A, et al: Glomerulonephritis with deposition of Australia antigen-antibody complexes in glomerular basement membrane. *Lancet* 2:234–237, 1972.
56. Sergent JS, Lockshin MD, Christian CL, et al: Vasculitis with hepatitis B antigenemia. *Medicine* 55:1–18, 1976.
57. Weyand CM, Hicok KC, Hunder GG, et al: The HLA-DRB1 locus as a genetic component in giant cell arteritis. *J Clin Invest* 90:2355–2361, 19992.
58. Zhang L, Jayne DRW, Zhao MH, et al: Distribution of MHC class II alleles in primary systemic vasculitis. *Kidney Int* 47:294–298, 1995.
59. Cochran CG, Weigle WO: The cutaneous reaction to soluble antigenantibody complexes: A comparison with the Arthus phenomenon. *J Exp Med* 108:591–604, 1958.
60. Dixon FJ, Vasquesz JJ, Weigle WO, et al: Pathogenesis of serum sickness. *Arch Pathol* 65:18–28, 1958.
61. Cochrane CG, Koffler D: Immune complex disease in experimental animals and man. *Adv Immunol* 16:185–264, 1973.
62. Kauffmann RH, Thompson J, Valentijn RM, et al: The clinical implications and the pathogenetic significance of circulating immune complexes in infective endocarditis. *Am J Med* 71:17–25, 1981.
63. Mackel SE, Tappeiner G, Brumfield H, et al: Circulating immune complexes in cutaneous vasculitis: Detection with Clq and monoclonal rheumatoid factor. *J Clin Invest* 64:1652–1660, 1979.

64. Copeman PWM, Ryan TJ: Cutaneous angiitis. Patterns of rashes explained by (1) flow properties of the blood, (2) anatomical disposition of vessels. *Br J Dermatol* 85:205–214, 1971.

65. Rich A: Hypersensitivity in disease, with special reference to polyarteritis nodosa, rheumatic fever, disseminated lupus erythematosus and rheumatoid arthritis. *Harvey Lect* 42:106–147, 1946.

66. Kniker WT, Cochrane CG: The localization of circulating immune complexes in experimental serum sickness: The role of vasoactive amines and hydrodynamic forces. *J Exp Med* 127:119–136, 1968.

67. Fisher ER, Bark J: Effect of hypertension on vascular and other lesions of serum sickness. *Am J Pathol* 39:665–675, 1961.

68. Copeman PWM: Investigations into the pathogenesis of acute cutaneous angiitis. *Br J Dermatol* 82:51–65, 1970.

69. Cochrane CG, Hawkins D: Studies on circulating immune complexes. (III) Factors governing the ability of circulating complexes to localize in blood vessels. *J Exp Med* 127:137–154, 1968.

70. Soter NA, Mihm M, Gigli I, et al: Cellular kinetics of cutaneous necrotizing angiitis in a patient with cold urticaria and dermatographism. *Clin Res* 23: 386A, 1975.

71. Cochrane PWM, Tyan TJ: Studies on the localization of circulating antigen-antibody complexes and other macromolecules in vessels. (1) Structural studies. *J Exp Med* 118:480–502, 1963.

72. Henson PM, Cochrane CG: Acute immune complex disease in rabbits: The role of complement and of a leukocyte-dependent release of vasoactive amine from platelets. *J Exp Med* 133:554–571, 1971.

73. Cochrane CG, Weigle WO, Dixon FJ: The role of polymorphonuclear leukocytes in the initiation and cessation of the Arthus vasculitis. *J Exp Med* 110: 481–494, 1959.

74. Kunkel SL, Thrall RS, Kunkel RG, et al: Suppression of immune complex vasculitis in rats by prostaglandin. *J Clin Invest* 64:1525–1529, 1979.

75. Benecerraf B, Sebestyen M, Cooper NS: The clearance of antigenantibody complexes from the blood by the reticulo-endothelial system. *J Immunol* 82: 131–137, 1959.

76. Salky MK, Mills D, DiLuzio NR, et al: Activity of the reticuloendothelial system in diseases of altered immunity. *J Lab Clin Med* 66:952–960, 1965.

77. Frank MM, Hamburger MI, Lawley TJ, et al: Defective reticuloendothelial system Fc-receptor function in systemic lupus erythematosus. *N Engl J Med* 300:518–523, 1979.

78. Hamburger MI, Moutsopoulos HM, Lawley TJ, et al: Sjogren's syndrome: A defect in reticuloendothelial system Fc-receptor-specific clearance. *Ann Intern Med* 91:534–538, 1979.

79. Lockwood CM, Worlledge S, Nicholas A, et al: Reversal of impaired splenic function in patients with nephritis or vasculitis (or both) by plasma exchange. *N Engl J Med* 300:524–530, 1979.

80. Parish WE: Studies on vasculitis. (III) Decreased formation of antibody to M protein, group A polysaccharide and to some exotoxins, in persons with cutaneous vasculitis after streptococcal infection. *Clin Allergy* 1:295–309, 1971.

81. Fauci AS: Vasculitis. In: McCarty DJ, ed. *Arthritis and Allied Conditions.* Philadelphia: Lea and Febiger; 1985.
82. Spector WG, Heesom N: The production of granulomata by antigenantibody complexes. *J Pathol* 98:31–39, 1969.
83. Cid MC, Grau JM, Casademont J, et al: Immunohistochemical characterization of inflammatory cells and immunologic activation markers in muscle and nerve biopsy specimens from patients with systemic polyarteritis nodosa. *Arthritis Rheum* 37:1055–1061, 1994.
84. Cid MC, Campo E, Ercilla G, et al: Immunohistochemical analysis of lymphoid and macrophage cell subsets and their immunologic activation markers in temporal arteritis. *Arthritis Rheum* 32:884–893, 1989.
85. Cid MC: New developments in the pathogenesis of systemic vasculitis. *Curr Opin Rheum* 8:1–11, 1996.
86. Abe J, Kotzin BL, Jujo K, et al: Selective expansion of T cells expressing T-cell receptor variable regions VB2 and VB8 in Kawasaki disease. *Proc Natl Acad Sci USA* 89:4066–4070, 1992.
87. Von der Woude FJ, Rasmussen N, Lobatto S, et al: Autoantibodies against neutrophils and monocytes: Tool for diagnosis and marker of disease activity in Wegener's granulomatosis. *Lancet* 1:425–429, 1985.
88. Gross WL, Ludeman G, Kieger G, et al: Anti-cytoplasmic antibodies in Wegener's granulomatosis. *Lancet* 1:806, 1986.
89. Lockwood CM, Bakes D, Jones S, et al: Association of alkaline phosphatase with an autoantigen recognized by circulating anti-neutrophil antibodies in systemic vasculitis. *Lancet* 1:716–720, 1987.
90. Gross WL, Csernok E: Immunodiagnostic and pathophysiologic aspects of antineutrophil cytoplasmic antibodies in vasculitis. *Curr Opin Rheum* 7:11–19, 1995.
91. Gross WL, Schmitt WH, Csernok E: ANCA and associated diseases: immunologic and pathogenetic aspects. *Clin Exp Immunol* 91:1–12, 1993.
92. Falk RJ, Terrell RS, Charles LA, et al: Anti-neutrophil cytoplasmic autoantibodies induce neutrophils to degranulate and produce oxygen radicals in vitro. *Proc Natl Acad Sci USA* 87:4115–4119, 1990.
93. Ewert BH, Jennette JC, Falk RJ: Anti-myeloperoxidase antibodies stimulate neutrophils to damage human endothelial cells. *Kidney Int* 41:375–383, 1992.
94. Brouwer E, Huitema MG, Klok PA, et al: Antimyeloperoxidase-associated proliferative glomerulonephritis: An animal model. *J Exp Med* 177:905–914, 1993.
95. Mrowka C, Csernok E, Bandel R, et al: An animal model of anti-PR3-associated glomerulonephritis (GN)—first results. *Clin Exp Immunol* 111(suppl):37, 1995.
96. van Vollenhoven RF: Adhesion molecules, sex steroids and the pathogenesis of vasculitis syndromes. *Curr Opin Rheum* 7:4–10, 1995.
97. von den Driesch P, Simon M: Cellular adhesion antigen modulation in purpura pigmentosa chronica. *J Am Acad Dermatol* 30:193–200, 1993.
98. Boehme MWJ, Schmitt WH, Youinou P, et al: Clinical relevance of elevated serum thrombomodulin and soluble E-selectin in patients with Wegener's granulomatosis and other systemic vasculitides. *Am J Med* 101:387–394, 1996.
99. Winkelmann RK, Ditto WB: Cutaneous and visceral syndromes of necrotizing or "allergic" angiitis: A study of 38 cases. *Medicine* 43:59–89, 1964.

100. Cream JJ, Gumpel JM, Peachey RDG: Henoch-Schönlein purpura in the adult: A study of 77 adults with anaphylactoid or Henoch-Schönlein purpura. *Q J Med* 156:461–484, 1970.
101. Lopez LR, Schocket AL, Stanford RE, et al: Gastrointestinal involvement in leukocytoclastic vasculitis and polyarteritis nodosa. *J Rheumatol* 7:677–684, 1980.
102. Gilliam JN, Smiley JD: Cutaneous necrotizing vasculitis and related disorders. *Ann Allergy* 37:328–339, 1976.
103. Sams WM, Thorne EG, Small P, et al: Leukocytoclastic vasculitis. *Arch Dermatol* 112:219–226, 1976.
104. Cupps TR, Springer RM, Fauci AS: Chronic, recurrent small-vessel cutaneous vasculitis: Clinical experience in 13 patients. *JAMA* 247:1194–1198, 1982.
105. Callen J, Ekenstam EAF: Cutaneous leukocytoclastic vasculitis: Clinical experience in 44 patients. *South Med J* 80:848–851, 1987.
106. McDuffie FC, Sams WM Jr, Maldonado JE, et al: Hypocomplementemia with cutaneous vasculitis and arthritis: Possible immune complex disease. *Mayo Clin Proc* 48:340–348, 1973.
107. Monroe EW: Urticaria and urticarial vasculitis. *Med Clin North Am* 64:867–883, 1980.
108. Zeiss CR, Bunch FX, Marder RJ, et al: A hypocomplementemic vasculitis urticarial syndrome: A report of new cases and definition of the disease. *Am J Med* 68:867–875, 1980.
109. Ballard HS, Eisinger RP, Gallo G: Renal manifestations of the Schönlein-Henoch syndrome in adults. *Am J Med* 49:328–335, 1970.
110. Koskimies O, Rapola J, Savilahti E, et al: Renal involvement in Henoch-Schönlein purpura. *Acta Paediatr Scand* 63:357–363, 1974.
111. Farine M, Poncell S, Geary DL, et al: Prognostic significance of urinary findings and renal biopsies in children with Henoch-Schönlein nephritis. *Clin Pediatr (Phila)* 25:257–259, 1986.
112. Martinez-Frontanilla LA, Haase GM, Ernster JA, et al: Surgical complications in Henoch-Schönlein purpura. *J Pediatr Surg* 19:434–436, 1984.
113. Belman AL, Leichner CR, Moshe SL, et al: Neurologic manifestations of Schönlein-Henoch purpura: Report of three cases and review of the literature. *Pediatrics* 75:687–692, 1985.
114. Casanueva B, Rodriguez Valverde V, Merino J, et al: Increased IgA producing cells in the blood of patients with active Henoch-Schönlein purpura. *Arthritis Rheum* 26:854–860, 1983.
115. Allen DM, Diamond LK, Howell DA: Anaphylactoid purpura in children (Henoch-Schönlein syndrome). *Am J Dis Child* 99:147–168, 1960.
116. Meltzer M, Franklin EC: Cryoglobulinemia: A study of 29 patients. *Am J Med* 80:828–836, 1966.
117. Brouet DC, Clauvel DP, Danon F, et al: Biologic and clinical significance of cryoglobulins: A report of 86 cases. *Am J Med* 57:775–788, 1974.
118. Gorevic PD, Kassab JH, Levo Y, et al: Mixed cryoglobulinemia: Clinical aspects and long-term follow-up of 40 patients. *Am J Med* 69:287–308, 1980.
119. Weinberger A, Berliner S, Pinkhas J: Articular manifestations of "essential" cryoglobulinemia. *Semin Arthritis Rheum* 10:224–229, 1981.

120. Tarantino A, DeVecchi A, Montagnino G, et al: Renal disease in essential mixed cryoglobulinemia. *Q J Med* 197:1–30, 1981.

121. Berkman EM, Orlin JB: Use of plasmapheresis and partial plasma exchange in the management of patients with cryoglobulinemia. *Transfusion* 20:171–178, 1980.

122. McLeod BC, Sassetti RJ: Plasmapheresis with return of cryoglobulin-depleted autologous plasma (cryoglobulinpheresis) in cryoglobulinemia. *Blood* 55: 866–870, 1980.

123. Durand JM, Cretel E, Kaplanski G, et al: Long-term results of therapy with interferon alpha for cryoglobulinemia associated with hepatitis C virus infection. *Clin Rheumatol* 13:123–125, 1994.

124. Arkin A: A clinical and pathological study of periarteritis nodosa: A report of five cases, one histologically healed. *Am J Pathol* 6:401–426, 1930.

125. Lieb ES, Restivo C, Paulus HE: Immunosuppressive and corticosteroid therapy of polyarteritis nodosa. *Am J Med* 67:941–947, 1979.

126. Fauci AS, Katz P, Haynes BF, et al: Cyclophosphamide therapy of severe systemic necrotizing vasculitis. *N Engl J Med* 301:235–238, 1979.

127. Cohen RD, Conn DL, Ilstrup DM: Clinical features, prognosis, and response to treatment in polyarteritis. *Mayo Clin Proc* 55:146–155, 1980.

128. Frohnert PP, Sheps SG: Long-term follow-up study of periarteritis nodosa. *Am J Med* 43:8–14, 1967.

129. Rose GA: The natural history of polyarteritis. *Br Med J* 4:1148–1152, 1957.

130. Nightingale EJ: The gastroenterological aspects of periarteritis nodosa. *Am J Gastroenterol* 31:152–161, 1959.

131. Ralston DE, Kvale WF: The renal lesions of periarteritis nodosa. *Mayo Clin Proc* 24:18–27, 1949.

132. White RH, Schambelan M: Hypertension, hyperreninemia, and secondary hyperaldosteronism in systemic necrotizing vasculitis. *Ann Intern Med* 92: 199–201, 1980.

133. Tocci PE, Lankford RW, Lynne CW: Spontaneous rupture of the kidney secondary to polyarteritis nodosa. *J Urol* 113:860–863, 1975.

134. Moore PM, Fauci AS: Neurologic manifestations of systemic vasculitis: A retrospective and prospective study of the clinicopathologic features and responses to therapy in 25 patients. *Am J Med* 71:517–521, 1981.

135. Wees SJ, Sunwoo IN, Oh SJ: Sural nerve biopsy in systemic necrotizing vasculitis. *Am J Med* 71:526–532, 1981.

136. Ford RG, Siekert RG: Central nervous system manifestations of periarteritis nodosa. *Neurology* 15:114–122, 1965.

137. Miller DH, Ormerod IE, Gibson A, et al: MR brain scanning in patients with vasculitis: Differentiation from multiple sclerosis. *Neuroradiology* 29:226–231, 1987.

138. Steven MM, Belch JJ, Sturrock RD: Destructive arthritis in a patient with cutaneous polyarteritis nodosa. *Arthritis Rheum* 29:812, 1986.

139. Belisario JC: Cutaneous manifestations in polyarteritis (periarteritis) nodosa. *Arch Dermatol* 82:526–532, 1960.

140. Travers RL, Allison DJ, Brettle RP, et al: Polyarteritis nodosa: A clinical and angiographic analysis of 17 cases. *Semin Arthritis Rheum* 8:184–199, 1979.

141. Diaz-Perez JL, Winkelmann RK: Cutaneous periarteritis nodosa. *Arch Dermatol* 110:407–414, 1974.
142. Wold LE, Baggenstoss AH: Gastrointestinal lesions of periarteritis nodosa. *Mayo Clin Proc* 24:28–35, 1949.
143. Fayemi AO, Ali M, Braun EV: Necrotizing vasculitis of the gallbladder and the appendix. *Am J Gastroenterol* 67:608–612, 1977.
144. Ford GA, Bradley JR, Appleton DS, et al: Spontaneous splenic rupture in polyarteritis nodosa. *Postgrad Med J* 62:965–966, 1986.
145. Lie JT: Nomenclature and classification of vasculitis: Plus ca change, plus cest la meme chose (editorial). *Arthritis Rheum* 37:181–186, 1994.
146. Golding DN, Letcher RG: Polyarteritis involving the lower limbs associated with periosteal new bone formation. *Br J Hosp Med* 36:59–61, 1986.
147. Leung AC, McLay A, Mosley J, et al: Polyarteritis group of systemic vasculitis: A new diagnostic criteria. *Scott Med J* 30:225–231, 1985.
148. Fauci AS, Doppman JL, Wolff SM: Cyclophosphamide-induced remissions in advanced polyarteritis nodosa. *Am J Med* 64:890–894, 1978.
149. Guillevin L, Lhote F: Distinguishing polyarteritis nodosa from microscopic polyangiitis and implications for treatment. *Curr Opin Rheum* 7:20–24, 1995.
150. Jennette JC, Falk RJ, Andrassy K, et al: Nomenclature of systemic vasculitides: Proposal of an international consensus conference. *Arthritis Rheum* 37:187–192, 1994.
151. Churg J, Strauss L: Allergic granulomatosis, allergic angiitis, and periarteritis nodosa. *Am J Pathol* 27:277–301, 1951.
152. Lie JT: The classification of vasculitis and reappraisal of allergic granulomatosis and angiitis (Churg-Strauss syndrome). *Mt Sinai J Med (NY)* 1986; 53:429–439.
153. Chumbley LC, Harrison EG, Jr., DeRemee RA : Allergic granulomatosis and angiitis (Churg-Strauss syndrome): Report and analysis of 30 cases. *Mayo Clin Proc* 52:477–484, 1977.
154. Tai PC, Holt ME, Denny P, et al: Deposition of eosinophil cationic protein in granulomas in allergic granulomatosis and vasculitis: The Churg-Strauss syndrome. *Br Med J (Clin Res)* 289:400–402, 1984.
155. Spry CJ, Tai PC, Barkans J: Tissue localization of human eosinophil cationic proteins in allergic diseases. *Int Arch Allergy Appl Immunol* 71:252–254, 1985.
156. Jessurun J, Azevedo M, Saldana M: Allergic angiitis and granulomatosis (Churg-Strauss syndrome): Report of a case with massive thymic involvement in a nonasthmatic patient. *Hum Pathol* 17:637–639, 1986.
157. Olsen KD, Neel H, III, DeRemee RA, et al: Nasal manifestations of allergic granulomatosis and angiitis (Churg-Strauss syndrome). *Otolaryngol Head Neck Surg* 88:85–89, 1980.
158. Robin JB, Schanzlin DJ, Meisler DM, et al: Ocular involvement in the respiratory vasculitides. *Surv Ophthalmol* 30:127–140, 1985.
159. Dagi LR, Currie J: Branch retinal artery occlusion in the Churg-Strauss syndrome. *J Clin Neuro Ophthalmol* 5:229–237, 1985.
160. Dicken CH, Winkelmann RK: The Churg-Strauss granuloma. Cutaneous, necrotizing, palisading granulomatous in vasculitis syndromes. *Arch Pathol Lab Med* 102:576–580, 1978.
161. Yonker RA, Katz P: Necrotizing granulomatous vasculitis with eosinophilic

infiltrates limited to the prostate: Case report and review of the literature. *Am J Med* 77:362–364, 1984.

162. Davidson AG, Thompson PJ, Davies J, et al: Prominent pericardial and myocardial lesions in the Churg-Strauss syndrome (allergic granulomatosis and angiitis). *Thorax* 38:793–795, 1983.

163. Sale S, Patterson R: Recurrent Churg-Strauss vasculitis with exophthalmos, hearing loss, nasal obstruction, amyloid deposits, hyperimmunoglobulinemia E, and circulating immune complexes. *Arch Intern Med* 141:1363–1365, 1981.

164. Kus J, Berjin C, Miller R, et al: Lymphocytic subpopulations in allergic granulomatosis and angiitis (Churg-Strauss syndrome). *Chest* 87:826–827, 1985.

165. MacFayden R, Tron B, Keshmiri M, et al: Allergic angiitis of Churg and Strauss syndrome: Response to pulse methylprednisolone. *Chest* 91:629–631, 1987.

166. Crawford WJ: Cogan's syndrome associated with polyarteritis nodosa: Report of three cases. *Postgrad Med J* 60:835–838, 1957.

167. Cooper BJ, Baca E, Patterson R: Allergic angiitis and granulomatosis: Prolonged remission induced by combined prednisone-azathioprine therapy. *Arch Intern Med* 138:367–371, 1978.

168. Fauci AS, Wolff SM: Wegener's granulomatosis: Studies in eighteen patients and a review of the literature. *Medicine* 52:535–561, 1973.

169. Wolff SM, Fauci AS, Horn RG, et al: Wegener's granulomatosis. *Ann Intern Med* 81:513–525, 1974.

170. Flye MW, Mundinger GH, Fauci AS: Diagnostic and therapeutic aspects of the surgical approach to Wegener's granulomatosis. *J Thorac Cardiovasc Surg* 77:331–337, 1979.

171. Cassan SM, Colers DT, Harrison EG: The concept of the limited forms of Wegener's granulomatosis. *Am J Med* 49:366–379, 1970.

172. DeRemee RA, Weiland LH, McDonald TJ: Respiratory vasculitis. *Mayo Clin Proc* 55:492–498, 1980.

173. Woodworth TG, Abuelo JG, Austin HA, III, et al: Severe glomerulonephritis with late emergence of classic Wegener's granulomatosis. *Medicine* 66:181–191, 1987.

174. Hensle TW, Mitchell ME, Crooks KK: Urologic manifestations of Wegener's granulomatosis. *Urology* 12:553–556, 1978.

175. Adelizzi RA, Schockley GK, Pietras JR: Wegener's granulomatosis with ureteric obstruction. *J Rheumatol* 13:448–451, 1986.

176. Cupps TR, Fauci AS: Wegener's granulomatosis. *Int J Dermatol* 19:76–80, 1980.

177. Reed WB, Jensen AK, Konwaler BE, et al: The cutaneous manifestations in Wegener's granulomatosis. *Arch Dermatol Venereal* 43:250–264, 1963.

178. Kroneman OC, Peuzner M: Failure of cyclophosphamide to prevent cerebritis in Wegener's granulomatosis. *Am J Med* 80:526–527, 1986.

179. Yamashita Y, Takahashi M, Bussaka H, et al: Cerebral vasculitis secondary to Wegener's granulomatosis: Computed tomography and angiographic findings. *J Comput Tomogr* 10:115–120, 1986.

180. Reza MJ, Dornfeld L, Goldberg LS, et al: Wegener's granulomatosis: Long-

term follow up of patients treated with cyclophosphamide. *Arthritis Rheum* 18:501–506, 1975.

181. Fauci AS, Haynes BF, Katz P, et al: Wegener's granulomatosis: Prospective clinical and therapeutic experience with 85 patients for 21 years. *Ann Intern Med* 98:76–85, 1983.

182. Strihou CY, Pirson Y, Vandenbroucke JM, et al: Haemodialysis and transplantation in Wegener's granulomatosis. *Br Med J* 2:93–94, 1979.

183. Steinman TL, Jaffee BF, Monaco AP, et al: Recurrence of Wegener's granulomatosis after kidney transplant: Successful reinduction of remission with cyclophosphamide. *Am J Med* 68:458–460, 1980.

184. Stegeman CA, Tervaert JWC, DeJong PE, et al: Trimethoprim-sulfamethoxazole(co-trimoxazole) for the prevention of relapses of Wegener's granulomatosis. *N Engl J Med* 335:16–20, 1996.

185. De Groot K, Reinhold-Keller E, Tatsis E, et al: Therapy for the maintenance of remission in sixty-five patients with generalized Wegener's granulomatosis. *Arthritis Rheum* 39:2052–2061, 1996.

186. Zvaifler NJ, Weintraub AM: Aortitis and aortic insufficiency in chronic rheumatic disorders: A reappraisal. *Arthritis Rheum* 6:241–245, 1973.

187. Paloheimo JA: Obstructive arteritis of the Takayasu's type: Clinical roentgenological and laboratory studies in 36 patients. *Acta Med Scand* 48(suppl):7–45, 1967.

188. Roth ML, Kissane MJ: Panaortitis and aortic valvulitis in progressive systemic sclerosis (scleroderma). *Am J Clin Pathol* 41:287–296, 1964.

189. Lande A, Berkman YM: Pathologic, clinical and arteriographic review. *Radiol Clin North Am* 41:287–296, 1976.

190. Lande A, Bard R, Rossi P, et al: Takayasu's arteritis: A worldwide entity. *NY State J Med* 76:1477–1482, 1976.

191. McKusick VA: A form of vascular disease relatively frequent in the Orient. *Am Heart J* 63:57–64, 1962.

192. Ueda J, Saito Y, Ito I, et al: Further immunological studies of aortitis syndrome. *Jpn Heart J* 12:1, 1971.

193. Weyand CM, Goronzy JJ: Molecular approaches toward pathologic mechanisms in giant cell arteritis and Takayasu's arteritis. *Curr Opin Rheum* 7:30–36, 1995.

194. Lupi-Herrera E, Sanchez-Torres G, Marushamer J, et al: Takayasu's arteritis: Clinical study of 107 cases. *Am Heart J* 93:94–103, 1977.

195. Nakato K, Ikeda M, Kimata S, et al: Takayasu's arteritis: Clinical report of eighty-four cases and immunological studies of seven cases. *Circulation* 35:1141–1155, 1967.

196. Ishikawa K: Natural history and classifications of occlusive thromboaortopathy (Takayasu's disease). *Circulation* 57:27–35, 1978.

197. Hall S, Barr W, Lie JT, et al: Takayasu's arteritis: A study of 32 North American patients. *Medicine* 64:89–99, 1985.

198. Mousa ARM, Marafie AA, Pajani AI: Cutaneous necrotizing vasculitis complicating Takayasu's arteritis with a review of cutaneous manifestations. *J Rheumatol* 12:607–610, 1985.

199. Nasu T: Aortitis syndrome: Pathologic aspect. *Gendai Iryo* 8:1143–1150, 1976.

200. Yamato M, Lecky JW, Hiramatsu K, et al: Takayasu's arteritis: Radiographic and angiographic findings in 59 patients. *Radiology* 162:329–334, 1986.
201. Inada K, Shimizu H, Kobayashi I, et al: Pulselessness disease and atypical coarctation of the aorta. *Arch Surg* 84:306–312, 1962.
202. Greene NB, Baughman RP, Kim CK: Takayasu's arteritis associated with interstitial lung disease and glomerulonephritis. *Chest* 89:605–606, 1986.
203. Hellman DB, Hardy K, Lindenfeld S, et al: Takayasu's arteritis associated with crescentic glomerulonephritis. *Arthritis Rheum* 30:451–454, 1987.
204. Hall S, Nelson AM: Takayasu's arteritis and juvenile rheumatoid arthritis. *J Rheumatol* 13:431–433, 1986.
205. Fraga A, Mintz G, Valle L, et al: Takayasu's arteritis: Frequency of systemic manifestations (study of 22 patients) and favorable response to maintenance steroid therapy with adrenocorticosteroids (12 patients). *Arthritis Rheum* 15: 617–624, 1972.
206. Lande A, Rossi P: The value of total aortography in the diagnosis of Takayasu's arteritis. *Radiology* 114:287–297, 1975.
207. Yamamoto S, Ogawa S, Kitano T, et al: Complete evaluation of the cardiovascular lesions in 24 patients with Takayasu's aortitis using four-image, intravenous digital subtraction angiography. *Am Heart J* 114:1426–1431, 1987.
208. Shelhamer JH, Volkman DJ, Parillo JE, et al: Takayasu's arteritis and its therapy. *Ann Intern Med* 103:121–126, 1985.
209. Lagneau P, Michel JB, Vuong PN: Surgical treatment of Takayasu's disease. *Ann Surg* 205:157–166, 1987.
210. Moro C, Tascon J, DeVega NG, et al: Takayasu's arteritis with surgically corrected severe aortic valvular regurgitation. *Vasc Surg* 13:357–361, 1979.
211. Cipriano PR, Silverman JF, Perlroth MG, et al: Coronary arterial narrowing in Takayasu's aortitis. *Am J Cardiol* 39:744–750, 1977.
212. Bloss RS, Duncan JM, Cooley DA, et al: Takayasu's arteritis: Surgical consideration. *Ann Thorac Surg* ??:27, 1979.
213. Mishima Y: Arterial insufficiency of the upper extremity with special reference to Takayasu's arteritis and Buerger's disease. *J Cardiovasc Surg* 23: 105–108, 1982.
214. Khalilullan M, Tyasi S, Lochan R, et al: Percutaneous transluminal balloon angioplasty of the aorta in patients with aortitis. *Circulation* 76:597–600, 1987.
215. Doug ZJ, Li SH, Lu XC: Percutaneous transluminal angioplasty in renovascular hypertension in arteritis: Experience in China. *Radiology* 162:447–479, 1987.
216. Grossman E, Morag B, Nussinovitch N, et al: Clinical use of captopril in Takayasu's disease. *Arch Intern Med* 44:95–96, 1984.
217. Hamilton CRJ, Shelley WM, Tumulty PA: Giant cell arteritis: Including temporal arteritis and polymyalgia rheumatica. *Medicine* 50:1–27, 1971.
218. Huston KA, Hunder GG: Giant cell (cranial) arteritis: A clinical review. *Am Heart J* 100:99–107, 1980.
219. Healey LA, Wilske KR: Manifestations of giant cell arteritis. *Med Clin North Am* 61:261–271, 1977.
220. Wilkinson IMS, Russell RWR: Arteries of the head and neck in giant cell arteritis: A pathological study to show the pattern of arterial involvement. *Arch Neurol* 27:378–391, 1972.

221. Parker F, Healey LA, Wilske KR, et al: Light and electron microscopic studies on human temporal arteries with special reference to alterations related to senescence, atherosclerosis and giant cell arteritis. *Am J Pathol* 79:57–80, 1975.
222. Waaler E, Tonder O, Milde E: Immunological and histological studies of temporal arteries from patients with temporal arteritis and/or polymyalgia rheumatica. *Acta Pathol Microbiol Scand* 79:55–63, 1976.
223. Hazelman BL, Goldstone A, Voak D: Association of polymyalgia rheumatica and giant cell arteritis with HLA-Bl. *Br Med J* 2:989–991, 1977.
224. Hazelman BL, MacLennan ICM, Esiri MM: Lymphocyte proliferation to artery antigen as a positive test in polymyalgia rheumatica. *Ann Rheum Dis* 34: 122–127, 1975.
225. Lowenstein MB, Bridgeford PH, Vasey FB, et al: Increased frequency of HLA DR3 and DR4 in polymyalgia rheumatica giant cell arteritis (abstract). *Arthritis Rheum* 25(suppl):S31, 1982.
226. Papionannou CC, Hunder GG, McDuffie FC: Cellular immunity in polymyalgia rheumatica and giant cell arteritis: Lack of response to muscle or artery homogenates. *Arthritis Rheum* 22:740–745, 1979.
227. O'Brien JP: Vascular accidents after actinic (solar) exposure: An aspect of the temporal arteritis/polymyalgia rheumatica syndrome. *Int J Dermatol* 26: 366–370, 1987.
228. Huston KA, Hunder GG, Lie JT, et al: Temporal arteritis: A 25-year epidemiologic, clinical, and pathologic study. *Ann Intern Med* 88:162–167, 1978.
229. Bengtsson B, Malmvall B: The epidemiology of giant cell arteritis including temporal arteritis and polymyalgia rheumatica: Indices of different clinical presentations and eye complications. *Arthritis Rheum* 24:899–904, 1981.
230. Kyle V, Silberman B, Silman A, et al: Polymyalgia rheumatica/giant cell arteritis in a Cambridge general practice. *Br Med J* 291:385–387, 1985.
231. Fauchald P, Rygvold O, Oystese B: Temporal arteritis and polymyalgia rheumatica, clinical and biopsy findings. *Ann Intern Med* 77:845–852, 1972.
232. Healey LA, Wilske KR: Presentation of occult giant cell arteritis. *Arthritis Rheum* 23:641–643, 1980.
233. Graham E, Holland A, Avery A, et al: Prognosis in giant cell arteritis. *Br Med J* 282:269–271, 1971.
234. Hamrin B, Jonsson M, Landberg T: Involvement of large vessels in polymyalgia rheumatica. *Lancet* 1:1193–1196, 1965.
235. Lie JT, Gordon LP, Titus JL: Juvenile temporal arteritis: Biopsy study of four cases. *JAMA* 234:496–499, 1975.
236. Ballou SP, Kahn MA, Kushner I: Giant cell arteritis in a black patient. *Ann Intern Med* 88:659–660, 1975.
237. Granato JE, Abben RP, May WS: Familial association of giant cell arteritis. *Arch Intern Med* 141:115–117, 1980.
238. Meadows SP: Temporal or giant cell arteritis. *Proc R Soc Med* 59:329–333, 1966.
239. Russell RWR: Giant cell arteritis: A review of 35 cases. *Q J Med* 59:471–489, 1959.
240. Dimant J, Ginzler E, Schlesinger M, et al: The clinical significance of Raynaud's phenomenon in systemic lupus erythematosus. *Arthritis Rheum* 22: 815–819, 1977.

241. Horton BT: Complications of temporal arteritis. *Br Med J* 1:105–106, 1966.

242. Hunder GG, Sheps SG: Intermittent claudication and polymyalgia rheumatica. *Arch Intern Med* 119:638–643, 1967.

243. Leong ASY, Alp MH: Hepatocellular disease in the giant cell arteritis/polymyalgia rheumatica syndrome. *Ann Rheum Dis* 40:92–95, 1981.

244. Olgilvie A, James PD, Toghill PJ: Hepatic artery involvement in polymyalgia rheumatica. *J Clin Pathol* 34:769–772, 1981.

245. Litwack KD, Bohan A, Silverman L: Granulomatous liver disease and giant cell arteritis. *J Rheumatol* 4:307–312, 1977.

246. McCormick HM, Neubuerger KT: Giant cell arteritis involving small meningeal and intracerebral vessels. *J Neuropathol Exp Neurol* 17:471–478, 1958.

247. Hitch JM: Dermatologic manifestations of giant cell (temporal, cranial) arteritis. *Arch Dermatol* 101:409–415, 1970.

248. Soderstrom CW, Seehafer JR: Bilateral scalp necrosis in temporal arteritis: A rare complication of Horton's disease. *Am J Med* 61:541–546, 1976.

249. Kinmont PDC, McCallum DI: Skin manifestations of giant cell arteritis. *Br J Dermatol* 76:299–308, 1964.

250. Sofferman RA: Cranial arteritis in otolaryngology. *Ann Otolaryngol* 89: 215–219, 1980.

251. Warren DA, Godfrey S, Olsen EGJ: Giant cell arteritis with peripheral neuropathy. *Lancet* 1:1010–1013, 1968.

252. Kaltreider HB, Talal N: The neuropathy of Sjogren's syndrome: Trigeminal nerve involvement. *Ann Intern Med* 70:751–762, 1969.

253. Paulley JW: Coronary ischaemia and occlusion in giant cell (temporal) arteritis. *Acta Med Scand* 208:257–263, 1980.

254. Goodman BWJ: Temporal arteritis. *Am J Med* 67:839–852, 1979.

255. Healey LA: Long-term follow-up of polymyalgia rheumatica: Evidence for synovitis. *Semin Arthritis Rheum* 13:322–328, 1985.

256. Hunder GG, Disney TF, Ward LE: Polymyalgia rheumatica. *Mayo Clin Proc* 44:849–875, 1969.

257. Kogstad OA: Polymyalgia rheumatica and its relation to arteritis temporalis. *Acta Med Scand* 178:591–598, 1965.

258. Jones JG, Hazelman BL: Prognosis and management of polymyalgia rheumatica. *Ann Rheum Dis* 40:1–5, 1981.

259. Strachan RW, How J, Brewsher PD: Masked giant cell arteritis. *Lancet* 1: 194–196, 1980.

260. Ghose MK, Shensa S, Lerner PI: Arteritis of the aged (giant cell arteritis) and fever of unexplained origin. *Am J Med* 60:429–436, 1976.

261. Bruk MI: Articular and vascular manifestations of polymyalgia rheumatica. *Ann Rheum Dis* 26:103–116, 1967.

262. Klein RG, Hunder GG, Stanson AW, et al: Large artery involvement in giant cell (temporal) arteritis. *Ann Intern Med* 83:806–812, 1975.

263. Pollock M, Blennerhassett JB, Clark AM: Giant cell arteritis and the subclavian steal syndrome. *Neurology* 23:653–657, 1973.

264. Ostberg G: On arteritis with special reference to polymyalgia rheumatica. *Acta Pathol Microbiol Scand* 237(suppl):1–59, 1973.

265. Coomes EN, Ellis RM, Kay AG: A prospective study of 102 patients with polymyalgia rheumatica syndrome. *Rheum Rehab* 15:270–276, 1976.

266. Petri JP, Sheppeard H: Giant cell arteritis diagnosed following arm claudication. *Aust NZ J Med* 14:275–276, 1984.
267. Swinson DR, Goodwill CJ, Talbot IC: Giant cell arteritis presenting as subclavian artery occlucion: A report of two cases. *Postgrad Med J* 52:525–529, 1976.
268. Hunder GG, Ward LE, Burbank MK: Giant cell arteritis producing an aortic arch syndrome. *Ann Intern Med* 66:578–582, 1967.
269. Kent DC, Arnold H: Aneurysm of the aorta due to giant cell aortitis. *J Thorac Cardiovasc Surg* 53:572–577, 1967.
270. Hepinstall RH, Porter KA, Barkley H: Giant cell (temporal) arteritis. *J Pathol Bacteriol* 67:507–519, 1954.
271. Austen WG, Blennerhassett JB: Giant cell arteritis causing an aneurysm of the ascending aorta and aortic regurgitation. *N Engl J Med* 272:80–83, 1954.
272. Salisbury RS, Hazelman BL: Successful treatment of dissecting aortic aneurysm due to giant cell arteritis. *Ann Rheum Dis* 40:507–508, 1981.
273. Bengtsson B, Malmvall B: Prognosis of giant cell arteritis including temporal arteritis and polymyalgia rheumatica: A follow-up study on ninety patients treated with corticosteroids. *Acta Med Scand* 209:339–345, 1981.
274. Thompson JR, Simmons CR, Smith LL: Polymyalgia rheumatica with bilateral subclavian artery occlusive disease. *Radiology* 101:595–596, 1971.
275. Frayha RA, Fahd S, Rizk G, et al: Pulseless disease of the elderly: An unusual presentation of giant cell (temporal) arteritis. *Rheumatol Rehabil* 21:36–41, 1982.
276. Espinoza LR, Espinoza CG: Temporal arteritis with normal E.S.R. (letter). *Arch Intern Med* 140:281–282, 1980.
277. Biller J, Ansconape J, Weinblatt ME, et al: Temporal arteritis associated with a normal sedimentation rate. *JAMA* 247:486–487, 1982.
278. Wong RL, Korn JH: Temporal arteritis without an elevated erythrocyte sedimentation rate: Case report and review of the literature. *Am J Med* 80:959–964, 1986.
279. Park JR, Jones JG, Hazelman BL: Relationship of the erythrocyte sedimentation rate to acute phase proteins in polymyalgia rheumatica and giant cell arteritis. *Ann Rheum Dis* 40:493–495, 1981.
280. Layfer LF, Banner BF, Huckman MS, et al: Temporal arteriography: Analysis of 21 cases and a review of the literature. *Arthritis Rheum* 21:780–784, 1978.
281. Horowitz HM, Pepe PF, Johnsrude IS, et al: Temporal arteriography and immunofluorescence as diagnostic tools in temporal arteritis. *J Rheumatol* 4: 76–85, 1977.
282. Sewell JR, Allison DJ, Tarin D, et al: Combined temporal arteriography and selective biopsy in suspected giant cell arteritis. *Ann Rheum Dis* 39:124–128, 1980.
283. Leu HJ, Garzoli G: Extracranial giant cell arteritis. *Pathol Microbiol* 43:187–191, 1975.
284. Frayha RA: Trichinosis-related polyarteritis nodosa. *Am J Med* 71:307–312, 1981.
285. Palm E: The ocular crises of the temporal artery syndrome (Horton). *Acta Ophthalmol* 36:208–243, 1948.
286. Kansu T, Corbett JJ, Savino P, et al: Giant cell arteritis with normal sedimentation rate. *Arch Neurol* 34:624–625, 1977.

287. Enos WF, Pierre RV, Rosenblatt JE: Giant cell arteritis detected by bone marrow biopsy. *Mayo Clin Proc* 56:381–383, 1981.

288. Klein RG, Campbell RJ, Hunder GG, et al: Skip lesions in temporal arteritis. *Mayo Clin Proc* 51:504–510, 1976.

289. Siemssen SJ: On the occurrence of necrotising lesions in arteritis temporalis: Review of literature with a note on the potential risk of a biopsy. *Br J Plastic Surg* 40:73–82, 1987.

290. Birkhead NC, Wagener HP, Shick RM: Treatment of temporal arteritis with adrenal corticosteroids: Results of fifty-five cases in which lesions were proven at biopsy. *JAMA* 163:821–827, 1957.

291. Hunder GG, Sheps SG, Allen GL, et al: Daily and alternate-day corticosteroid regimens in treatment of giant cell arteritis: Comparison in a prospective study. *Ann Intern Med* 82:613–618, 1975.

292. Bengtsson B, Malmvall B: An alternate-day corticosteroid regimen in maintenace therapy of giant cell arteritis. *Acta Med Scand* 209:347–350, 1981.

293. Beevers DG, Harpur JE, Turk KAD: Giant cell arteritis-the need for prolonged treatment. *J Chron Dis* 26:571–584, 1973.

294. Hamilton EBD: Nail studies in rheumatoid arthritis. *Ann Rheum Dis* 19:167–173, 1960.

295. Andersson R, Malmvall B, Bengtsson BA: Long-term corticosteroid treatment in giant cell arteritis. *Acta Med Scand* 220:465–469, 1986.

296. Rosenfeld SI, Kosmovsky GS, Klingele TG, et al: Treatment of temporal arteritis with ocular involvement. *Am J Med* 80:143–145, 1986.

297. Easterbrook WM, Baxter DW, Martin JR: Temporal arteritis developing during indomethacin therapy of polymyalgia rheumatica. *Can Med Assoc* 97:296–299, 1967.

298. Wadman B, Werner I: Therapeutic hazards of phenylbutazone and oxyphenbutazone in polymyalgia rheumatica. *Lancet* 1:597–598, 1'967.

299. Utsinger PD: Treatment of steroid non-responsive giant cell arteritis (GCA) with cytoxan (abstract). *Arthritis Rheum* 25(suppl):00, 1982.

300. Hernandezgarcia C, Soriano C, Morado C, et al: Methotrexate treatment in the management of giant cell arteritis. *Scand J Rheumatol* 23:295–298, 1994.

301. deSilva M, Hazelman BL: Azathioprine in giant cell arteritis/polymyalgia rheumatica: A double-blind study. *Ann Rheum Dis* 45:136–138, 1986.

302. Doury P, Pattin S, Eulry F, et al: The use of dapsone in the treatment of giant cell arteritis and polymyalgia rheumatica. *Arthritis Rheum* 26:689–690, 1983.

303. Wendling D, Hovy B, Blanc D: Cyclosporin: A new adjuvant therapy for giant cell arteritis? *Arthritis Rheum* 28:1078–1079, 1985.

304. Rivers SP, Baur GM, Inahara T, et al: Arm ischemia secondary to giant cell arteritis. *Am J Surg* 143:554–558, 1982.

305. Schneider HA, Yonker RA, Katz P, et al: Rheumatoid vasculitis: Experience with 13 patients and review of the literature. *Semin Arthritis Rheum* 14:280–286, 1985.

306. Dequeker J, Rosberg G: Digital capillaritis in rheumatoid arthritis. *Acta Rheum Scand* 13:299–307, 1967.

307. Laine VAI, Vainio KJ: Ulceration of the skin in rheumatoid arthritis. *Acta Rheum Scand* 1:113–118, 1955.

308. O'Quinn SE, Kennedy CB, Baker DT: Peripheral vascular lesions in rheumatoid arthritis. *Arch Dermatol* 92:489–494, 1965.
309. Wilkinson M, Kirk J: Leg ulcers complicating rheumatoid arthritis. *Scott Med J* 10:175–182, 1965.
310. Scott DGI, Bacon PA, Tribe CR: Systemic rheumatoid vasculitis: A clinical and laboratory study of 50 cases. *Medicine* 60:288–297, 1981.
311. Schmid FR, Cooper NS, Ziff M: Arteritis in rheumatoid arthritis. *Am J Med* 30:56–83, 1961.
312. Sokoloff L, Bunim JJ: Vascular lesions in rheumatoid arthritis. *J Chron Dis* 5: 668–687, 1957.
313. Weisman M, Zvaifler N: Cryoglobulinemia in rheumatoid arthritis: Significance in serum of patients with rheumatoid vasculitis. *J Clin Invest* 56: 725–739, 1975.
314. Scott DGI, Bacon PA, Allen C, et al: IgG rheumatoid factor, compliment and immune complexes in rheumatoid synovitis and vasculitis: Comparative and serial studies during cytotoxic therapy. *Clin Exp Immunol* 43:54–63, 1981.
315. Bywaters EGL, Scott JT: The natural history of vascular lesions in rheumatoid arthritis. *J Chron Dis* 16:905–914, 1963.
316. Bywaters EGL: Peripheral vascular obstruction in rheumatoid arthritis and its relationship to other vascular lesions. *Ann Rheum Dis* 16:84–103, 1957.
317. Glass D, Soter NA, Schur PH: Rheumatoid vasculitis. *Arthritis Rheum* 19: 950–952, 1976.
318. Stolman LP, Rosenthal D, Yaworski R, et al: Pyoderma gangrenosum and rheumatoid arthritis. *Arch Dermatol* 111:1020–1023, 1975.
319. Holt PJA, Davies MG, Saunders KC, et al: Pyoderma gangrenosum: Clinical and laboratory findings in 115 patients with special reference to polyarthritis. *Medicine* 59:114–133, 1980.
320. Scott JT, Hourihane DO, Doyle FH, et al: Digital arteritis in rheumatoid disease. *Ann Rheum Dis* 20:224–234, 1961.
321. Pallis CA, Scott JT: Peripheral neuropathy in rheumatoid arthritis. *Br Med J* 1:1141–1147, 1965.
322. Abel T, Andrew BS, Cunningham PH, et al: Rheumatoid vasculitis: Effect of cyclophosphamide on the clinical course and levels of circulating immune complexes. *Ann Intern Med* 93:407–413, 1980.
323. Cruickshank B: The arteritis of rheumatoid arthritis. *Ann Rheum Dis* 13: 136–146, 1954.
324. Conn DL, McDuffie FC, Dyck PJ: Immunopathologic study of sural nerves in rheumatoid arthritis. *Arthritis Rheum* 15:135–143, 1972.
325. Sokoloff L, Wilens AL, Bunim JJ: Arteritis of striated muscle in rheumatoid arthritis. *Am J Pathol* 27:157–173, 1951.
326. Voyles WF, Searles RP, Bankhurst AD: Myocardial infarction caused by rheumatoid arthritis. *Arthritis Rheum* 23:860–863, 1980.
327. Susmano A, Muenster JJ, Javid H, et al: Coronary arteritis in rheumatoid arthritis. *Arch Intern Med* 132:241–244, 1973.
328. Ramos M, Mandybiu TI: Cerebral vasculitis in rheumatoid arthritis. *Arch Neurol* 32:271–275, 1975.
329. Edwards JCW: Relationship between pressure and digital vasculitis. *Ann Rheum Dis* 39:138–140, 1980.

330. Gordon DA, Stein JL, Border I: The extra-articular features of rheumatoid arthritis: A systematic analysis of 127 cases. *Am J Med* 54:445–452, 1973.
331. Sokoloff L, McCluskey RT, Bunim JT: Vascularity of the early subcutaneous nodule of rheumatoid arthritis. *Arch Pathol* 55:475–495, 1953.
332. Mongan ES, Cass RM, Jacox RF, et al: A study of the relation of seronegative and seropositive rheumatoid arthritis to each other and to necrotizing vasculitis. *Am J Med* 47:23–35, 1969.
333. Theofilopoulos AN, Burtonboy G, LoSpalluto JJ, et al: IgM rheumatoid factor and low molecular weight IgM: An association with vasculitis. *Arthritis Rheum* 17:272–284, 1974.
334. Stage DE, Mannik M: 7S gM-globulin in rheumatoid arthritis: Evaluation of its clinical significance. *Arthritis Rheum* 14:440–450, 1971.
335. Scott DGI, Bacon PA, Bothamley JE, et al: Plasma exchange in rheumatoid arthritis. *J Rheumatol* 8:433–439, 1981.
336. Allen C, Elson DJ, Scott DGI, et al: IgG antiglobulins in rheumatoid arthritis and other arthritides: Relationship with clinical features and other parameters. *Ann Rheum Dis* 40:127–131, 1981.
337. Nydegger UE, Zubler RH, Gabay R, et al: Circulating complement breakdown products in patients with rheumatoid arthritis: Correlation between C3d, circulating immune complexes and clinical activity. *J Clin Invest* 59: 862–868, 1977.
338. Venebles PJW, Erhardt CC, Maini RN: Antibodies to extractable nuclear antigens in rheumatoid arthritis: Relationship to vasculitis and circulating immune complexes. *Clin Exp Immunol* 39:146–153, 1980.
339. Brubaker B, Winkelstein A: Plasma exchange in rheumatoid vasculitis. *Vox Sang* 41:295–301, 1981.
340. Erhardt CC, Mumford P, Maini RN: The association of cryoglobulinaemia with nodules, vasculitis and fibrosing alveolitis in rheumatoid arthritis and their relationship to serum Clq binding activity and rheumatoid factor. *Clin Exp Immunol* 38:408–413, 1979.
341. Starz TW, Medsger TA, Eisenbeis CH, et al: Sural nerve biopsies in rheumatoid arthritis: Light microscopic and immunofluorescence findings in 13 patients (abstract). *Arthritis Rheum* 19:823–824, 1976.
342. Rapoport RJ, Kozin F, Mackel SE, et al: Cutaneous vascular immunofluorescence in rheumatoid arthritis: Correlation with circulating immune complexes and vasculitis. *Am J Med* 68:325–331, 1980.
343. Conn DL, Schroeter AL, McDuffie FC: Cutaneous vessel immune deposits in rheumatoid arthritis. *Arthritis Rheum* 19:15–20, 1976.
344. Ferguson RH, Slocum CH: Peripheral neuropathy in rheumatoid arthritis. *Bull Rheum Dis* 11:251–254, 1961.
345. Jaffe IA: The treatment of rheumatoid arthritis and necrotizing vasculitis with penicillamine. *Arthritis Rheum* 13:436–443, 1970.
346. DeSeze S, Debeyre N, Bedoiseau M, et al: Polyarthritis rheumatoides malignes avec vasculitidies: Traitement par les medicaments a visse immuno-depressive. Etude de 5 cas. *Rev Rheum* 35:406–415, 1968.
347. Nicholls A, Snaith ML, Maini RN, et al: Controlled trial of azathioprine in rheumatoid vasculitis (abstract). *Ann Rheum Dis* 32:589–591, 1973.
348. Scott DG, Bacon PA: Intravenous cyclophosphamide plus methylpredniso-

lone in treatment of systemic rheumatoid vasculitis. *Am J Med* 76:377–384, 1984.

349. Russell AS, Davis P, Percy JS: Plasma exchange in rheumatoid arthritis? *J Rheumatol* 8:364–366, 1981.

350. Upchurch KS, Heller K, Bress NM: Low dose methotrexate therapy for cutaneous vasculitis of rheumatoid arthritis. *J Am Acad Dermatol* 17:355–359, 1987.

351. Kay S, Nanearrow JD: Spontaneous healing and relief of pain in a patient with intractable vasculitic ulceration of the lower limb following an intravenous infusion of prostacyclin: A case report. *Br J Plast Surg* 37:175–178, 1984.

352. Mintz G, Fraga A: Arteritis in systemic lupus erythematosus. *Arch Intern Med* 116:55–66, 1965.

353. Estes D, Christian CL: The natural history of systemic lupus erythematosus by prospective analysis. *Medicine* 50:85–95, 1971.

354. Tuffanelli DL, Dubois EL: Cutaneous manifestations of systemic lupus erythematosus. *Arch Dermatol* 90:377–386, 1964.

355. Caero F, Michielson FMC, Bernstein R, et al: Systemic lupus erythematosus in childhood. *Ann Rheum Dis* 40:325–331, 1981.

356. Grigor R, Edmonds J, Lewkonia R, et al: Systemic lupus erythematosus: A prospective analysis. *Ann Rheum Dis* 37:121–128, 1978.

357. Alarcon-Segovia D, Osmundson PJ: Peripheral vascular syndromes associated with systemic lupus erythematosus. *Ann Intern Med* 62:9047–919, 1965.

358. Shaffer B, James GW, Scully JP, et al: Systemic lupus erythematosus: Some cutaneous manifestations related to the diffuse collagenous diseases. *Am J Med Sci* 221:314–430, 1951.

359. Provost TT, Zone JJ, Synkowski D, et al: Unusual cutaneous manifestations of systemic lupus erythematosus: (I) Urticaria-like lesions: Correlation with clinical and serological abnormalities. *J Invest Dermatol* 75:495–499, 1980.

360. Desser KB, Sartiano GP, Cooper JL: Lupus livedo and cutaneous infarction. *Angiology* 20:261, 1969.

361. Barker LP: Disseminated lupus erythematosus with leg ulcers. *Arch Dermatol Syph* 66:758–759, 1952.

362. Brogadir SP, Myers AR: Chronic lower leg ulceration in systemic lupus erythematosus. *J Rheumatol* 6:204–209, 1979.

363. Gladstein GS, Rynes RI, Parhami N, et al: Gangrene of foot secondary to systemic lupus erythematosus with large vessel vasculitis. *J Rheumatol* 6:549–553, 1979.

364. Dubois EL, Arterberry JD: Gangrene as a manifestation of systemic lupus erythematosus. *JAMA* 181:366–374, 1962.

365. Kelley RE, Stokes N, Reyes P, et al: Cerebral transmural angiitis and ruptured aneurysm: A complication of systemic lupus erythematosus. *Arch Neurol* 37:526–527, 1980.

366. Ellis GG, Verity MA: Central nervous system involvement in systemic lupus erythematosus: A review of neuropathologic findings in 57 cases, 1955–1977. *Semin Arthritis Rheum* 8:212–221, 1979.

367. Andrianakos AA, Duffy J, Suzuki M, et al: Transverse myelopathy in systemic lupus erythematosus: Reports of 3 cases and review of the literature. *Ann Intern Med* 83:616–624, 1975.

368. Stoddard CJ, Kay PH, Simms JM, et al: Acute abdominal complications of systemic lupus erythematosus. *Br J Surg* 65:625–628, 1978.
369. Hoffman BI, Katz WA: The gastrointestinal manifestations of systemic lupus erythematosus: A review of the literature. *Semin Arthritis Rheum* 9:237–247, 1980.
370. Hermann G: Intussusception secondary to mesenteric arteritis. *JAMA* 200: 74–75, 1967.
371. Weiser MM, Andres GA, Brentjens JR, et al: Systemic lupus erythematosus and intestinal venulitis. *Gastroenterology* 81:570–579, 1981.
372. Aronson AJ, Ordonez NG, Diddie KR, et al: Immune-complex deposition in the eye in systemic lupus erythematosus. *Arch Intern Med* 139:1312–1313, 1979.
373. Haupt H, Moore GW, Hutchins GM: The lung in systemic lupus erythematosus: Analysis of the pathologic changes in 120 patients. *Am J Med* 71:791–798, 1981.
374. Rothfield NF, McCluskey RT, Baldwin DS: Renal disease in systemic lupus erythematosus. *N Engl J Med* 269:537–544, 1963.
375. Longstreth PL, Korobkin M, Paluvinskias AJ: Renal micro-aneurysms in patient with systemic lupus erythematosus. *Radiology* 113:65–66, 1974.
376. Benisch BM, Perrez N: Coronary artery vasculitis and myocardial infarction with systemic lupus erythematosus. *NY State J Med* 74:873–874, 1974.
377. Abramowsky CR, Vegas ME, Swinehart G, et al: Decidual vasculopathy of the placenta in lupus erythematosus. *N Engl J Med* 303:668–672, 1980.
378. Schocket AL, Lain D, Kohler PF, et al: Immune complex vasculitis as a cause of ascites and pleural effusion in systemic lupus erythematosus. *J Rheumatol* 5:33–38, 1978.
379. Peck B, Hoffman GS, Franck WA: Thrombophlebitis in systemic lupus erythematosus. *JAMA* 240:1729–1730, 1987.
380. Case records of the Massachusetts General Hospital 1–162. *N Engl J Med* 266: 42–49, 1962.
381. Golden RL: Livedo reticularis in systemic lupus erythematosus. *Arch Dermatol* 87:299–301, 1963.
382. Fraga A, Mintz G: Splinter hemorrhages in SLE. *Arthritis Rheum* 9:648–649, 1966.
383. Rudusky BM: Recurrent Osler's nodes in systemic lupus erythematosus. *Angiology* 20:33–37, 1969.
384. Lloyd W, Schur PH: Immune complexes, complement, and anti-DNA in exacerbations of systemic lupus erythematosus (SLE). *Medicine* 60:208–217, 1981.
385. Kirsner AV, Diller JG, Sheon RP: Systemic lupus erythematosus with cutaneous ulceration: Correlation of immunologic factors with therapy and clinical activity. *JAMA* 217:821–823, 1971.
386. Gladman DD, Urowitz MB, Keystone EC: Serologically active clinically quiescent systemic lupus erythematosus: A discordance between clinical and serologic features. *Am J Med* 66:210–215, 1979.
387. Goltz RW, Smith NG: Recurrent lower leg ulcers in lupus erythematosus. *Minn Med* 41:348–349, 1958.
388. Shingu M, Hurd ER: Sera from patients with systemic lupus erythematosus reactive with human endothelial cells. *J Rheumatol* 8:581–586, 1981.

389. Tuffanelli DL, Kay DM: Morphological and immunological studies of necrotizing vasculitis in systemic lupus erythematosus (SLE) (abstract). *Clin Res* 17:278, 1969.
390. Johnson GD, Edmonds JP, Hoborow EJ: Precipitating antibody to DNA detected by two-stage electroimmunodiffusion. *Lancet* 2:883–885, 1973.
391. Tedesco F, Silvani CM, Agelli M, et al: A lupus-like syndrome in a patient with deficiency of the sixth component of complement. *Arthritis Rheum* 24:1438–1440, 1981.
392. Bowie WEJ, Thompson JH, Pacusi CA, et al: Thrombosis in systemic lupus erythematosus despite circulating anticoagulants. *J Clin Invest* 62:416–430, 1963.
393. Gilliam JN, Cheatum DE, Hurd ER, et al: Immunoglobulin in clinically uninvolved skin in systemic lupus erythematosus: Association with renal disease. *J Clin Invest* 53:1434–1440, 1974.
394. Rothfield NF: Dermal-epidermal junction deposits in non-lesional skin of patients with systemic lupus erythematosus reflects clinical and serologic disease activity (abstract). *Arthritis Rheum* 22:652–653, 1979.
395. Klemperer P, Pollack AD, Baehr G: Pathology of disseminated lupus erythematosus. *Arch Pathol* 32:569–631, 1941.
396. Yasue T: Livedoid vasculitis and central nervous system involvement in systemic lupus erythematosus. *Arch Dermatol* 122:66–70, 1986.
397. Cheah JS: Systemic lupus erythematosus in a Chinese woman presenting with gangrene of the fingers. *Aust NZ J Med* 3:197–199, 1973.
398. Kimberly RP, Lockshin MD, Sherman RL, et al: High-dose intravenous methylprednisolone pulse therapy in systemic lupus erythematosus. *Am J Med* 70:817–824, 1981.
399. Eyanson S, Passo MH, Aldo-Benson MA, et al: Methylprednisolone pulse therapy for nonrenal lupus erythematosus. *Ann Rheum Dis* 39:377–380, 1980.
400. Dubois EL: Antimalarials in the management of discoid and systemic lupus erythematosus. *Semin Arthritis Rheum* 8:33–51, 1978.
401. Ruzicka T, Goerz G: Systemic lupus erythematosus and vasculitic urticaria. Effect of dapsone and complement levels. *Dermatologica* 162:203–205, 1981.
402. Paulus HE, Pearson CM, Pitts WJ: Aortic insufficiency in five patients with Reiter's syndrome: A detailed clinical and pathologic study. *Am J Med* 53:464–472, 1972.
403. Graham DC, Smythe HA: The carditis and aortitis of ankylosing spondylitis. *Bull Rheum Dis* 9:171–174, 1958.
404. Good AE: Reiter's disease: A review with special attention to cardiovascular and neurologic sequellae. *Semin Arthritis Rheum* 3:253–286, 1974.
405. Clark WS, Kulka JP, Bauer W: Rheumatoid aortitis with aortic regurgitation: An unusual manifestation of rheumatoid arthritis (including spondylitis). *Am J Med* 22:580–592, 1957.
406. Ansell BM, Bywaters EGL, Doniach I: The aortic lesions of ankylosing spondylitis. *Br Heart J* 20:507–515, 1958.
407. Pirani CL, Benner GA: Rheumatoid arthritis: A report of three cases progressing from childhood and emphasizing certain systemic manifestations. *Hosp Jt Dis Bull* 12:335–367, 1951.

408. Weed CL, Kulander BG, Mazzarella JA, et al: Heart block in ankylosing spondylitis. *Arch Intern Med* 117:800–806, 1966.
409. Schilder DP, Harvery WP, Hufnagel CA: Rheumatoid spondylitis and aortic insufficiency. *N Engl J Med* 255:11–17, 1956.
410. Stewart SR, Robbins DL, Castles JJ: Acute fulminant aortic and mitral insufficiency in ankylosing spondylitis. *N Engl J Med* 299:1448–1449, 1978.
411. Weintraub AM, Zvaifler NJ: Rheumatoid heart disease: A clinical as well as pathologic entity (abstract). *Arthritis Rheum* 5:327–328, 1962.
412. Csonka GW, Litchfield JW, Oates JK, et al: Cardiac lesions in Reiter's disease. *Br Med J* 1:243–247, 1961.
413. Rodnan GP, Benedek TG, Sharer JA, et al: Reiter's syndrome and aortic insufficiency. *JAMA* 189:889–894, 1964.
414. Cliff JM: Spinal bony bridging and carditis in Reiter's disease. *Ann Rheum Dis* 30:171–179, 1971.
415. Ball GV, Hathaway B: Ankylosing spondylitis with widespread arteritis. *Arthritis Rheum* 9:737–745, 1966.
416. Somer T, Siltanen P: Aneurysm of the descending thoracic aorta, amyloidosis and renal cell carcinoma in a patient with ankylosing spondylitis. *Am J Med* 49:408–415, 1970.
417. Duvernoy WFC, Schatz IJ: Rheumatoid spondylitis associated with aneurysmal dilatation of the entire thoracic aorta. *Henry Ford Hosp Med Bull* 14:309–312, 1966.
418. La Bresh RA, Lally EV, Sharma SC, et al: Two dimensional echocardiographic detection of preclinical aortic root abnormalities in rheumatoid variant disease. *Am J Med* 78:908–912, 1985.
419. Roberts WC, Hollinsworth JF, Bulkley BH, et al: Combined mitral and aortic regurgitation in ankylosing spondylitis. Angiographic and anatomic features. *Am J Med* 56:237–243, 1974.
420. Malette WG, Eisenman B, Danielson GK, et al: Rheumatoid spondylitis and aortic insufficiency: An operable combination. *J Thorac Cardiovasc Surg* 57:471–474, 1969.
421. McAdam LP, O'Hanlan MA, Bluestone R, et al: Relapsing polychondritis: Prospective study of 23 patients and a review of the literature. *Medicine* 55:193–215, 1976.
422. Hughes RAC, Berry CL, Seifert M, et al: Relapsing polychrondritis: Three cases with a clinico-pathological study and literature review. *Q J Med* 163:363–380, 1972.
423. Arkin CR, Masi AT: Relapsing polychondritis: Review of current status and case report. *Semin Arthritis Rheum* 5:41–62, 1975.
424. Anderson B: Ocular lesions in relapsing polychrondritis and other rheumatoid syndromes. *Am J Ophthalmol* 64:35–50, 1967.
425. Damiani JM, Leving HL: Relapsing polychrondritis. Report of ten cases. *Laryngoscope* 89:929–946, 1979.
426. Chang-Miller A, Okamura M, Torres VE, et al: Renal involvement in relapsing polychondritis. *Medicine* 60:202–217, 1987.
427. Prentice RL, Gatonby PA, Dagleish AG, et al: Relapsing polychondritis associated with recurrent oral ulceration. *J Rheumatol* 11:559–561, 1984.

428. Esdaile J, Hawkins D, Gold P, et al: Vascular involvement in relapsing poly-chondritis. *Can Med Assoc J* 116:1019–1022, 1977.
429. Cipriano PR, Alonso DR, Baltaxe HA, et al: Multiple aortic aneurysms in relapsing polychondritis. *Am J Cardiol* 37:1097–1102, 1976.
430. Pearson CM, Kroening R, Verity MA, et al: Aortic insufficiency and aortic aneurysm in relapsing polychondritis. *Trans Assoc Am Physiol* 80:71–89, 1967.
431. Hainer JW, Hamilton GW: Aortic abnormalities in relapsing polychondritis: Report of a case with dissecting aortic aneurysm. *N Engl J Med* 280:1166–1168, 1969.
432. Somers G, Potvliege P: Relapsing polychondritis: Relation to periarteritis nodosa. *Br Med J* 2:603–604, 1978.
433. Weinberger A, Myers AR: Relapsing polychondritis associated with cuta-neous vasculitis. *Arch Dermatol* 115:980–981, 1979.
434. Small P, Black M, Davidman M, et al: Wegener's granulomatosis and relaps-ing polychondritis: A case report. *J Rheumatol* 7:915–918, 1980.
435. Jouanen ED, Alarcon-Segovia D: Chondritis of the ear in Wegener's granulo-matosis. *Arthritis Rheum* 20:1286–1288, 1977.
436. Herman JH, Dennis MV: Immunopathologic studies in relapsing polychon-dritis. *J Clin Invest* 52:549–558, 1973.
437. Rajapakse DA, Bywaters EGL: Relapsing polychrondritis and pulseless dis-ease. *Br Med J* 4:488–489, 1973.
438. Barjon P, Bouder C, Pelisser JG, et al: Polychondrite chronique recidivante (a propos d'une observation). *J Med Montpeller* 2:197–198, 1967.
439. Foidert J-M, Abe S, Martin GR, et al: Antibodies to type II collagen in relaps-ing polychondritis. *N Engl J Med* 299:1203–1207, 1978.
440. Bergfield WF: Relapsing polychondritis with positive direct immunofluores-cence. *Arch Dermatol* 114:127, 1978.
441. Valenzuela R, Cooperrider PA, Gogate P, et al: Relapsing polychondritis: Immunomicroscopic findings in cartilage of ear biopsy specimens. *Hum Pa-thol* 11:19–22, 1980.
442. Michet CJ, McKenna CH, Luthra HS, et al: Relapsing polychondritis: Survival and predictive role of early disease manifestations. *Ann Intern Med* 104:74–78, 1986.
443. Kremer J, Gates SA, Parhami N: Relapsing polychondritis: Excellent response to naproxen and aspirin. *J Rheumatol* 6:719–720, 1979.
444. Ridgeway HB, Hansotia PL, Schorr WF: Relapsing polychondritis: Unusual neurological findings and therapeutic efficacy of dapsone. *Arch Dermatol* 115:43–45, 1979.
445. Askari AD: Colchicine for treatment of relapsing polychondritis. *J Am Acad Dermatol* 10:507–510, 1984.
446. Svenson KL, Holmdahl R, Klareskog L, et al: Cyclosporin A treatment in a case of relapsing polychondritis. *Scand J Rheumatol* 13:329–333, 1984.
447. D'Angleo WA, Fries JF, Masi AT, et al: Pathologic observations in systemic sclerosis (scleroderma): A study of fifty-eight autopsy cases and fifty-eight matched controls. *Am J Med* 46:428–440, 1969.
448. Lee JE, Haynes JM: Carotid arteritis and cerebral infarction due to sclero-derma. *Neurology* 17:18–22, 1967.

449. Norton WL, Nardo JM: Vascular disease in progressive systemic sclerosis (scleroderma). *Ann Intern Med* 73:317–324, 1970.

450. Clinico Pathologic Conference: Scleroderma (progressive systemic sclerosis). *Am J Med* 36:301–314, 1964.

451. Blunt RJ, Porter JM: Raynaud's syndrome. *Semin Arthritis Rheum* 10:281–308, 1981.

452. Jaffe I: Nifedipine in digital ulceration in scleroderma. *Arthritis Rheum* 25:1267–1269, 1982.

453. Martin MFR, Dowd PM, Ring EFJ: Prostaglandin E1 infusions for vascular insufficiency in progressive systemic sclerosis. *Ann Rheum Dis* 40:350–354, 1981

454. D'Angelo WA: Progressive systemic sclerosis. Management I. Introduction and general commentary. *Clin Rheum Dis* 5:263–276, 1979.

455. Banker BQ, Victor M: Dermatomyositis (systemic angiopathy) of childhood. *Medicine* 45:261–289, 1966.

456. Niakan E, Pitner SE, Whitaker JN, et al: Immunosuppressive agents in corticosteroid-refractory childhood dermatomyositis. *Neurology* 30:286–291, 1980.

457. Crowe WE, Bove KE, Lecinson JE, et al: Clinical and pathogenetic implications of histopathology in childhood polydermatomyositis. *Arthritis Rheum* 25:126–139, 1982.

458. Pachman LM, Cooke N: Juvenile dermatomyositis: A clinical and immunologic study. *J Pediatr* 96:226–234, 1980.

459. Pachman LM: Juvenile dermatomyositis. *Pediatr Clin North Am* 33:1097–1117, 1988.

460. Carpenter S, Karpati G, Rothman S, et al: The childhood type of dermatomyositis. *Neurology* 26:952–562, 1976.

461. Hochberg MC, Feldman D, Stevens MB: Adult onset polymyositis/dermatomyositis: An analysis of clinical and laboratory features and survival in 76 patients with a review of the literature. *Semin Arthritis Rheum* 15:168–178, 1986.

462. Sharp GC, Irvin WS, Tan EM, et al: Mixed connective tissue disease: An apparent distinct rheumatic disease syndrome associated with a specific antibody to an extractable nuclear antigen (ENA). *Am J Med* 52:148–159, 1972.

463. Nimelstein SH, Brody S, McShane D, et al: Mixed connective tissue disease: A subsequent evaluation of the original 25 patients. *Medicine* 59:239–248, 1980.

464. Bennett RM, O'Connell DJ: Mixed connective tissue disease: A clinicopathologic study of 20 cases. *Semin Arthritis Rheum* 10:25–51, 1980.

465. Singsen BH, Swanson VL, Bernstein BH, et al: A histologic evaluation of mixed connective tissue disease in childhood. *Am J Med* 68:710–717, 1980.

466. Haynes DC, Gershwin ME: The immunopathology of progressive systemic sclerosis (PSS). *Semin Arthritis Rheum* 11:331–351, 1982.

467. Tsokos M, Lazarou SA, Moutsopoulos HM: Vasculitis in primary Sjogren's syndrome: Histologic classification and clinical presentation. *Am J Clin Pathol* 88:26–31, 1987.

468. Provost TT, Vasily D, Alexander E: Sjogren's syndrome: Cutaneous, immunologic and nervous system manifestations. *Neurol Clin* 5:405–425, 1987.

469. Alexander E, Provost TT: Sjogren's syndrome: Association of cutaneous vasculitis with central nervous system disease. *Arch Dermatol* 123:801–810, 1987.
470. Kawasaki T: Mucocutaneous lymph node syndrome: Clinical observation of 50 cases (Japanese). *Jpn J Allergy* 16:178–222, 1967.
471. Morens DM, O'Brien RJ: Kawasaki disease in the United States. *J Infect Dis* 137:91–93, 1978.
472. Melish ME, Hicks RM, Larson EJ: Mucocutaneous lymph node syndrome in the United States. *Am J Dis Child* 130:599–607, 1976.
473. Melish ME: Kawasaki syndrome: A 1986 perspective. *Rheum Dis Child* 13: 7–17, 1987.
474. Glanzer JM, Galbraith WB, Jacobs JP: Kawasaki disease in a 28-year old man. *JAMA* 244:1604–1606, 1980.
475. Odom RB, Olson EG: Mucocutaneous lymph node syndrome. *Arch Dermatol* 113:339–340, 1977.
476. Tanaka N, Sakimoto K, Naoe S: Kawasaki disease: Relationship with infantile polyarteritis nodosa. *Arch Pathol Lab Med* 100:81–86, 1976.
477. Amano S, Hazama F, Hamashima Y: Pathology of Kawasaki disease: (II) Distribution and incidence of the vascular lesions. *Jpn Circ J* 43:741–748, 1979.
478. Kata H, Koike S, Tanaka C, et al: Coronary heart disease in children with Kawasaki disease. *Jpn Circ J* 43:469–475, 1979.
479. Canter CE, Bower RJ, Strauss AW: A typical Kawasaki disease with aortic aneurysm. *Pediatrics* 68:885–888, 1981.
480. Lipson HM, Ament ME, Fonkalsrud EW: Ruptured hepatic artery aneurysm and coronary artery aneurysms with myocardial infarction in a 14 year-old boy: New manifestations of mucocutaneous lymph node syndrome. *J Pediatr* 98:933–936, 1981.
481. Mercer S, Carpenter B: Surgical complications of Kawasaki disease. *J Pediatr Surg* 16:444–448, 1981.
482. Fukushige J, Nihill M, McNamara DG: Spectrum of cardiovascular lesions in mucocutaneous lymph node syndrome: Analysis of eight cases. *Am J Cardiol* 45:98–107, 1980.
483. Teixeira OHP, Pong AH Vlad P: Amputating gangrene in Kawasaki disease. *Can Med Assoc J* 127:132–134, 1982.
484. Westphalen MA, Mc Grath MA, Kelly W, et al: Kawasaki disease with severe peripheral ischaemia: Treatment with prostaglandin E infusion. *Clin Lab Observ* 112:431–433, 1987.
485. Miller DL, Reinig JW, Volkman DJ: Vascular imaging with MRI: Inadequacy in Takayasu's arteritis compared with angiography. *AJR* 146:949–954, 1986.
486. Koren G, Macleod M: Difficulty in achieving therapeutic serum concentrations of salicylate in Kawasaki disease. *J Pediatr* 105:991, 1984.
487. Furnsho K, Nakano H, Shinomiya K, et al: High-dose intravenous gammaglobulin for Kawasaki disease. *Lancet* 8411:1055–1057, 1984.
488. Newburger JW, Takahashi M, Burns JC, et al: The treatment of Kawasaki syndrome with intravenous gamma globulin. *N Engl J Med* 315:341–347, 1986.
489. Nagashima M, Matsushima M, Matsuoka H, et al: High dose gammaglobulin therapy for Kawasaki disease. *J Pediatr* 110:710–712, 1987.
490. Calabrese LH, Duna GF, Lie JT: Review: Vasculitis in the central nervous system. *Arthritis Rheum* 40:1189–1201, 1997.

491. Sigal LH: The neurologic presentation of vasculitis and rheumatologic syndromes. *Medicine* 66:157–180, 1987.

492. Cogan DG: Syndrome of nonsyphilitic interstitial keratitis and vestibuloauditory symptoms. *Arch Ophthalmol* 33:144–149, 1945.

493. Haynes BF, Kaiser-Kupfer MI, Mason P, et al: Cogan's syndrome: Studies in thirteen patients, long-term follow-up, and a review of the literature. *Medicine* 59:426–441, 1980.

494. Cheson BD, Bluming AZ, Alroy J: Cogan's syndrome: A systemic vasculitis. *Am J Med* 60:549–555, 1976.

495. Bicknell JM, Holland JV: Neurologic manifestations of Cogan's syndrome. *Neurology* 28:278–281, 1978.

496. Pinals RS: Cogan's syndrome with arthritis and aortic insufficiency. *J Rheumatol* 5:294–298, 1978.

497. Eisenstein B, Tanbenhaus M: Nonsyphilitic interstitial keratitis and bilateral deafness (Cogan's syndrome) associated with cardiovascular disease. *N Engl J Med* 258:1076–1079, 1958.

498. Cogan DG, Dickersin GR: Nonsyphilitic interstitial keratitis with vestibuloauditory symptoms: A case with fatal aortitis. *Arch Opthalmol* 71:172–175, 1964.

499. Gelfand ML, Kantor T, Gorstein F: Cogan's syndrome with cardiovascular involvement: Aortic insufficiency. *Bull NY Acad Med* 48:647–660, 1972.

500. Vollertsen RS, Mc Donald TJ, Younge BR, et al: Cogan's syndrome: 18 cases and a review of the literature. *Mayo Clin Proc* 61:344–361, 1986.

501. Behcet H: Uba rezidivierende apthose, durch ein Virus revursachte Geschwure am und, am Auge und an der Genitalien. *Dermatol Wochenschr* 105:1152–1157, 1937.

502. Jorizzo JL: Behcet's disease: An update based on the 1985 International Conference in London. *Arch Dermatol* 122:556–558, 1986.

503. Chajek T, Fainaru M: Behcet's disease: Report of 41 cases and a review of the literature. *Medicine* 54:179–196, 1975.

504. Shimizu T, Ehrlich GE, Inaba G, et al: Behcet's disease (Behcet's Syndrome). *Semin Arthritis Rheum* 8:223–260, 1979.

505. O'Duffy DJ, Godstein NP: Neurologic involvement in seven patients with Behcet's disease. *Am J Med* 61:170–178, 1976.

506. Oshima Y, Shimizu T, Yokohari R, et al: Clinical studies on Behcet's syndrome. *Ann Rheum Dis* 22:36–45, 1963.

507. Pallis CA, Fudge BJ: The neurological complications of Behcet's syndrome. *Arch Neurol Psych* 75:1–14, 1956.

508. Jorizzo JL: Behcet's disease. *Neurol Clin* 5:427–440, 1987.

509. Shikano S: Ocular pathology of Behcet's syndrome. In: Monacelli M, ed. *Symposium on Behcet's Disease*. Rome: S. Karger AG; 1966, pp. 111–136.

510. O'Duffy DJ, Carney JA: Behcet's disease: Report of 10 cases, 3 with new manifestations. *Ann Intern Med* 75:561–570, 1971.

511. Hamza M: Large artery involvement in Behcet's disease. *J Rheumatol* 14:554–559, 1987.

512. Enoch BA: Gangrene in Behcet's syndrome. *Br Med J* 3:54, 1969; .

513. Mowat AG, Hothersall TE: Gangrene in Behcet's syndrome. *Br Med J* 2:636, 1969.

514. Hirohata S, Takeuchi A, Miyamoto T: Association of cerebrospinal fluid IgM

index with central nervous system involvement in Behcet's disease. *Arthritis Rheum* 29:793–796, 1986.

515. Nussenblatt RB, Palestine AG, Chan CC, et al: Effective use of cyclosporin therapy for Behcet's disease. *Arthritis Rheum* 28:671–679, 1985.

516. Binder AL, Graham EM, Sanders MD, et al: Cyclosporin A in the treatment of severe Behcet's uveitis. *Br J Rheumatol* 26:285–291, 1987.

517. Hamuryudau V, Moral F, Yurdakul S, et al: Systemic interferon alpha-2b treatment in Behcet's syndrome. *J Rheumatol* 21:1098–1100, 1994.

518. Pacor ML, Biasi D, Lunardi C, et al: Cyclosporin in Behcet's disease: Results in 16 patients after 24 months of therapy. *Clin Rheumatol* 13:224–227, 1994.

519. Buerger L: Thromboangiitis obliterans: A study of the vascular lesions leading to presenile spontaneous gangrene. *Am J Med Sci* 136:567–580, 1908.

520. Fisher CM: Cerebral thromboangiitis obliterans (including a critical review of the literature). *Medicine* 36:169–209, 1957.

521. Wessler S, Ming SC, Gurewich B, et al: A critical evaluation of thromboangiitis obliterans: The case against Buerger's disease. *N Engl J Med* 262:1149–1160, 1960.

522. McKusick BA, Harris WS, Ottesen OE, et al: Buerger's disease: A distinct clinical and pathologic entity. *JAMA* 181:5–12, 1962.

523. Szilagyi DE, DeRusso FJ, Elliot JPJ: Thromboangiitis obliterans: Clinico-angiographic correlations. *Arch Surg* 88:824–835, 1964.

524. Schatz IJ, Fine G, Eyler WR: Thromboangiitis obliterans. *Br Heart J* 28:84–91, 1966.

525. McPherson JR, Jergens JL, Gifford RW, Jr: Thromboangiitis obliterans and atherosclerosis obliterans. *Ann Intern Med* 59:288–296, 1963.

526. Wessler S: Buerger's disease revisited. *Surg Clin North Am* 49:703–713, 1969.

527. Inada K, Hayashi M, Okatani T: Chronic occlusive arterial disease of the lower extremity in Japan. With special reference to Buerger's disease. *Arch Surg* 88:454–460, 1964.

528. McKusick VA, Harris WS, Ottesen OE, et al: Arteriographic observations, with special reference to involvement of the upper extremities and the differentiation from atherosclerosis and embolism. *Bull Johns Hopkins Hosp* 110:145–176, 1962.

529. Shionoya S, Ban I, Nakata Y, et al: Diagnosis, pathology, and treatment of Buerger's disease. *Surgery* 75:695–700, 1974.

530. Nielubowicz J, Rosnowski A, Pruszynski B, et al: Natural history of Buerger's disease. *J Cardiovasc Surg* 21:629–640, 1980.

531. Goodman RM, Elian B, Mozes M, et al: Buerger's disease in Israel. *Am J Med* 39:601–615, 1965.

532. Symposium on Buerger's disease. 19th Congress of the European Society of Cardiovascular Surgery (Warsaw, July 2, 1970). *J Cardiovasc Surg* 14:1–51, 1973.

533. Wong J, Lam STK, Ong GB: Buerger's disease: A review of 105 patients. *Aust N Z J Surg* 48:382–387, 1978.

534. Hill GL: A rational basis for the management of patients with the Buerger syndrome. *Br J Surg* 61:476–481, 1974.

535. Hiertonn T, Lund F, Philipson J: Thromboangiitis obliterans in women. Gangrene; blood vessel graft. *Angiology* 7:233–242, 1956.

536. Cabezas-Moya R, Dragstedt LR: An extreme example of Buerger's disease. *Arch Surg* 101:632–634, 1970.

537. O'Dell JL Jr, Mankin RS, et al: Thromboangiitis obliterans (Buerger's disease) and smokeless tobacco. *Arthritis Rheum* 30:1054–1056, 1987.

538. Flesh LH, Kihm RH, Ciccio S: Radionuclide imaging of aortic involvement in Buerger's disease: Case report. *J Nucl Med* 18:125–127, 1977.

539. Hirai M, Shionoya S: Intermittent claudication in the foot and Buerger's disease. *Br J Surg* 65:210–213, 1978.

540. Quenneville JG, Prat A, Gossard D: Sublingual-splinter hemorrhage in early sign of thromboangiitis obliterans. *Angiology* 32:424–432, 1981.

541. Biller J, Asconape J, Challa BR, et al: A case for cerebral thromboangiitis obliterans. *Stroke* 12:686–689, 1981.

542. Deitch EA, Sikkema WW: Intestinal manifestations of Buerger's disease: Case report and literature review. *Am Surg* 7:326–328, 1981.

543. Sobel RA, Ruebner BH: Buerger's disease involving the celiac artery. *Hum Pathol* 10:112–115, 1979.

544. Hirai M, Shionoya S: Arterial obstruction of the upper limb in Buerger's disease: Its incidence and primary lesion. *Br J Surg* 66:124–128, 1979.

545. Giler SH, Zelikovski A, Goren G, et al: Aneurysm of the radial artery in a patient with Buerger's disease. *Vasa* 8:147–149, 1979.

546. Williams G: Recent views on Buerger's disease. *J Clin Pathol* 22:573–578, 1969.

547. Smolen JS, Youngchiyud U, Weidinger P, et al: Autoimmunological aspects of thromboangiitis obliterans (Buerger's disease). *Clin Immunol Immunopathol* 11:168–177, 1978.

548. Gulati SM, Singh KS, Thusoo TK, et al: Immunological studies in thromboangiitis obliterans (Buerger's disease). *J Surg Res* 27:287–293, 1979.

549. Eisen ME, Tyson MC, Michael S, et al: Adhesiveness of blood platelets in arteriosclerosis obliterans, thromboangiitis obliterans, acute thrombophlebitis, chronic venous insufficiency and arteriosclerotic heart disease. *Circulation* 3:271–274, 1951.

550. Kobayashi H, Mishima Y: Platelet aggregability in chronic arterial occlusive diseases of the extremities. *Thromb Res* 20:363–373, 1980.

551. Craven JL, Cotton RC: Haematological differences between thromboangiitis obliterans and atherosclerosis. *Br J Surg* 54:862–867, 1967.

552. McLoughlin GA, Helsby CR, Evans CC, et al: Association of HLA-A9 and HLA-B5 with Buerger's disease. *Br Med J*; 2:1165–1166, 1976.

553. deMoerloose PH, Jeannet M, Mitimanoff P, et al: Evidence for an HLA-linked resistance gene in Buerger's disease. *Tissue Antigens* 14:169–173, 1979.

554. Gupta RL, Papiha SS: ABO blood groups and serum proteins in thromboangiitis obliterans (Buerger's disease). *Hum Hered* 28:285–292, 1978.

555. Lie JT: Thromboangiitis obliterans (Buerger's disease) in an elderly man after cessation of cigarette smoking: A case report. *Angiology* 38:864–867, 1987.

556. Nakata Y, Suzuki S, Kawai S, et al: Effects of lumbar sympathectomy on thromboangiitis obliterans. *J Cardiovasc Surg* 16:415–425, 1975.

557. Shionoya S, Ban I, Nakata Y, et al: Surgical treatment of Buerger's disease. *J Cardiovasc Surg* 21:77–84, 1980.

558. Shionoya S, Ban I, Nakata Y, et al: Vascular reconstruction in Buerger's disease. *Br J Surg* 1976; 63:841–846, 1980.

559. Hoshino S, Nakayama K, Igari T, et al: Long-term results of omental trans-plantation for chronic occlusive arterital disease. *Int Surg* 68:47–50, 1983.
560. Szczeklik A, Gryglewski RJ, Nizankowski R, et al: Prostacyclin in the therapy of peripheral arterial disease. *Adv Prostaglandin Thromboxane Leukot Res*7: 687–689, 1980; .
561. Olsson AG, Thyresson N: Healing of ischaemic ulcers by intravenous prosta-glandin E in a woman with thromboangiitis obliterans. *Acta Derm Vernereol (Stockh)* 58:467–472, 1985.
562. Brassai S, Kovalszki P, Pop GH, et al: Hypervolemic treatment of the chronic obliterative arteriopathies of extremitis. *Med Interna* 24:37–41, 1986.

18

Current Techniques for Thoracoscopic Sympathectomy

Samuel S. Ahn, MD, Kyung M. Ro, BS, and J. Patrick Johnson, MD

Anesthesia

Thoracoscopic sympathectomy is performed under general endotracheal anesthesia using a double lumen endotracheal tube with the ipsilateral lung deflated and nonventilated. Standard intraoperative monitoring techniques should be used. The patient is placed in the standard lateral decubitis position with the arm abducted and the ipsilateral chest hyperextended to provide optimal exposure of the pleural space (Figure 1). The operating table is flexed with the abducted ipsilateral arm positioned at a 90° angle on a mechanical armrest to maximize expansion of the intercostal space. Should it be necessary, this position will also allow for immediate conversion to an open thoracotomy.

Instruments

The instruments and equipment required for successful implementation of the thoracoscopic sympathectomy include the following: (1) an endoscopic video monitor with an 8- to 10-mm diameter rigid laparoscope with an available 0° and 30° angled lens; (2) a 5-mm diameter blunt-tipped scissors with an electrocautery attachment; (3) a 5-mm diameter suction/irrigator with an electrocautery hook apparatus; (4) a 10-mm diameter

From Machleder HI, (ed): *Vascular Disorders of the Upper Extremity*. Third Revised Edition. Futura Publishing Company, Inc., Armonk, NY, © 1998.

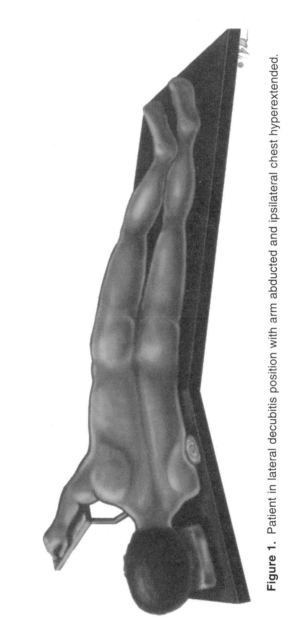

Figure 1. Patient in lateral decubitis position with arm abducted and ipsilateral chest hyperextended.

curved grasper; (5) a 10-mm diameter right-angled clamp; (6) a 10-mm diameter laparoscopic clip applier; and (7) a 10-mm diameter laparoscopic fan-shaped retractor.

Ports

All port incisions require a 1- to 1.5-cm skin incision and blunt dissection with a curved clamp through the muscles and pleura into the thorax. Three ports are recommended: one endoscope port and two instrument ports (Figure 2). The thoracoports are soft, flexible rubber tubes that are inserted through the chest wall. The endoscope port extends through the

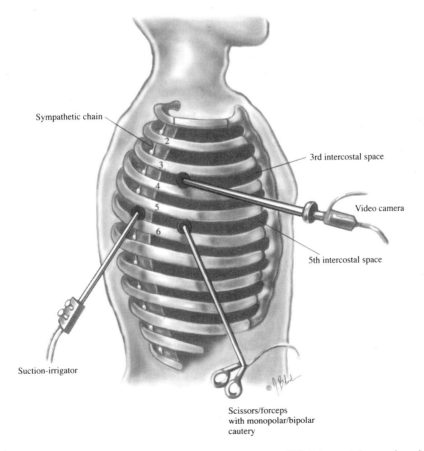

Figure 2. Diagram of port placement: one endoscope (fifth intercostal space) and two intrument ports (third and fourth intercostal space).

fifth or sixth intercostal space in the mid-axillary line. The remaining two instrument ports are placed in the posterior axillary line in the same intercostal space and in the third or fourth intercostal space in the anterior axillary line, respectively. If an additional port is neccessary for lung retraction, this should be placed in the fifth intercostal space along the anterior axillary line.

Steps for the Procedure

1. Insert the endoscope through the port located in the fifth or sixth intercostal space in the mid-axillary line to allow for optimal visualization of the upper thoracic cavity. The 0° endoscope will suffice for most procedures, but the 30° endoscope should be readily available.

2. With scope assistance, insert two instrument ports, one in the fifth or sixth intercostal space in the posterior axillary line and the other in the third or fourth intercostal space in the anterior axillary line.

3. Coagulate any adhesions of the lung to the parietal pleura to allow proper retraction of the lung. Opacification of the pleura, which is often seen in older patients due to pleural scarring, impedes visualization of the sympathetic chain.

4. Mechanically collapse and deflate the ipsilateral lung. The fan retractor can be used if additional collapse and retraction of the ipsilateral lung is required.

5. Identify ribs 1 through 4 and the intercostal nerves inferior to the ribs that course over the mid-portion of the vertebral body.

6. Identify the sympathetic ganglia and chain located dorsal to the vetebral body. The sympathetic chain will appear as a slightly pinkish-white, glistening, raised longitudinal structure that courses over the neck of the ribs (Figure 3).

7. The superior aspect of the sympathetic chain and the extent of surgical dissection is identified by visualization of the subclavian artery. The azygous and subclavian vein and the highest intercostal artery and veins should be promptly identified to avoid damaging them during subsequent dissection.

8. The sympathectomy procedure begins with the incision of the pleura over the sympathetic chain at T4. The pleural incision is extended over the length of the sympathetic chain from T4 to the superior cervical ganglion. The sympathetic chain is then mobilized and lifted from its bed (Figure 3).

9. Cut each rami communicantes of the corresponding sympathetic ganglia, T2–4 (Figure 4).

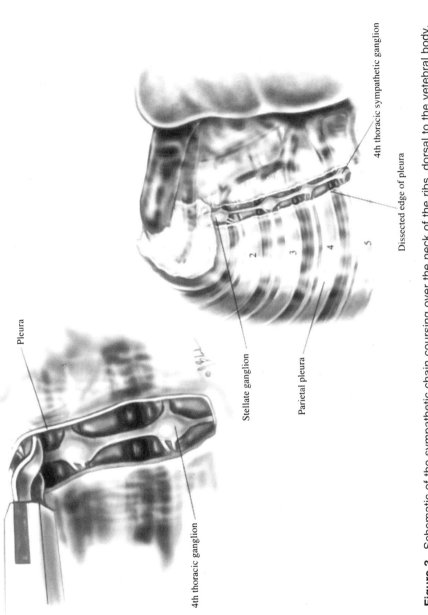

Figure 3. Schematic of the sympathetic chain coursing over the neck of the ribs, dorsal to the vetebral body.

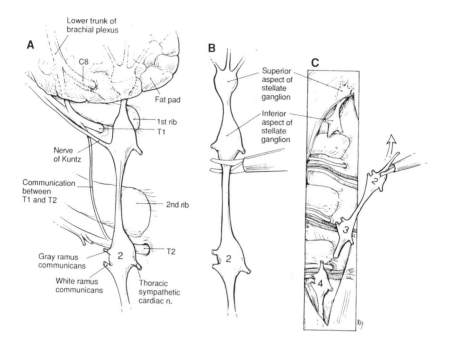

Figure 4. Diagram of the dissected rami communicante and corresponding sympathetic ganglia.

10. Identify and cut the nerve of Kuntz. This is a large branch of the T1 ramus that runs parallel and lateral to the trunk of the sympathetic chain at the inferior aspect of the superior stellate ganglion (Figure 4A). Failure to divide this nerve will result in incomplete denervation of the upper extremity. The nerve of Kuntz helps identify T1, the lower portion of the stellate ganglion; the upper portion of the stellate ganglion is below a yellowish fat pad at the pleural cavity that envelops the subclavian artery.

11. Dissect below the inferior aspect of the stellate ganglion above the T1 ramus along with the rami communicantes coursing in the caudal direction from the stellate ganglion (Figure 4B). The stellate ganglion and the rami coursing in the rostral direction should be left intact (Figure 4C). Injury or traction to the upper portion of the stellate ganglion should be avoided to minimize the risk of developing Horner's syndrome.

12. Divide immediately below the T4 ganglion, while avoiding the underlying intercostal vessels. Failure to avoid the intercostal vessels may result in bleeding, which can be controlled by suction, electrocautery or cottonball stick pressure.

13. The sympathetic chain should be excised just below the T1 ganglion and sent to pathology for histological confirmation (Figure 5).
14. Irrigate the dissection bed and control any bleeding points with electrocautery or clips.

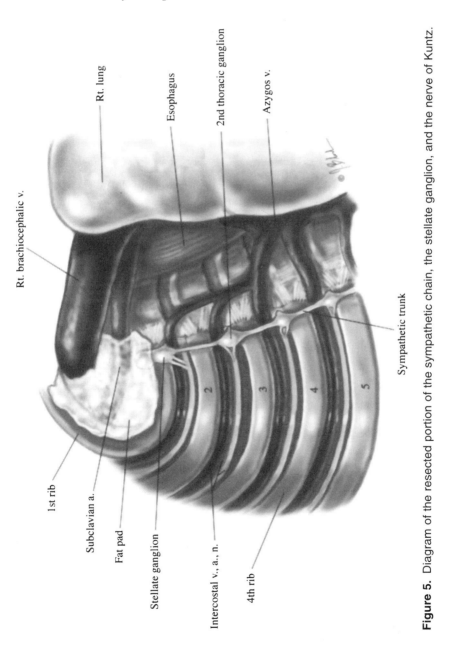

Figure 5. Diagram of the resected portion of the sympathetic chain, the stellate ganglion, and the nerve of Kuntz.

15. Remove the instrument ports and insert the endoscope to inspect the intercostal vessels for hemostasis.
16. Insert a small chest tube (16F) through one of the thoracoscope ports and position it under scope visualization.
17. Reinflate the lung using 30 to 40 mm Hg positive pressure and confirm adequate inflation with the endoscope. Incomplete reinflation of the collapsed apical lobe will result in postoperative complications from atelectasis and pneumothorax. A small apical pneumothorax can be treated conservatively.
18. Close the incision in two layers using absorbable sutures followed by steri-strips.

The procedure requires 1 to 2 hours, with an average time of 1.5 hours. The operating time is a direct reflection of the surgeon's experience and the anatomy and complexity of the patient.

Postoperative Care

A chest tube should be placed to −15 cm water suction and water-sealed immediately after the operation. Obtain a chest x-ray film to rule out possible pneumothorax or pleural effusions. If no air leaks are present, the chest tube can be removed in the recovery room; however, if air leaks do occur, the chest tube should not be removed. An air leak in the lung parenchyma will result in a persistent pneumothorax and can be remedied with a large negative pressure tube until all air leaks have been completely sealed. Oral analgesics are adequate for most patients. Hospital stay is usually 1 day.

Index